AF751067

RESEARCH DIRECTIONS IN TUMOR ANGIOGENESIS

Edited by **Jianyuan Chai**

Research Directions in Tumor Angiogenesis
http://dx.doi.org/10.5772/56020
Edited by Jianyuan Chai

Contributors

Massimo Mattia Santoro, Vera Mugoni, Takaaki Sasaki, Yoshinori Minami, Yoshinobu Ohsaki, Veronika Sysoeva, Mathias Francois, Jeroen Overman, Mani Valarmathi, Qigui Li, Mark Hickman, Peter Weina, Jianyuan Chai, Ramani Ramchandran, Jill Gershan, Andrew Chan, Magdalena Chrzanowska-Wodnicka, Bryon Johnson, Qing Miao

Published by InTech

Janeza Trdine 9, 51000 Rijeka, Croatia

Copyright © 2013 InTech

All chapters are distributed under the Creative Commons Attribution 3.0 license, which allows users to download, copy and build upon published articles even for commercial purposes, as long as the author and publisher are properly credited, which ensures maximum dissemination and a wider impact of our publications. However, users who aim to disseminate and distribute copies of this book as a whole must not seek monetary compensation for such service (excluded InTech representatives and agreed collaborations). After this work has been published by InTech, authors have the right to republish it, in whole or part, in any publication of which they are the author, and to make other personal use of the work. Any republication, referencing or personal use of the work must explicitly identify the original source.

Notice

Statements and opinions expressed in the chapters are these of the individual contributors and not necessarily those of the editors or publisher. No responsibility is accepted for the accuracy of information contained in the published chapters. The publisher assumes no responsibility for any damage or injury to persons or property arising out of the use of any materials, instructions, methods or ideas contained in the book.

Publishing Process Manager Iva Lipovic
Technical Editor InTech DTP team
Cover InTech Design team

Additional hard copies can be obtained from orders@intechopen.com

Research Directions in Tumor Angiogenesis, Edited by Jianyuan Chai
p. cm.
ISBN 978-953-51-0963-1

We are IntechOpen, the world's leading publisher of Open Access books

Built by scientists, for scientists

4,200+
Open access books available

116,000+
International authors and editors

125M+
Downloads

151
Countries delivered to

Our authors are among the
Top 1%
most cited scientists

12.2%
Contributors from top 500 universities

CLARIVATE ANALYTICS
BOOK CITATION INDEX
INDEXED

WEB OF SCIENCE™

Selection of our books indexed in the Book Citation Index
in Web of Science™ Core Collection (BKCI)

Interested in publishing with us?
Contact book.department@intechopen.com

Numbers displayed above are based on latest data collected.
For more information visit www.intechopen.com

For EU product safety concerns:
IN TECH d.o.o., Prolaz Marije Krucifikse Kozulić 3, 51000 Rijeka, Croatia,
info@intechopen.com or visit our website at intechopen.com.

Meet the editor

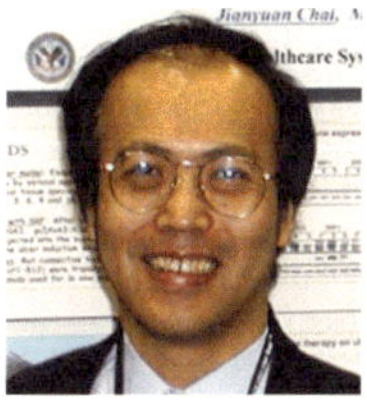

Dr. Chai received his Ph.D. from the City University of New York in 1998 and completed his post-doctoral training at Harvard University in 2001. Currently, he is a Principal Investigator of the U.S. Department of Veterans Affairs and a faculty member of the Department of Medicine at the University of California in Irvine. He directs the Laboratory of GI Injury and Cancer at the VA Long Beach Healthcare System in California and also serves as the IACUC Chairman at this facility. Dr. Chai has published over 30 research articles and 7 book chapters in diverse areas including protozoology, arachnology, cardiology and gastroenterology. His current research focuses on acid reflux induced esophageal cancer. He holds professional membership with AGA, AHA, and ASBMB, has been an editorial board member of 6 journals and a reviewer for multiple journals and grants.

Contents

Preface

As a process of extension of the vascular network within human body, angiogenesis plays a fundamental role to support cell survival, because all cells need oxygen and nutrients to operate and blood circulation is the only way to provide them. In human adults, angiogenesis mainly takes place in two conditions, wound healing and tumor progression. During wound healing, angiogenesis supports new tissue growth to repair the wound; therefore, it is beneficial to the body and should be promoted. In tumor progression, on the other hand, angiogenesis is hijacked to serve the mutated cells for their multiplication and therefore, it should be inhibited. This book focuses on the second situation – angiogenesis in tumor progression. However, since the molecular and cellular interactions under both conditions are essentially identical, the content of the book is suitable for all the readers who are interested in angiogenesis.

The book includes eight chapters written by highly experienced scholars from several nations. The first chapter, **"Transcriptional modulation of tumor induced angiogenesis"**, by Overman & Francois *(University of Queensland, Australia)*, gives a comprehensive introduction on how angiogenesis at the molecular and cellular levels is initiated and regulated during tumorigenesis as comparing to a normal biological system. Despite the similarity in the molecules involved in both conditions, including transcription factors, angiogenic factors, and cell proliferation/migration factors, the key difference is the balance among these molecules. In a normal biological system, angiogenesis is highly organized in a spatial-and-temporal manner. In tumors, however, the uncontrollably replicating cancer cells create an extremely hypoxic environment, which induces a persistent production of angiogenic factors that allow angiogenesis to go on and on. As a consequence, the vasculature generated during tumorigenesis is leaky and immature because it never has the time or molecular/cellular mass to become completed. In a way this makes metastasis easier, because the cancer cells can effortlessly enter into the circulatory system through the porous vessel wall and invade other organs.

The imbalance of angiogenic factors during tumorigenesis starts with the disproportional activation of transcription factors, which are reviewed in the second chapter, **"Role of serum response factor in endothelial cells during hypoxia"**, by Chai *(University of California, USA)*. The best known transcription factors in tumor angiogenesis are hypoxia-inducible factor (HIF) and p53. They both can be activated by oxygen shortage. While HIF activates angiogenic factors like vascular endothelial growth factor (VEGF) to promote tumor cell survival, p53 is doomed to kill the cells through up-regulation of apoptotic factors like BAX, which is why p53 is often found mutated in the vast majority of tumor cells. Although these two transcription factors appear to be the enemies to each other, sometimes they also shake hands under the table. For instance, HIF has been reported in several occasions to help p53 to induce cell death under severe hypoxia. I guess, if you can't beat them, it won't be a bad idea to join them. In addition to the commonly known transcription factors involved in angiogenesis, this chapter also brings a new member into the light, i.e., Serum Response Factor (SRF). This is a much more powerful regulator than either HIF or p53, and some even call it the master regulator. SRF directly controls nearly 1% of the known human genes, and through these gene derivatives SRF may have influence on a quarter of the entire human genome. This chapter presents convincing data to show that SRF regulates hypoxia-induced angiogenesis through multi-levels and therefore could be an excellent target for cancer gene therapy.

The activation of HIF not only initiates VEGF production, the best known angiogenic stimulator, but also directs the gene transcription of two other molecules, endothelial nitric oxide synthase (eNOS) and inducible nitric oxide synthase (iNOS), both responsible for the generation of nitric oxide (NO-), one of the key reactive oxygen species (ROS) in the body. The next chapter, **"Manipulating REDOX signaling to block tumor angiogenesis"**, by Mugoni & Santoro *(University of Torino, Italy)*, summarizes all the known ROS and dissects how they influence tumor angiogenesis. The level of ROS in the tumor microenvironment can be a determining factor for the fate of a tumor. A moderate amount of these free radicals can help to maintain normal blood pressure, protect endothelial cell integrity, and support angiogenesis, while high level of ROS can cause endothelial cell death and thereby stop tumor angiogenesis. Therefore, manipulation of ROS level could be an alternative approach to control tumor progression.

Although angiogenesis is performed by endothelial cells, other cells also contribute to the process. In Chapter 4, **"Accessory cells in tumor angiogenesis"**, Minami et al *(Asahikawa Medical University, Japan)* introduce a major helper of endothelial cells during angiogenesis, the pericytes. Endothelial cells form the inner lining of the blood vessels, while pericytes wrap around the endothelial cells from the outside and provide molecular and cellular support to stabilize the newly formed microvasculature. Although pericytes are usually absent in tumor vasculature due to the accelerating angiogenic activities, this chapter provides several strategies to increase the local population of pericytes to counteract the tumor angiogenesis, which may be advanced to promising therapeutic approaches in the near future.

In the following chapter, **"Endothelial and accessory cell interactions in neuroblastoma tumor microenvironment"**, Gershan et al *(Medical College of Wisconsin, USA)* present a special case of tumor biology – neuroblastoma, and give a thorough review on its development, molecular and cellular interactions, and therapeutic strategies. Of particular interest is the point that "tumors are wounds that never heal", which precisely reflects the truth about tumors. From molecular and cellular point of view, these two events are almost identical. Molecules up-regulated during wound healing are often found elevated in a tumor microenvironment. Wound healing requires cell proliferation, migration and differentiation, and so does tumor progression. Angiogenesis provides fundamental support for wound healing as well as for tumor growth. The only difference, as the team points out, is that wound healing is a highly orchestrated event in which the activations of cells and molecules are regulated spatially and temporally. Once the wound is healed, all of these molecular and cellular activities return to their normal physiological levels. Tumors, on the other hand, sustain the high molecular and cellular activities eternally, which is like an open wound.

In the next chapter, **"T-cadherin stimulates melanoma cell proliferation and mesenchymal stromal cell recruitment, but inhibits angiogenesis in a mouse melanoma model"**, Rubina et al *(M.V. Lomonosov Moscow State University, Russia)*present original data on the role of T-cadherin in melanoma angiogenesis. T-cadherin is a membrane-associated protein and its real function remains largely unknown. While its up-regulation has been associated with high grade astrocytomas, in the majority of cancers including melanoma, T-cadherin is down-regulated or completely lost. Overexpression of T-cadherin in endothelial cells correlates with a migratory phenotype, which usually suggests a positive role in angiogenesis. However, this study found in a melanoma model that the number of microvessels is reduced when T-cadherin is expressed, supporting an argument that T-cadherin might inhibit angiogenesis.

Using natural products to treat chronic diseases is always the top choice in cancer therapy, because they are cheap and less toxic compared to the synthetic drugs. In the next chapter, **"The use of artemisinin compounds as angiogenesis inhibitors to treat cancer"**, Li et al *(Walter Reed Army Institute of Research, USA)* introduce such a compound, artemisinin, an extract from the plant sagewort. Artemisinin is the first line treatment recommended by WHO for malaria. However, an increasing amount of data indicates an anti-cancer effect, particularly against tumor angiogenesis. Li et al give a thorough review on artemisinin and its derivatives in cancer and non-cancer context, and provide valuable perspectives for the future research direction.

The final chapter of the book, **"3-D microvascular tissue constructs for exploring concurrent temporal and spatial regulation of postnatal neovasculogenesis"**, by Valarmathi et al *(University of South Carolina, USA)*, demonstrates a marvelous research technique to study neovasculogenesis in vitro, the three-dimensional collagen scaffold. Depending on the culture medium provided, bone marrow stromal cells can differentiate into either endothelial cells or smooth muscle cells in front of your eyes and form tube-like network within the scaffold, mimicking the vasculature formation in vivo. Although the study is on neovasculogenesis, meaning generating microvessels from stem cells, the technique can be easily applied to angiogenesis studies using differentiated endothelial cells. The beautiful images generated from confocal immunostaining, transmission and scanning electron microscope provide a perfect end for this book.

Jianyuan Chai, Ph.D.
Laboratory of GI Injury and Cancer
VA Long Beach Healthcare System and
University of California
Long Beach, California
USA

Chapter 1

Transcriptional Modulation of Tumour Induced Angiogenesis

Jeroen Overman and Mathias François

Additional information is available at the end of the chapter

http://dx.doi.org/10.5772/54055

1. Introduction

This chapter provides a summary of the current literature addressing key processes and transcriptional regulators of endothelial cell fate during embryonic blood vascular and lymphatic vascular development, and discusses the implications of these processes/regulators during tumour vascularization. First, we will address normal embryonic development of the vascular systems at the molecular and cellular level. With these fundamental processes recognized, the second part the chapter will focus on how these regulators face dysregulation during tumorigenesis and how they consequently facilitate abnormal vessel growth.

2. Blood vessel development in the embryo

During embryogenesis, the development of the vasculature occurs prior to the onset of blood circulation, and is initiated by *de novo* formation of endothelial cells (EC) from mesoderm derived precursor cells. In a succession of morphogenic events, intricate transcriptional programs orchestrate the further differentiation, proliferation and migration of blood endothelial cells (BECs) to establish the vascular systems (fig. 1). This includes assembly of individual ECs into linear structures and the formation of lumen to facilitate the flow of blood; the designation of arterial, venous, capillary and later lymphatic endothelial cell identity; and the remodelling, coalescence and maturation of the primary vascular plexus to form large heterogeneous interlaced structures, that warrants a contiguous and fully functional blood- and lymphatic vascular system.

INTECH
open science | open minds

© 2013 The Author(s). Licensee InTech. This chapter is distributed under the terms of the Creative Commons Attribution License http://creativecommons.org/licenses/by/3.0), which permits unrestricted use, distribution, and reproduction in any medium, provided the original work is properly cited.

2.1. Embryonic blood vessel morphogenesis

2.1.1. Endothelial specification and initial blood vessel formation

De novo generation of the first EC precursors in mammals occurs in the extra-embryonic mesoderm. The mesoderm is a hotbed for cell specification in the embryo, and the pluripotent haemangioblast ancestor of EC precursors (angioblasts) also gives rise to haematopoietic lineages and ostensibly even smooth muscle cells (SMC)[1-5]. In addition, ECs have been shown to share a common precursor with mesenchymal stem/stromal cells (MSC), the so-called mesenchymoangioblast[6], and it has been suggested that other precursors can propagate endothelial cell lineages in the yolk sac. Together these observations signify the differentiation potential of these precursor cells, and impending consequences for plasticity during later remodelling and pathologies[7-9]. During vasculogenesis, defined as *de novo* generation of embryonic blood vessels, these pluripotent mesodermal progenitor cells acquire an endothelial cell (EC) precursor- or blood cell (BC) precursor- phenotype, and subsequently co-localize and aggregate in the mesoderm to form blood islands[10-12], with the EC precursors flattened around the edges and the BC precursors in the centre to generate the haematopoietic lineages[11-13].

2.1.2. Blood vascular lumen formation

To initiate the formation of actual vessel-like structures, the angioblasts assemble into arterial and venous cords, and in doing so form the primitive vascular plexus. These nascent rope-like threads have a solid core and are consequently not yet able to facilitate the flow of blood. This functional feature requires the heart of the cord to be tunnelled out, to give way to a central continuous lumen along the length of the nascent vessel. The transition of EC cords into vascular tubes is a process that necessitates defined EC-polarity, and a delicate interplay between adhesion and contractility. Polarity is essential for the distribution of membrane junction proteins and the definition of apical/luminal (inside) and basal/abluminal (outside) surfaces. This is harmonized by the interplay between adhesion and contractility, through the regulating of physical force propensity that accounts for the EC-flattening against the extracellular matrix[14-16].

Two principal cellular mechanisms have been described to explain for the formation of *de novo* blood vascular lumen: cord hollowing and cell hollowing[13, 16, 17]. Both mechanisms rely on the accumulation of vacuoles, but a fundamental difference between them is revealed in the distinct nature and location of vacuole accumulation, which is usually determined by vessel type and size. Cord hollowing is characterized by the creation of an extracellular luminal space within a cylindrical EC-cord. This involves the loss of apical cell adhesion between the central- but not peripheral- ECs, and results in a lumen diameter that is enclosed by multiple ECs[14-16, 18, 19]. Cell hollowing on the other hand involves the intracellular fusion of vacuoles within a single EC to give rise to a cytoplasmic lumen that spans the length of the cell, and typically results in vessels that have single-EC lining[17, 20]. The aorta in the mouse embryo for example relies on extracellular lumen formation as do most major vessels[15], while intracellular lumen formation is generally the designated mechanism for smaller vessels.

http://dx.doi.org/10.5772/54055

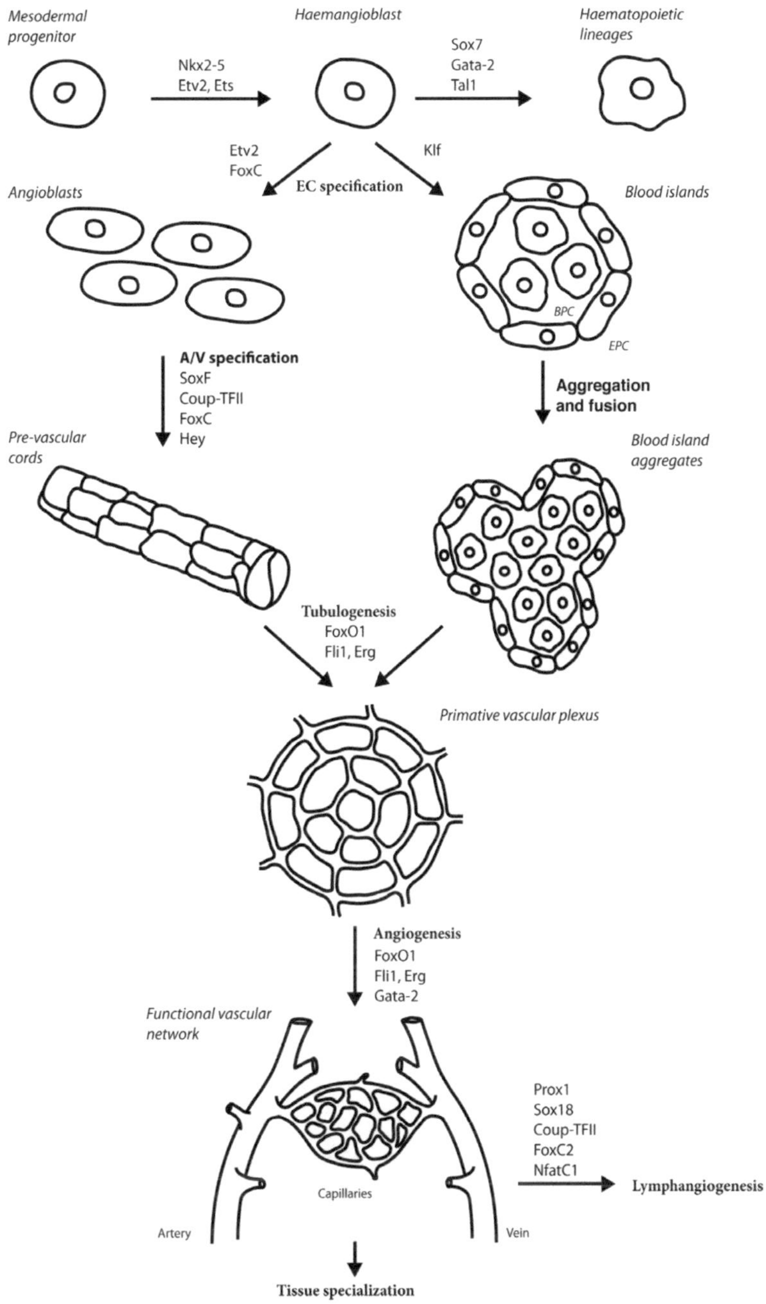

Figure 1. *Embryonic morphogenesis of the blood vasculature.* Mesodermal progenitor cells give rise the vascular endothelium through a series of steps that progressively specify ECs. In the mesoderm, angioblasts (EC-precursors) are formed and aggregate into cords or blood island, which later arrange into the primitive vascular plexus. Angiogenic remodelling of the primary plexus gives rise to a functional vascular network, from where the lymphatic vascular system eventually develops.

2.1.3. Angiogenesis and blood vessel maturation

The institution of a continuous blood vascular lumen is a milestone for the developing vascular system and paramount for further vascular development, as it permits the flow of blood. The nascent blood vessels that constitute this primitive vascular network will subsequently expand, and then functionalize, into an extensive and more intricate systemic vasculature, in two processes respectively known as angiogenesis and vessel maturation. Angiogenesis describes the processes of branching, expansion and remodelling of the primitive vasculature in response to pro-angiogenic signals. This is different from vasculogenesis in that the ECs are not generated by *de novo* differentiation of stem cells, but rather depend on the proliferation and migration of pre-existing vascular ECs. Vessel maturation on the other hand describes the functionalization of nascent blood vessels, and is characterized by mural cell ensheathment of the vessel walls. The continuous mêlée between angiogenesis and vessel maturation – wherein vessel maturation blocks angiogenic growth, and visa versa – ensures optimal systemic blood vascular performance.

Vascular remodelling conventionally occurs through sprouting- and intussusception angiogenesis, and together with vessel maturation gives rise to organ specific vascular beds. Intussusception angiogenesis is a process of vessel invagination wherein vessels ultimate divide and split – which requires appreciably high levels of polarization and localized en masse loss of cell junctions. Sprouting angiogenesis is visibly distinct from intussusception, and unsurprisingly involves the sprouting of a subset of ECs from the vascular wall to protrude into a primed ECM. In this discrete set of ECs, the cell-cell contacts are loosened to promote a motile phenotype. The actual stromal invasion requires enzymatic degradation of the basement membrane and ECM. There is a remarkably strict hierarchy amongst the distinct EC-types in angiogenic sprouts, as a single tip-cell (TC) leads the way, and a host of stalk-cells (SC) follow[21]. Filopodia protrude from the TC that sense the microenvironment for attractive and repulsive signals to guide their migration, and to eventually fuse with adjacent vessels (anastomosis), while SCs contribute principally to the recruitment of pericytes and lumen preservation, while at the same time maintaining the connection between the TC and parent vessel.

Once the newly formed blood vasculature has extended and webbed to an appropriate level, the temporal pro-angiogenic signal will fade and the nascent vessel will be disposed to maturation. Blood vessels maturation primarily requires the recruitment of pericytes and SMCs, to ensheath and stabilize the vessel wall. This mural cell coverage strengthens the cell-cell contacts, decreases vessel permeability, and assures control over vessel diameter and therefore blood flow. Also, pericytes supress EC proliferation and promote EC survival, resulting in a long EC life and a quiescent state, which is typical for mature and functional vessels. Pericytes also subsidize the construction of the vessel basement membrane and deposit various ECM components into the stroma, to generate an angiogenesis incompetent milieu.

The whole process of vessel maturation is strikingly dynamic and intermittently reversible. Mature ECs can, conversely to quiescence, be activated by pro-angiogenic signals, upon which pericytes detach, cell-junctions are loosened, and the ECM is primed for angiogenic growth. In the adult, these processes are recapitulated during pathophysiological conditions as a means to maintain vessel perfusion and tissue oxygenation in a dynamic milieu. Pro-angiogenic signals can, for example, originate from inflammation and hypoxia as a transient cue, or from a more broadly encompassing and tenacious source such as a neoplasm. The latter type of molecular (dys-) regulation results in abnormal vessel formation, and will be discussed later in this chapter, once the transcriptional basis for EC specification and angiogenesis has been established.

2.2. Transcriptional basis of blood vascular endothelial cell differentiation

The complexity and significance of the numerous morphological events contributing to blood vessel formation, as are highlighted above, underline the necessity for scrupulous regulation to ensure that these processes occur in a spatiotemporally controlled fashion with a high level of precision over EC behaviour (fig. 2). Copious amounts of transcription factors are at the foundation of these coordinating programs, to guide the dynamic gene expression profiles at different stages of embryonic EC fate determination and vascular development (fig. 1), which are later – at least partially – recapitulated during vessel growth in the adult.

2.2.1. Ets transcription factors regulate mesodermal specification of endothelial and haematopoietic lineages

The E-twenty-six (ETS) family is a large group of proteins, with close to thirty members in human and mouse, that achieves transcriptional regulation by binding clusters of ETS binding motifs on gene enhancers and promoters[22]. In itself, this conserved core DNA sequence, 5′-GGA(A/T)-3′, offers little binding specificity between Ets members, and is by no means exclusive to endothelial-associated genes. Similarly, Ets expression extends beyond the vascular endothelium. Even so, multiple Ets members are of crucial importance for vascular development by regulating endothelial gene transcription. The way this is accomplished despite these seemingly ubiquitous features, is illustrated by the presence of multiple ETS motifs in large number of enhancers and promoters that regulate specific EC gene transcription. There is also a combination of distinct Ets members being expressed in cells that are programmed to attain or maintain an EC phenotype. It is thus proposed that the combinatorial effort of these transcription factors accounts for the tight control over EC differentiation[23, 24]. Complementary to interaction within the Ets family, recent studies indicate that Ets members also affiliate with other partner proteins to this end, and that multiple Ets members form a transcriptional network with associated partner proteins such as Tal1 and GATA-2 to regulate EC differentiation[25]. Another method by which specificity and function is thought to be regulated is post-translational modification, such as phosphorylation, sumoylation and acetylation[26], while regions flanking the ETS motif on the DNA have also been shown to affect the binding specificity of some Ets members[22].

The exact mechanisms by which the individual or combinatorial Ets expression profiles achieve endothelial gene regulation remain largely unknown, but several Ets members have been identified in recent years to be critical at different stages during EC specification, vasculogenesis and angiogenic remodelling. For example, mouse null-embryos for the ETS translocation variant 2 (Etv2/Er71/Etsrp71) transcription factor do not form blood island due to lack of EC and HPC specification, and are embryonic lethal with severe blood and vascular defects[27, 28]. Friend leukemia integration 1 (Fli-1), another Ets member, has alternatively been shown to be essential during the establishment of the vascular plexus but not for endothelial specification[29]. Phylogenetically and functionally close to Fli-1 is ETS related gene (Erg)[30]. This particular Ets member acts slightly later during vascular development and is associated predominantly with angiogenesis, by controlling a host of processes such as EC junction dynamics and migration[31, 32].

Etv2 has in recent years arisen as the master transcriptional regulator of endothelial cell fate in mouse and zebrafish, because its function is absolutely critical for endothelial specification, with Etv2-null embryos failing to express vital endothelial markers and being devoid of ECs. Expression patterns have shown that Etv2 mainly functions in the embryonic mesoderm and blood islands at around 7.5 dpc (days post coitum) in mice, and is transiently present in larger vessels until at least 9.5 dpc[28, 33]. Mesodermally expressed Etv2 does not only direct specification towards EC lineages, but is also indispensible for the development of haematopoietic cells. In support of this, the endodermal stem cell precursors common to HPCs and ECs, halt differentiating towards haematopoietic or EC lineages prematurely in Etv2-null mice, in vascular endothelial growth factor (VEGF) receptor-2 (VEGFR2)-positive cells [28]. The vascular endothelial growth factor receptor-2 (VEGFR-2/Flk1), receptor to VEGF-A and considered to be one of the most potent transducers of pro-angiogenic signalling, is thus not regulated by Etv2 in the mouse embryo. By contras, it has previously been reported that the zebrafish orthologue of Etv2, Etsrp, is required for the expression of the zebrafish VEGFR-2 orthologue, kdr[33], and the VEGFR-2 enhancer contains an ETS motif[34].

Other endothelial genes have been shown to be transcriptionally regulated by Etv2, confirming its essential role in early vasculogenesis (refer to table 1). For example, the angiopoietin (Ang) receptor tyrosine kinase with immunoglobin-like and EGF-like domains-1 (Tie2) gene is a direct target of Etv2, and is an important vascular marker that regulates angiogenesis[27]. Endothelial transcription factor GATA-2 is also a likely downstream target of Etv2[23, 28]. Similar to Etv2, GATA-2 is involved in both haemangioblast and endothelial development, and GATA-2 is severely downregulated in Etv2-null embryos[28]. Downstream targets of GATA-2 include VEGFR-2[35] and ANG-2[36], and several other genes that encode endothelial proteins, such as Kruppel-like factor-2 (KLF2), Ets variant- (Etv6) and myocyte enhancer factor-2 (MEF2C), have been identified to be occupied by transcription factor GATA-2[37], hence might be indirectly affected by Etv2 loss of function.

The bulk of transcriptional regulation by Etv2, however, is though to be achieved through recognition of the composite FOX:ETS motif, which is exclusive to endothelial-specific enhancers, and is present in approximately 23% of all endothelial genes[24]. Members of both the forkhead and Ets transcription factor families, in particular the forkhead box protein C2 (FoxC2) and Etv2, synergistically bind this motif to activate endothelial gene expression[24]. In vivo studies in Xenopus and zebrafish embryos have identified this motif within the enhancer of 11 important endothelial genes, being Mef2c, VEGFR-2, Tal1, Tie2, VE-cadherin (Cdh5), ECE1, VEGFR-3 (Flt-4), PDGFRβ, FoxP1, NRP1 and NOTCH4[24]. Not all of these molecular players are individually discussed in this chapter, but it is clear that the FOX:ETS motif is prevalent in endothelial enhancers and appreciably regulate endothelial gene transcription. In support of this, forced activity of both Etv2 and Foxc2 induces ectopic expression of vascular markers VEGFR-2, Tie2, Tal1, NOTCH4 and VE-cadherin, while conversely, a mutation in the FOX:ETS motif disrupts Etv2/FoxC2 function and ablates endothelial specific LacZ expression in mice[24].

Upstream regulation of Etv2 has been an additional focus of recent studies, to further understand the mechanisms whereby endocardial and endothelial fate is determined and to trace back the transcriptional programs even further. In mice, the homeobox transcription factor Nkx2-5 has been shown to directly bind the Etv2 promoter and transactivate its expression in endothelial progenitor cells within the heart *in vitro* and *in vivo*[27]. In zebrafish, Etsrp was identified to be downstream of Foxc1a/b (FoxC1/C2 homologues found in zebrafish) in angioblast development[38]. These factors were shown to be able to bind the upstream Etsrp enhancer *up1*, and the knockdown of Foxc1a/b results in loss of *up1* enhancer activity to drive transcription[38]. This supports the collaborative role of forkhead transcription factors and Etv2 in endothelial gene expression, and adds a dimension to the transcriptional network.

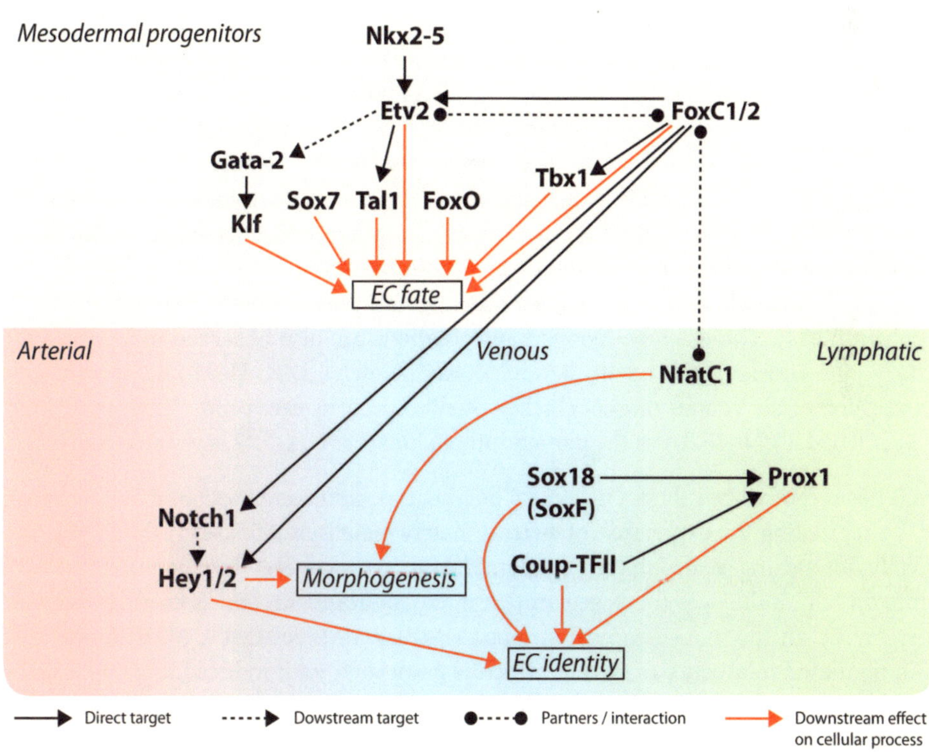

Figure 2. Transcriptional hierarchy orchestrating embryonic vascular development. Endothelial cell specification is an intricate process that relies on extensive crosstalk between transcription factors. Downstream of their transcriptional regulation are signalling molecules that shape the cells and define EC identity and morphogenesis.

2.2.2. Fox transcription factors regulate arteriovenous specification and angiogenesis

It is clear that forkhead transcription factor FoxC2 has an important role during EC specification, through the collaboration with Etv2 at early stages of embryogenesis. Notably, FoxO1 is also able to operate synergistically with Etv2 by binding the FOX:ETS motif[24]. However, not unlike Etv2, FoxO and FoxC transcription factors also direct FOX:ETS independent endothelial gene transcription, which is crucial for vascular development.

Endothelial cells are specified in FoxO1-null mice, and thus differentiate beyond the VEGFR2^{+} stage of Etv2-null embryos. However, embryonic lethality occurs only slightly later due to a severe angiogenic defect, characterized by disorganized and few vessels by E9.5, with low expression of some crucial vascular markers[39]. Amongst those downregulated is the arterial marker Eprin-B2, a key regulator of VEGFR3 receptor internalization and transducer of VEGF-C/PI3K/Akt signalling, so it is hypothesized that FoxO1 regulates angiogenesis by controlling VEGF responsiveness[39-41]. What further underlines the importance of FoxO1 is the elaborate control over its the transcriptional activity, which is regulated on many levels by posttranscriptional modifications, interaction with co-activators or co-repressors, and absolute FoxO1 protein levels, to regulate localization, DNA-binding activity, and function[42].

FoxC1 and FoxC2 are, in addition to their role in Etv2-mediated endothelial specification, required for endothelial cells to acquire an arterial cell phenotype[43]. Both FoxC transcription factors directly activate the transcription of the arterial cell fate promoters Notch1 and Delta-like 4 (Dll4), and overexpression of FoxC genes results in concomitant induction of Notch and Dll4 expression *in vitro*[43]. Notch signalling has been shown to be essential for arteriovenous (A/V) specification, by mediating the transcription of Hairy/enhancer-of-split related with YRPW motif protein 1 and 2 (Hey1/2). Null-mice for either Notch1 or Hey1/2 have severe vascular defects, with impaired remodelling and general loss of arterial markers such as Ephrin-B2[44]. These arteriovenous malformations are also observed in FoxC1/2 double homozygous knockout mice, with loss of Notch1, Notch4, Dll4, Hey2 and ephrinB2, while transcription of the venous marker chicken ovalbumin upstream promoter transcription factor 2 (COUP-TFII/NR2F2) and the pan-endothelial marker VEGFR2 is not affected[43].

FoxC1 has recently been shown to control ECM composition and basement membrane integrity, by regulating the expression of several matrix metalloproteinases (MMPs)[45], and genetically interacting with laminin α-1(lama1)[46], respectively. The homeostasis of these factors directly influences the vasculature's microenvironment, and is of great relevance to angiogenesis. In the mouse corneal stroma, MMP1a, MMP3, MMP9, MMP12 and MMP12 are upregulated in absence of FoxC1, which is associated with induced angiogenesis by the excessive degradation of the ECM and increased bioavailability of VEGF[45]. The crosstalk between VEGF signalling and forkhead transcription factors is thus a recurring observation, although it is unclear if and how they physically interact. Expression levels of collagens Col1a1, Col3a1, Col4a1 seem unaffected by loss of FoxC1[45], suggesting that FoxC1 does not directly contribute so structural basement membrane or stromal components. However, as mentioned, FoxC1 does interact with lama1 to support basement membrane integrity and vascular stability during vascular development in zebrafish, with FoxC1 morphants having severe basement membrane defects similar to that reported for lama1[46].

The divergent roles of FoxC1/2 are not limited to orchestration blood vascular development, and concomitantly also control the development of the lymphatic vascular system. Naturally occurring mutations in the human FoxC2 gene are associated with hereditary lymphedema-distichiasis (LD) syndrome, an autosomal dominant disorder which is characterized by accumulation of interstitial flood leading to swelling (lymphedema), and aberrant eyelash growth (distichiasis)[47]. Clinical studies have revealed that patient with LD have impaired lymphatic valve function[48], and *in vivo* mouse studies have shown that lymphatic valves do not form properly in FoxC2-nul mutants[49]. Also, the smooth muscle coverage of lymphatic collector vessels is increased in FoxC2 heterozygous mice, which is inherent to LD, owing to an increased expression of platelet derived growth factor β (Pdgfβ) *in vivo*[49]. Hence, it has been suggested that FoxC2 regulates lymphatic vessel maturation, and possibly lymphatic sprouting, by interacting with growth factors and transcription factors that regulate lymphatic development. Notably, the lymphatic endothelial cell (LEC) receptor VEGFR3 is thought to be upstream of FoxC2, linking pro-lymphangiogenic VEGF signalling to FoxC2 activity[49], which supports the observation that FoxC2 mutants have increased vSMC-mediated LEC maturation. FoxC2 has since been shown to cooperate with the master regulator of LEC commitment prospero homeobox protein 1 (Prox1) during lymphatic valve formation in controlling the activity of gap junction protein connexin37 (Cx37) and nuclear factor of activated T-cells cytoplastmic-1 (NFATc1)[50]. In this context, NFATc1 activity is controlled by VEGF-C that leads to FoxC2 interaction[51]. Compound FoxC1 heterozygous; FoxC2 homozygous mice further have lymphatic sprouting defects during the earliest stages of lymphangiogenesis[43].

Taken together, this suggests that FoxC signalling has critical roles during lymphangiogenesis and lymphatic maturation in addition to A/V specification and angiogenesis, through cooperation with lymphatic specific transcription factors.

2.2.3. Members SOXF transcription factors determine A/V specification and lymphangiogenenic switch

The three members of the SOXF group – SOX7, SOX17 and SOX18 – are all endogenously expressed in ECs during vascular development[52], and several key functions of these transcription factors have been described over the years. This includes regulation of A/V specification, angiogenesis, lymphangiogenesis and red blood cell specification, but also other roles perceivably not associated with the blood or lymphatic vasculature, such as hair follicle development and endoderm differentiation.

SOXF transcription factors belong to the SRY-box (SOX) family that is comprised of 20 members. SOX members are all characterized and identified by their highly homologous 79 amino acid high-mobility group (HMG) domain, which was first discovered in their founding member sex-determining region Y (SRY)[53]. This typical SOX element binds the heptameric consensus sequence 5′-(A/T)(A/T)CAA(A/T)G-3′[54], to induce DNA bending and regulate the expression of a broad collection of genes during embryonic development[55]. Specificity and functional differentiation between SOX-groups and individual members is accomplished by additional operative elements on the SOX transcription factors, and through association with partner proteins[54, 56, 57]. Their coexpression and HMG domain homology, however, does suggest that functional redundancies or cooperative roles apply for members within the same SOX group. However, of the SOXF group only SOX18 is endogenously expressed during lymphatic vascular development in LEC precursors[58].

SOX18 function in vascular development has received considerable attention since the naturally occurring *ragged* mouse mutation, the mural counterpart of the human syndrome hypotrichosis-lymphedema-telangiecstasia (HLT) and underlying cause of severe cardiovascular and hair follicle defects, was identified in the Sox18 gene ($Sox18^{Ra}$)[59]. This mutation produces a truncated form of SOX18 that acts in a dominant negative fashion and fails to recruit essential co-factors, and is therefor unable to induce target gene transcription[56, 59]. The defects in the *ragged* mice are much more severe than the observed phenotype of Sox18-null mice[59], as truncated SOX18 competes with redundant SOXF members to occupy the same site on the DNA. This supports the notion that redundancies exist amongst SOXF transcription factors, and in fact it has been shown that SOX7 and SOX17 can activate SOX18 targets by binding to SOX18 promoter elements[58].

In the zebrafish embryo, individual knockdown of either SOX7 or SOX18 causes no obvious vascular defects, while the SOX7/18 double knockdown is characterized by partial loss of circulation, ectopic shunts between the main artery and vein, cardiac oedema, blood pooling, and a general loss of A/V specification[60, 61]. Indeed, SOX7 and SOX18 were found to be coexpressed in ECs and their precursors, and their combined loss of function resulted in reduction of arterial markers Ephrin-B2, notch3 and Dll4 and ectopic expression of the venous endothelial marker VEGFR3 in the dorsal aorta (DA)[60, 61].

Several direct SOX18 vascular target genes have been described, notably the genes encoding the tight junction component claudin-5[62] and the vascular adhesion molecule VCAM-1[63], which are both essential for vascular integrity and endothelial activation during angiogenesis. SOX18 also directly activates the expression of MMP7, EphrinB2, interleukin receptor 7 (IL-7R)[64] and Robo4[65] *in vitro*. Robo4 expression *in vivo* is correspondingly under control of Sox7/18 activity in the mouse caudal vein, and in the intersegmental vessels (ISV) of zebrafish embryos[65]. Archetypically, Robo4 functions in axon guidance, but has more recently been identified as an important coordinator of EC migration during spouting angiogenesis in zebrafish[66]. *In vitro* assays have further shown that compound SOX17 heterozygous; SOX18-null primary ECs have a sprouting and vascular remodelling defect[67].

SOX18-null mice, although devoid of any obvious blood vascular defects, are characterized by the lack of lymphatic vasculature. This is inherent to the *Ragged* mouse, and describes a nonredundant role for SOX18 in mouse lymphatic endothelial differentiation[68]. At the onset of lymphangiogenesis, SOX18 is coexpressed with COUP-TFII and drives the expression of Prox1 in a subset of endothelial cells lining the wall of the CV. These LECs form the basis of the lymphatic vasculature, and absolutely require transient SOX18 and COUP-TFII activity to induce Prox1 transcription[68, 69].. SOX18-null and COUP-TFII-null mice do not express Prox1 in the embryonic CV, are devoid of LECs, and consequently have a total lack of lymph sacs and lymphatic vasculature[68, 69]. However, after the initial LEC specification, Prox1 expression becomes independent of SOX18, and later COUP-TFII, but itself remains critical for lymphatic remodelling and maintenance of LEC identity[68, 69].

3. Blood vessel development in solid tumours

Tumour cells are characterized by chronic proliferation and immortality, due to mutations in genes that regulate cell cycle, homeostasis and cell death[70]. As a solid tumour grows, it is evident that the need for oxygen and nutrients increases correspondingly, and waste materials need to be carried off in escalating amounts, which rationalizes the commonly observed tumour-induced neo-vascularisation. To accomplish this remarkable feat, tumour cells exploit many of the vascular signalling pathways that are activated during embryogenesis, but without tight spatiotemporal control (fig. 3). Vascular architecture and integrity is therefore often compromised, promoting malign features of progressive tumours, such as metastatic behaviour.

3.1. Characteristics of the tumour vasculature

Due to the high oxygen demand and great metabolic activity of tumour cells, the peritumoral region usually becomes hypervascularised. However, this does not truly solve the problem for tumour cells, as in their gluttony they induce constitutive pro-angiogenic signalling that fails to generate a functional vascular network (fig. 3ab). The balance between pro-angiogenic signalling and the subsequent maturation of the newly formed nascent vessels is key for proper circulation and perfusion. Typically, vessel maturation is inadequate in tumour tissue, owing to persistent presence of pro-angiogenic factors. The overabundance of pro-angiogenic signalling originates in part from the tumour directly, but is also a result of the chronic hypoxic and acidic state of the tumour microenvironment. In addition, tumours often trigger and maintain a chronic inflammatory response, wherein cells of the innate and adaptive immune system – mostly macrophages, neutrophils, mast cells and lymphocytes – infiltrate the tumour stoma and crosstalk with ECs to activate quiescent ECs and sustain pro-angiogenic signalling. Although an immune response can in fact reject certain tumours, malignant tumours and their microenvironment can generally evade immune cell mediated destruction, and instead recruit them to their angiogenic campaign[70, 71].

However, tumour angiogenesis proceeds in an unorganized tempest of random sprouting because the guiding signals in the stroma are disorganized, and sprouting cells are unable to filter out any consistent cues. Abnormal shunts, including arteriovenous anastomoses, are commonly observed due to abrogated intervascular communication leading to bi-directional blood flow and impaired perfusion[72]. Tumours are highly diverse due to their tissue of origin and the heterogeneity of the mutations underlying their tumorigenic state. The type and degree of tumour vessel abnormality is correspondingly context dependent, but there are some general traits that tumour vessels share. These regard to overall vascular organization and hierarchy as a network, immediate manifestation of maturation deficiencies, and morphology of vascular ECs.

While the dysregulation of angiogenesis causes overall hypervascularization, vessels are distributed unevenly throughout the peritumoral region, with very low vascular density in some areas. Moreover, large tumours instigate high tissue pressure that can compress and constrict vessels, and vessel diameter thus becomes independent of blood flow rate[73]. Normally, high interstitial pressure is an important queue for lymphatic vessel to drain off the excess fluid, but this function is perturbed in tumour tissue and extravasated fluid is not the sole cause of pressure rise[74, 75]. Where larger blood vessels in normal tissue branch into gradually decreasing size vessels and eventually thin-walled capillaries, this obvious hierarchy is often lost in tumour vasculature, and heterogeneous vessel subtypes are randomly distributed throughout the tumour vascular bed[76, 77]. This affects, but not truly reflects, their functional status.

Where normal vascular endothelial cells line up in the vessel wall to create a continuous barrier to maintain tissue fluid homeostasis and allow the selective diffusion and transport of certain molecules, the tumour vasculature is characterized by loss of EC polarity and cell-cell adhesion that results in an incontinuous and leaky vessel wall. This is aggravated by the loosening of EC-associated mural cells, who fail attach tightly to ECs in the presence of constitutive pro-angiogenic signalling, which in turn leads to reduced vessel stability and incoherent deposition of basement membrane- and ECM components[78, 79]. These resultant vessels cannot maintain a trans-vascular pressure gradient, because excessive amounts of fluid leak into the interstitial space through the porous vessels. Furthermore, tumour cells can gain entrance to the vascular system, for either transport throughout the circulation, or incorporation into the vessel wall.

The entry of tumour cells into the vasculature is a primary facilitator of distant metastasis formation, and is importantly applicable for both blood vessel and lymphatic vessels (fig 3b). It is of note that the lymphatic system is specifically designed to not only transport immune cells, but also to absorb, and drain off, fluid and larger molecules. Therefore, lymphatic capillaries are inadvertently effective in the uptake of tumour cells, and regional lymph node metastasis is a common indication of malignant tumour progression that is used a prognostic tool in human cancer patients[80, 81].

Overall, tumour cells seem to be able to initiate a chronic state of angiogenesis and lymphangiogenesis, but in doing so fail to create normal functional vascular networks. The signalling programmes that underlie these tumour-induced malformations may often have their foundation at a transcription level, with balance in transcriptional networks tipped towards proliferation of both tumour- and vascular EC proliferation and migration.

3.2. Cellular origin of the tumour derived endothelium

The vascular expansion that rapid growing tumours induce requires great numbers of vascular EC to form these structures. Tumours engage in three distinct strategies to wheel in these recruits and promote angiogenesis. The most obvious pro-angiogenic signalling pathway is that which leads to proliferation of a pre-existing vasculature, as it occurs in embryonic remodelling and normal vascularization in the adult. However, tumours also promote the mobilization and specification of bone marrow derived cells (BMDCs). In addition, tumour cells themselves can transdifferentiate into ECs to be incorporated into the tumour vasculature (fig. 3)[82].

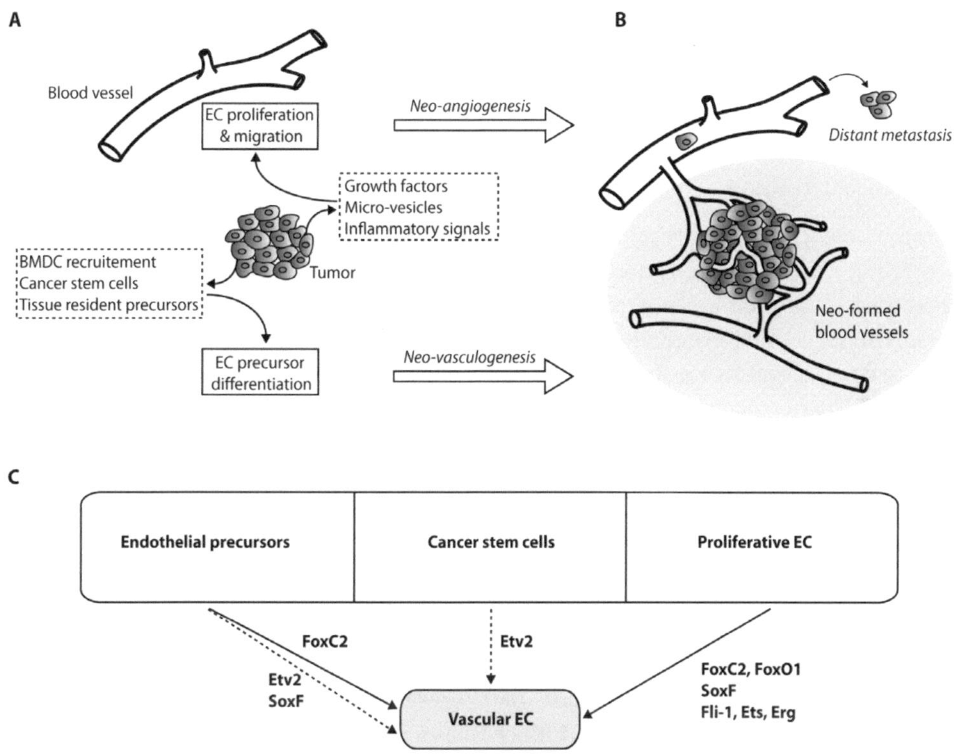

Figure 3. Tumour vascularization strategies originating from TF-dysregulation. **(A)** As it grows, a tumour adapts several techniques to induce vascularization, either though proliferation of preexcisting peritumoral vessels or by promoting differentiation of non-EC into vascular endothelium. **(B)** The peritumoral and intratumoral regions get hypervascularized by the pro-angiogenic and pro-vasculogenic signals that the tumour instigates, which facilitates vessel intravasation metastatis through the vasculature. **(C)** Transciptional dysregulation underlies the angiogenic and vasculogenic signalling that tumour emanate.

Proliferation of the existing vasculature proceeds for a large part through VEGF signalling. The VEGF signalling axis controls angiogenic- and lymphangiogenic sprouting through regulation of cell proliferation and migration, with a set of several VEGF ligands and VEGFR receptors. VEGF-A is particularly angiogenic, while VEGF-C and VEGF-D are primarily lymphangiogenic. The downstream effect however is much dependant on the VEGFR they bind, with several possible combinations and dynamic receptor homodimerization, heterodymerization or co-receptor (NRPs) interaction adding to the complexity. In general, VEGF-A binds to VEGFR1 or VEGFR2 with the former interaction being anti-angiogenic to due high affinity but low downstream tyrosine kinase activity, and the latter being pro-angiogenic. VEGF-C and VEGF-D on the other hand primarily bind the lymphangiogenic VEGFR3 receptor or VEGFR2-3 heterodimers to promote lymphangiogenesis. Hence, VEGFs, their receptors, and regulatory proteins upstream of VEGF – or signalling molecules that crosstalk with VEGF – are beguiling (lymph-)angiogenic players[83, 84].

Recently, light has been shed on tumour signalling to neighbouring endothelium, which convolutes this classical growth factor signalling. Microvesicles released from tumour cells can transport genetic material and signalling molecules directly into endothelial (progenitor) cells that can make epigenetic modification to regulatory genes and otherwise alter expression patterns[85-88]. These microvesicles can also originate from non-tumour cells, such as EPC, to activate angiogenic programmes in vascular ECs[89, 90]. This demonstrates that cells residing in the tumour stroma are altered at a more fundamental level to contribute to tumour vascularization.

Although angiogenesis is the prevailing concept that accounts for tumour vascularization, it is becoming ever more prevalent that vasculogenesis has a significant contribution to vessel formation in tumours. EPCs, and other BMDCs such as tumour associated macrophages (TAMs), mesenchymal progenitor cells (MPC), monocytes, are thought to participate in tumour vascularization in varying degrees, and are common components of the tumour stroma [91-95]. These cells can actively be recruited to the site of neovascularization [96], and reside there to promote angiogenesis or differentiate into vascular EC themselves. This process is further propagated by chronic inflammation of the tumour microenvironment[97]. Furthermore, tissue resident stem cells may contribute to angiogenesis as was shown to be the case in renal cancinoma's[98].

Adding to the mechanism of vasculogenesis and the role of stem cells, is an active role for tumour cells themselves. A heterogeneous malignant tumour is often characterized by subpopulations of cancer stem cells (CSCs) that have great self-renewal and differentiation capacity, similar to normal stem cells[99, 100]. These CMCs have the ability to acquire an endothelial progenitor phenotype, and function as vascular ECs, which benefits tumour vascularization and proliferation[101, 102]. This practise is generally dependent on conditions such as hypoxia, where tumour cells find themselves in acute need of supply and transdifferentiate in vascular progenitors[103-105]. Vascular mimicry is a remarkable demonstration of this CSC-trait. Tumour cells in this process align into channel-like structures, gain EC gene expression, acquire and EC phenotype, and roughly function as blood vessel (fig. 3B). Suggested mechanisms by which tumour cells can differentiate into vascular progenitor include signalling through VEGF and IKKβ [102, 106].

3.3. Dysregulation of transcriptional angiogenic pathways

3.3.1. Ets transcription factors

Many Ets transcription factors have a suggested or confirmed role in tumour angiogenesis and progression. Probably the most obvious Ets members to be involved in tumorigenesis are Fli1 and ERG, which have been acknowledged for their role in embryonic angiogenesis and vasculogenesis in a previous section of this chapter, but also ETS1/2 and several members of the ternary complex factor (TCF) subfamily. These transcription factors have been shown to be overexpressed in tumour cells of divergent cancer types, and to facilitate tumour progression, vascularization and invasion by regulation of growth factor responsiveness and MMP expression [107-112] (fig. 3C).

With the recently discovery of tumour associated vascular ECs, however, it is imminent that key players of cell fate determination contribute to tumour induced neo-vascularization. The master regulator of endothelial and haematopoietic cell specification, Etv2, is only transiently expressed during embryonic development, as further angiogenesis generally occurs through proliferation of pre-existing vasculature. As Etv2 activity is absolutely critical for the specification of ECs, it is conceivable that transdifferentiation of tumour cells and specification and/or mobilization of bone marrow derived progenitors, requires Etv2 activity in tumour angiogenesis[91] (fig. 3c).

Although little is known about the actual expression levels of Etv2 in tumour cells or their microenvironment, several direct target genes or other downstream Etv2 targets are upregulated in tumour tissue. The Ang-2/Tie-2 system, for example, is often strongly activated in endothelial cells of tumour associated remodelling vessels, leading to increased angiogenesis and proliferation[93, 113-115]. MMPs are known to facilitate a broad range of vascular events by ECM remodelling and paving the tumour stroma to promote angiogenesis, and MMP overexpression is instrumental to progression of distinct cancer types[116, 117]. Etv2 can also directly activate the MMP-1 promoter, and MMP-1 is often overexpressed in cancer as are many others[118-121].

Other Etv2 targets, many of which carry the FOX:ETS motif in their promoter, are ubiquitously dysregulated during tumour angiogenesis[122-126]. It is not clear whether this is Etv2-dependent, but it has been shown that Etv2 activity can induce ectopic expression of these genes in embryonic development, and it is conceivable that Etv2 function is recapitulated and exploited in tumour vasculogenesis and angiogenesis. This could explain the transdifferentiation capacity of tumour cells that contribute to the vascular progenitor population, and the recruitment of BMDCs as Etv2 activity specifies EC and haematopoietic lineages from stem cells in the mesoderm. In addition, putative Etv2 targets during tumour angiogenesis have extensive crosstalk with growth factor signalling, which further endorses the suggested role and significance of Etv2 in this process[127].

3.3.2. Forkhead transcription factors

The presence and role of FoxC2 in tumour angiogenesis has been fairly well characterized over the past few years, and it has been shown that the expression of FoxC2 in tumour endothelium coincides with neovascularization. This further supports the notion of Etv2 recurrence during tumour vascularization because of the synergistic function between these transcription factors in regulating endothelial genes expression through the FOX:ETS motif.

FoxC2 overexpression is associated with aggressive human cancers, and has been shown to be overexpressed in mammary breast cancer cells *in vitro* where it directly promotes a metastasis phenotype[128]. More recently, FoxC2 was detected in the tumour ECs of human and mouse melanomas, and it therefore hypothesized that FoxC2 directly contributes to tumour angiogenesis[129]. In a B16 melanoma mouse model, the high expression level of FoxC2 in tumour cells and endothelium correlates with the induced expression of a set of angiogenic factors, such as Notch ligand Dll4, MMP-2, Pdgfβ and VEGF. Deleting one copy of FoxC2 causes reduction of their expression levels, and these FoxC2 heterozygous mutants also display reduced angiogenesis and correspondingly perturbed tumour growth with signs of tumour necrosis [129]. This is in line with the roles of the suggested targets of FoxC2 in tumour neovascularization[127, 130], and the pro-migratory and angiogenic phenotype of FoxC2 overexpressing ECs[129, 131] (fig 3c).

Tumour-induced endothelial to mesenchymal transition can promote FoxC2 expression, which feeds back into further mesenchymal differentiation[128, 132]. This can for a part explain the pro-tumorigenic character of FoxC2, as it increases the ability of tumour ECs to migrate and proliferate, and prevents entry of tumour ECs into a quiescent state. Interestingly, FoxC2 heterozygous mutant mice indeed show a reduced amount of tumour-associated fibroblasts, corroborating this hypothesis[129]. FoxC2 may further contribute to tumour angiogenesis by recruiting mesenchymal stem cells[133], or endothelial progenitor cells [134], although this has yet to be determined.

Interestingly, FoxC1 is also upregulated in some tumour but its role in in tumour angiogenesis is unclear, as deletion of one copy of FoxC 1in mice does not seem to affect melanoma tumour growth or angiogenesis[129]. Also, neither FoxC1 nor FoxC2 explicitly affect tumour lymphangiogenesis as lymphatic marker Lyve-1 and Prox1 expression levels are independent of FoxC1/2 activity in melanoma tumours[129].

FoxO transcription factors operate, in contrast to FoxC1, as tumour suppressors[135-137]. Their function in mediating PI3K-AKT and HIF signalling make them key regulators of cell cycle and apoptosis, and therefore, inactivation of FoxO's is frequently observed in cancer[136, 138-141]. Mouse studies have revealed that FoxOs display functional redundancy in tumour suppression and vascular homeostasis, and triple FoxO knockout (FoxO1, FoxO3, FoxO4) mice develop aggressive tumours with a poor survival rate, and have widely altered expression levels of EC-survival and vascular genes[137]. FoxO1 is required for embryonic vascular development, and its inactivation in cancer has repercussions on tumour vascularization, which is confirmed by vascular remodelling defects in FoxO1-null mice and their established crosstalk with VEGF-signalling[39]. This instigates a paradox wherein tumour cells gain 'immortality' through FoxO inactivation, and simultaneously seem to lose vessel functionalization via the same mechanism[39, 141-143].

On a particular note, FoxO3 depletion in tumour cells can attenuate migration due to reduction in MMP expression, leading to decreased tumour size[144]. Henceforth, the compound FoxO alterations in tumours, and modifications to specific Fox members, must be further explored to fully appreciate the contexts dependent roles of these transcription factors.

3.3.3. SoxF transcription factors

SOXF is expressed transiently in the developing endothelium and then again during pathological conditions, such as wound healing where SOX18 is reexpressed in the capillary endothelium[145], and in tumorigenesis where SOX18 is reexpressed in the tumour stroma[146], including the blood and lymphatic vasculature[52, 147]. Recently, SOXF transcription factors have emerged as novel prognostic markers during gastric cancer progression, as SOX7, SOX17 and particularly SOX18 are frequently overexpressed in gastric tumour tissue of human cancer patients, and survival rates are considerably lower for patients with SOX18 positive tumours [146].

The role of Sox18 in tumour angiogenesis has been studied in SOX18-null, and SOXF loss of function (SOX18 dominant negative mutant-) mice. These studies revealed that melanoma tumours grow more slowly in absence of SOX18 protein or function *in vivo*, with a corresponding reduction in tumour associated microvessel density[52] (fig. 3c). This was further illustrated *in vitro*, where ECs and human breast cancer cells with the dominant negative form of SOX18 proliferate poorly, and tube formation of ECs is impaired, which could be improved by overexpressing functional SOX18[52].

SOX18 has also been shown to directly facilitate the metastatic spread of tumour cells to the sentinel lymph node in mice[147]. This is likely to be achieved by promoting neolymphangiogenesis in the tumour microenvironment and thereby paving the way for tumour cell migration towards the draining lymph node. During tumour growth, SOX18 has been shown to be reexpressed in LECs and is suggested to promote lymphatic vascular expansion[147]. Indeed, SOX18 heterozygous mutant mice have reduced lymphatic vessel density, which is accompanied by a decrease in lymphatic drainage and sentinel lymph node metastasis[147].

Taken together, these observations allocate an important role to SOX18 and possibly other SOXF transcription factors in regulation tumour vascularization. A recent finding descibes that SOX18 expression in tumour tissue is regulated on an epigenetic level by multiple states of promoter-methylation, which underlines the intricacy and divergency of transcriptional programmes in tumours[148]. With a role for SOXF members in arteriovenous specification, angiogenesis and lymphangiogenesis, their dysregulation in tumour settings might be a parameter influencing the heterogeneity and overabundance of tumour vasculature.

4. Concluding remarks

The blood and lymphatic vascular systems are crucial in higher vertebrates for the transport of fluids, oxygen, signalling molecules, immune cells, waste material and other components that maintain homeostasis in the body. These systems develop very early on during embryonic development and are orchestrated by a finely tuned combination of transcriptional regulators that can flick cell fate switches.

The transcriptional networks that underlie EC specification are usually transient or at least very well ordered in the embryo, but this all changes in tumour settings where they are distorted and exploited to induce chronic angiogenesis and vasculogenesis. Although most attention in therapeutic cancer research over the years has gone to growth factor signalling or other downstream players of proliferation, migration and morphogenesis there seems to be an emerging paradigm shift in studying both prognostic and therapeutic potential of fundamental transcription factors. The ETS, Forkhead, and SOXF transcription factors discussed in this overview are in many ways associated with tumour proliferation and vascularization. Studies in developmental biology have laid the groundwork for further study of transcription factors dysregulation in tumours. Remarkably, there is a high level over crosstalk with traditional VEGF signalling either through increased VEGF bio-availability, transduction, or responsiveness within these transcriptional networks.

In the years to come, these transcription factors will expectantly further develop as prognostic tools for tumorigenesis and possibly arise as molecular targets for treatment of malignant tumours. At the very least, studying these fundamental regulators in cancer will add to our understanding of tumour origins and the tools they utilize to achieve proliferation, angiogenesis, and malignancy.

Author details

Jeroen Overman and Mathias François

*Address all correspondence to: m.francois@imb.uq.edu.au

Institute for Molecular Bioscience, The University of Queensland, Brisbane, Australia

References

[1] Choi, K., et al., *A common precursor for hematopoietic and endothelial cells.* Development, 1998. 125(4): p. 725-732.

[2] Huber, T.L., et al., *Haemangioblast commitment is initiated in the primitive streak of the mouse embryo.* Nature, 2004. 432(7017): p. 625-30.

[3] Vogeli, K.M., et al., *A common progenitor for haematopoietic and endothelial lineages in the zebrafish gastrula.* Nature, 2006. 443(7109): p. 337-9.

[4] Shin, M., H. Nagai, and G. Sheng, *Notch mediates Wnt and BMP signals in the early separation of smooth muscle progenitors and blood/endothelial common progenitors.* Development, 2009. 136(4): p. 595-603.

[5] Lancrin, C., et al., *The haemangioblast generates haematopoietic cells through a haemogenic endothelium stage.* Nature, 2009. 457(7231): p. 892-5.

[6] Vodyanik, M.A., et al., *A mesoderm-derived precursor for mesenchymal stem and endothelial cells.* Cell Stem Cell, 2010. 7(6): p. 718-29.

[7] Friedl, P. and S. Alexander, *Cancer invasion and the microenvironment: plasticity and reciprocity.* Cell, 2011. 147(5): p. 992-1009.

[8] Kirschmann, D.A., et al., *Molecular pathways: vasculogenic mimicry in tumor cells: diagnostic and therapeutic implications.* Clin Cancer Res, 2012. 18(10): p. 2726-32.

[9] Oliver, G. and R.S. Srinivasan, *Endothelial cell plasticity: how to become and remain a lymphatic endothelial cell.* Development, 2010. 137(3): p. 363-72.

[10] Sabin, F.R., *Preliminary note on the differentiation of angioblasts and the method by which they produce blood-vessels, blood-plasma and red blood-cells as seen in the living chick. 1917.* J Hematother Stem Cell Res, 2002. 11(1): p. 5-7.

[11] Ferkowicz, M.J. and M.C. Yoder, *Blood island formation: longstanding observations and modern interpretations.* Exp Hematol, 2005. 33(9): p. 1041-7.

[12] Haar, J.L. and G.A. Ackerman, *A phase and electron microscopic study of vasculogenesis and erythropoiesis in the yolk sac of the mouse.* Anat Rec, 1971. 170(2): p. 199-223.

[13] Xu, K. and O. Cleaver, *Tubulogenesis during blood vessel formation.* Semin Cell Dev Biol, 2011. 22(9): p. 993-1004.

[14] Zovein, A.C., et al., *Beta1 integrin establishes endothelial cell polarity and arteriolar lumen formation via a Par3-dependent mechanism.* Dev Cell, 2010. 18(1): p. 39-51.

[15] Strilic, B., et al., *The molecular basis of vascular lumen formation in the developing mouse aorta.* Dev Cell, 2009. 17(4): p. 505-15.

[16] Xu, K., et al., *Blood vessel tubulogenesis requires Rasip1 regulation of GTPase signaling.* Dev Cell, 2011. 20(4): p. 526-39.

[17] Kamei, M., et al., *Endothelial tubes assemble from intracellular vacuoles in vivo.* Nature, 2006. 442(7101): p. 453-6.

[18] Blum, Y., et al., *Complex cell rearrangements during intersegmental vessel sprouting and vessel fusion in the zebrafish embryo.* Dev Biol, 2008. 316(2): p. 312-22.

[19] Wang, Y., et al., *Moesin1 and Ve-cadherin are required in endothelial cells during in vivo tubulogenesis.* Development, 2010. 137(18): p. 3119-28.

[20] Davis, G.E. and C.W. Camarillo, *An alpha 2 beta 1 integrin-dependent pinocytic mechanism involving intracellular vacuole formation and coalescence regulates capillary lumen and tube formation in three-dimensional collagen matrix.* Exp Cell Res, 1996. 224(1): p. 39-51.

[21] Jakobsson, L., et al., *Endothelial cells dynamically compete for the tip cell position during angiogenic sprouting.* Nat Cell Biol, 2010. 12(10): p. 943-53.

[22] Wei, G.H., et al., *Genome-wide analysis of ETS-family DNA-binding in vitro and in vivo.* EMBO J, 2010. 29(13): p. 2147-60.

[23] Pham, V.N., et al., *Combinatorial function of ETS transcription factors in the developing vasculature.* Dev Biol, 2007. 303(2): p. 772-83.

[24] De Val, S., et al., *Combinatorial regulation of endothelial gene expression by ets and forkhead transcription factors.* Cell, 2008. 135(6): p. 1053-64.

[25] Pimanda, J.E., et al., *Gata2, Fli1, and Scl form a recursively wired gene-regulatory circuit during early hematopoietic development.* Proc Natl Acad Sci U S A, 2007. 104(45): p. 17692-7.

[26] Charlot, C., et al., *A review of post-translational modifications and subcellular localization of Ets transcription factors: possible connection with cancer and involvement in the hypoxic response.* Methods Mol Biol, 2010. 647: p. 3-30.

[27] Ferdous, A., et al., *Nkx2-5 transactivates the Ets-related protein 71 gene and specifies an endothelial/endocardial fate in the developing embryo.* Proc Natl Acad Sci U S A, 2009. 106(3): p. 814-9.

[28] Kataoka, H., et al., *Etv2/ER71 induces vascular mesoderm from Flk1+PDGFRalpha+ primitive mesoderm.* Blood, 2011. 118(26): p. 6975-86.

[29] Hart, A., et al., *Fli-1 is required for murine vascular and megakaryocytic development and is hemizygously deleted in patients with thrombocytopenia.* Immunity, 2000. 13(2): p. 167-77.

[30] Hollenhorst, P.C., et al., *Genome-wide analyses reveal properties of redundant and specific promoter occupancy within the ETS gene family.* Genes Dev, 2007. 21(15): p. 1882-94.

[31] Birdsey, G.M., et al., *Transcription factor Erg regulates angiogenesis and endothelial apoptosis through VE-cadherin.* Blood, 2008. 111(7): p. 3498-506.

[32] Birdsey, G.M., et al., *The transcription factor Erg regulates expression of histone deacetylase 6 and multiple pathways involved in endothelial cell migration and angiogenesis.* Blood, 2012. 119(3): p. 894-903.

[33] Lee, D., et al., *ER71 acts downstream of BMP, Notch, and Wnt signaling in blood and vessel progenitor specification.* Cell Stem Cell, 2008. 2(5): p. 497-507.

[34] Kappel, A., et al., *Identification of vascular endothelial growth factor (VEGF) receptor-2 (Flk-1) promoter/enhancer sequences sufficient for angioblast and endothelial cell-specific transcription in transgenic mice.* Blood, 1999. 93(12): p. 4284-92.

[35] Mammoto, A., et al., *A mechanosensitive transcriptional mechanism that controls angiogenesis.* Nature, 2009. 457(7233): p. 1103-8.

[36] Simon, M.P., R. Tournaire, and J. Pouyssegur, *The angiopoietin-2 gene of endothelial cells is up-regulated in hypoxia by a HIF binding site located in its first intron and by the central factors GATA-2 and Ets-1.* J Cell Physiol, 2008. 217(3): p. 809-18.

[37] Linnemann, A.K., et al., *Genetic framework for GATA factor function in vascular biology.* Proc Natl Acad Sci U S A, 2011. 108(33): p. 13641-6.

[38] Veldman, M.B. and S. Lin, *Etsrp/Etv2 is directly regulated by Foxc1a/b in the zebrafish angioblast.* Circ Res, 2012. 110(2): p. 220-9.

[39] Furuyama, T., et al., *Abnormal angiogenesis in Foxo1 (Fkhr)-deficient mice.* J Biol Chem, 2004. 279(33): p. 34741-9.

[40] Wang, Y., et al., *Ephrin-B2 controls VEGF-induced angiogenesis and lymphangiogenesis.* Nature, 2010. 465(7297): p. 483-6.

[41] Matsukawa, M., et al., *Different roles of Foxo1 and Foxo3 in the control of endothelial cell morphology.* Genes Cells, 2009. 14(10): p. 1167-81.

[42] Calnan, D.R. and A. Brunet, *The FoxO code.* Oncogene, 2008. 27(16): p. 2276-88.

[43] Seo, S., et al., *The forkhead transcription factors, Foxc1 and Foxc2, are required for arterial specification and lymphatic sprouting during vascular development.* Dev Biol, 2006. 294(2): p. 458-70.

[44] Fischer, A., et al., *The Notch target genes Hey1 and Hey2 are required for embryonic vascular development.* Genes Dev, 2004. 18(8): p. 901-11.

[45] Seo, S., et al., *Forkhead box transcription factor FoxC1 preserves corneal transparency by regulating vascular growth.* Proc Natl Acad Sci U S A, 2012. 109(6): p. 2015-20.

[46] Skarie, J.M. and B.A. Link, *FoxC1 is essential for vascular basement membrane integrity and hyaloid vessel morphogenesis.* Invest Ophthalmol Vis Sci, 2009. 50(11): p. 5026-34.

[47] Fang, J., et al., *Mutations in FOXC2 (MFH-1), a forkhead family transcription factor, are responsible for the hereditary lymphedema-distichiasis syndrome.* Am J Hum Genet, 2000. 67(6): p. 1382-8.

[48] Mellor, R.H., et al., *Mutations in FOXC2 are strongly associated with primary valve failure in veins of the lower limb.* Circulation, 2007. 115(14): p. 1912-20.

[49] Petrova, T.V., et al., *Defective valves and abnormal mural cell recruitment underlie lymphatic vascular failure in lymphedema distichiasis.* Nat Med, 2004. 10(9): p. 974-81.

[50] Sabine, A., et al., *Mechanotransduction, PROX1, and FOXC2 cooperate to control connexin37 and calcineurin during lymphatic-valve formation.* Dev Cell, 2012. 22(2): p. 430-45.

[51] Norrmen, C., et al., *FOXC2 controls formation and maturation of lymphatic collecting vessels through cooperation with NFATc1.* J Cell Biol, 2009. 185(3): p. 439-57.

[52] Young, N., et al., *Effect of disrupted SOX18 transcription factor function on tumor growth, vascularization, and endothelial development.* J Natl Cancer Inst, 2006. 98(15): p. 1060-7.

[53] Bowles, J., G. Schepers, and P. Koopman, *Phylogeny of the SOX family of developmental transcription factors based on sequence and structural indicators.* Dev Biol, 2000. 227(2): p. 239-55.

[54] Hosking, B.M., et al., *Trans-activation and DNA-binding properties of the transcription factor, Sox-18.* Nucleic Acids Res, 1995. 23(14): p. 2626-8.

[55] Wegner, M., *From head to toes: the multiple facets of Sox proteins.* Nucleic Acids Res, 1999. 27(6): p. 1409-20.

[56] Hosking, B.M., et al., *SOX18 directly interacts with MEF2C in endothelial cells.* Biochem Biophys Res Commun, 2001. 287(2): p. 493-500.

[57] Wilson, M. and P. Koopman, *Matching SOX: partner proteins and co-factors of the SOX family of transcriptional regulators.* Curr Opin Genet Dev, 2002. 12(4): p. 441-6.

[58] Hosking, B., et al., *Sox7 and Sox17 are strain-specific modifiers of the lymphangiogenic defects caused by Sox18 dysfunction in mice.* Development, 2009. 136(14): p. 2385-91.

[59] Pennisi, D., et al., *Mutations in Sox18 underlie cardiovascular and hair follicle defects in ragged mice.* Nat Genet, 2000. 24(4): p. 434-7.

[60] Cermenati, S., et al., *Sox18 and Sox7 play redundant roles in vascular development.* Blood, 2008. 111(5): p. 2657-66.

[61] Herpers, R., et al., *Redundant roles for sox7 and sox18 in arteriovenous specification in zebrafish.* Circ Res, 2008. 102(1): p. 12-5.

[62] Fontijn, R.D., et al., *SOX-18 controls endothelial-specific claudin-5 gene expression and barrier function.* Am J Physiol Heart Circ Physiol, 2008. 294(2): p. H891-900.

[63] Hosking, B.M., et al., *The VCAM-1 gene that encodes the vascular cell adhesion molecule is a target of the Sry-related high mobility group box gene, Sox18.* J Biol Chem, 2004. 279(7): p. 5314-22.

[64] Hoeth, M., et al., *The transcription factor SOX18 regulates the expression of matrix metalloproteinase 7 and guidance molecules in human endothelial cells.* PLoS One, 2012. 7(1): p. e30982.

[65] Samant, G.V., et al., *Sox factors transcriptionally regulate ROBO4 gene expression in developing vasculature in zebrafish.* J Biol Chem, 2011. 286(35): p. 30740-7.

[66] Bedell, V.M., et al., *roundabout4 is essential for angiogenesis in vivo.* Proc Natl Acad Sci U S A, 2005. 102(18): p. 6373-8.

[67] Matsui, T., et al., *Redundant roles of Sox17 and Sox18 in postnatal angiogenesis in mice.* J Cell Sci, 2006. 119(Pt 17): p. 3513-26.

[68] Francois, M., et al., *Sox18 induces development of the lymphatic vasculature in mice.* Nature, 2008. 456(7222): p. 643-7.

[69] Srinivasan, R.S., et al., *The nuclear hormone receptor Coup-TFII is required for the initiation and early maintenance of Prox1 expression in lymphatic endothelial cells.* Genes Dev, 2010. 24(7): p. 696-707.

[70] Hanahan, D. and R.A. Weinberg, *Hallmarks of cancer: the next generation.* Cell, 2011. 144(5): p. 646-74.

[71] Schreiber, R.D., L.J. Old, and M.J. Smyth, *Cancer immunoediting: integrating immunity's roles in cancer suppression and promotion.* Science, 2011. 331(6024): p. 1565-70.

[72] Pries, A.R., et al., *The shunt problem: control of functional shunting in normal and tumour vasculature.* Nat Rev Cancer, 2010. 10(8): p. 587-93.

[73] Kamoun, W.S., et al., *Simultaneous measurement of RBC velocity, flux, hematocrit and shear rate in vascular networks.* Nat Methods, 2010. 7(8): p. 655-60.

[74] Padera, T.P., et al., *Pathology: cancer cells compress intratumour vessels.* Nature, 2004. 427(6976): p. 695.

[75] Heldin, C.H., et al., *High interstitial fluid pressure - an obstacle in cancer therapy.* Nat Rev Cancer, 2004. 4(10): p. 806-13.

[76] Eberhard, A., et al., *Heterogeneity of angiogenesis and blood vessel maturation in human tumors: implications for antiangiogenic tumor therapies.* Cancer Res, 2000. 60(5): p. 1388-93.

[77] Yu, J.L., et al., *Heterogeneous vascular dependence of tumor cell populations.* Am J Pathol, 2001. 158(4): p. 1325-34.

[78] Morikawa, S., et al., *Abnormalities in pericytes on blood vessels and endothelial sprouts in tumors.* Am J Pathol, 2002. 160(3): p. 985-1000.

[79] Gerhardt, H. and H. Semb, *Pericytes: gatekeepers in tumour cell metastasis?* J Mol Med (Berl), 2008. 86(2): p. 135-44.

[80] Alitalo, K., T. Tammela, and T.V. Petrova, *Lymphangiogenesis in development and human disease.* Nature, 2005. 438(7070): p. 946-53.

[81] Achen, M.G., B.K. McColl, and S.A. Stacker, *Focus on lymphangiogenesis in tumor metastasis.* Cancer Cell, 2005. 7(2): p. 121-7.

[82] Soda, Y., et al., *Transdifferentiation of glioblastoma cells into vascular endothelial cells.* Proc Natl Acad Sci U S A, 2011. 108(11): p. 4274-80.

[83] Adams, R.H. and K. Alitalo, *Molecular regulation of angiogenesis and lymphangiogenesis.* Nat Rev Mol Cell Biol, 2007. 8(6): p. 464-78.

[84] Lohela, M., et al., *VEGFs and receptors involved in angiogenesis versus lymphangiogenesis.* Curr Opin Cell Biol, 2009. 21(2): p. 154-65.

[85] Skog, J., et al., *Glioblastoma microvesicles transport RNA and proteins that promote tumour growth and provide diagnostic biomarkers.* Nat Cell Biol, 2008. 10(12): p. 1470-6.

[86] Valadi, H., et al., *Exosome-mediated transfer of mRNAs and microRNAs is a novel mechanism of genetic exchange between cells.* Nat Cell Biol, 2007. 9(6): p. 654-9.

[87] Balaj, L., et al., *Tumour microvesicles contain retrotransposon elements and amplified oncogene sequences.* Nat Commun, 2011. 2: p. 180.

[88] Millimaggi, D., et al., *Tumor vesicle-associated CD147 modulates the angiogenic capability of endothelial cells.* Neoplasia, 2007. 9(4): p. 349-57.

[89] Deregibus, M.C., et al., *Endothelial progenitor cell derived microvesicles activate an angiogenic program in endothelial cells by a horizontal transfer of mRNA.* Blood, 2007. 110(7): p. 2440-8.

[90] Collino, F., et al., *Microvesicles derived from adult human bone marrow and tissue specific mesenchymal stem cells shuttle selected pattern of miRNAs.* PLoS One, 2010. 5(7): p. e11803.

[91] Li Calzi, S., et al., *EPCs and pathological angiogenesis: when good cells go bad.* Microvasc Res, 2010. 79(3): p. 207-16.

[92] Joyce, J.A. and J.W. Pollard, *Microenvironmental regulation of metastasis.* Nat Rev Cancer, 2009. 9(4): p. 239-52.

[93] De Palma, M., et al., *Tie2 identifies a hematopoietic lineage of proangiogenic monocytes required for tumor vessel formation and a mesenchymal population of pericyte progenitors.* Cancer Cell, 2005. 8(3): p. 211-26.

[94] Gao, D., et al., *Endothelial progenitor cells control the angiogenic switch in mouse lung metastasis.* Science, 2008. 319(5860): p. 195-8.

[95] Karnoub, A.E., et al., *Mesenchymal stem cells within tumour stroma promote breast cancer metastasis.* Nature, 2007. 449(7162): p. 557-63.

[96] Grunewald, M., et al., *VEGF-induced adult neovascularization: recruitment, retention, and role of accessory cells.* Cell, 2006. 124(1): p. 175-89.

[97] Mantovani, A., et al., *Cancer-related inflammation.* Nature, 2008. 454(7203): p. 436-44.

[98] Bruno, S., et al., *CD133+ renal progenitor cells contribute to tumor angiogenesis.* Am J Pathol, 2006. 169(6): p. 2223-35.

[99] Fang, D., et al., *A tumorigenic subpopulation with stem cell properties in melanomas.* Cancer Res, 2005. 65(20): p. 9328-37.

[100] Pezzolo, A., et al., *Oct-4+/Tenascin C+ neuroblastoma cells serve as progenitors of tumor-derived endothelial cells.* Cell Res, 2011. 21(10): p. 1470-86.

[101] Gao, J.X., *Cancer stem cells: the lessons from pre-cancerous stem cells.* J Cell Mol Med, 2008. 12(1): p. 67-96.

[102] Alvero, A.B., et al., *Stem-like ovarian cancer cells can serve as tumor vascular progenitors.* Stem Cells, 2009. 27(10): p. 2405-13.

[103] Yao, X.H., Y.F. Ping, and X.W. Bian, *Contribution of cancer stem cells to tumor vasculogenic mimicry.* Protein Cell, 2011. 2(4): p. 266-72.

[104] El Hallani, S., et al., *A new alternative mechanism in glioblastoma vascularization: tubular vasculogenic mimicry.* Brain, 2010. 133(Pt 4): p. 973-82.

[105] Shen, R., et al., *Precancerous stem cells can serve as tumor vasculogenic progenitors.* PLoS One, 2008. 3(2): p. e1652.

[106] Kusumbe, A.P., A.M. Mali, and S.A. Bapat, *CD133-expressing stem cells associated with ovarian metastases establish an endothelial hierarchy and contribute to tumor vasculature.* Stem Cells, 2009. 27(3): p. 498-508.

[107] Nakayama, T., et al., *Expression of the Ets-1 proto-oncogene in human gastric carcinoma: correlation with tumor invasion.* Am J Pathol, 1996. 149(6): p. 1931-9.

[108] Alipov, G., et al., *Overexpression of Ets-1 proto-oncogene in latent and clinical prostatic carcinomas.* Histopathology, 2005. 46(2): p. 202-8.

[109] Saeki, H., et al., *Concurrent overexpression of Ets-1 and c-Met correlates with a phenotype of high cellular motility in human esophageal cancer.* Int J Cancer, 2002. 98(1): p. 8-13.

[110] Pourtier-Manzanedo, A., et al., *Expression of an Ets-1 dominant-negative mutant perturbs normal and tumor angiogenesis in a mouse ear model.* Oncogene, 2003. 22(12): p. 1795-806.

[111] Potikyan, G., et al., *EWS/FLI1 regulates tumor angiogenesis in Ewing's sarcoma via suppression of thrombospondins.* Cancer Res, 2007. 67(14): p. 6675-84.

[112] Carver, B.S., et al., *Aberrant ERG expression cooperates with loss of PTEN to promote cancer progression in the prostate.* Nat Genet, 2009. 41(5): p. 619-24.

[113] Mitsuhashi, N., et al., *Angiopoietins and Tie-2 expression in angiogenesis and proliferation of human hepatocellular carcinoma.* Hepatology, 2003. 37(5): p. 1105-13.

[114] Peters, K.G., et al., *Expression of Tie2/Tek in breast tumour vasculature provides a new marker for evaluation of tumour angiogenesis.* Br J Cancer, 1998. 77(1): p. 51-6.

[115] Staton, C.A., et al., *Angiopoietins 1 and 2 and Tie-2 receptor expression in human ductal breast disease.* Histopathology, 2011. 59(2): p. 256-63.

[116] Littlepage, L.E., et al., *Matrix metalloproteinases contribute distinct roles in neuroendocrine prostate carcinogenesis, metastasis, and angiogenesis progression.* Cancer Res, 2010. 70(6): p. 2224-34.

[117] Egeblad, M. and Z. Werb, *New functions for the matrix metalloproteinases in cancer progression.* Nat Rev Cancer, 2002. 2(3): p. 161-74.

[118] Murray, G.I., et al., *Matrix metalloproteinase-1 is associated with poor prognosis in colorectal cancer.* Nat Med, 1996. 2(4): p. 461 2.

[119] Sauter, W., et al., *Matrix metalloproteinase 1 (MMP1) is associated with early-onset lung cancer.* Cancer Epidemiol Biomarkers Prev, 2008. 17(5): p. 1127-35.

[120] Pallavi, S.K., et al., *Notch and Mef2 synergize to promote proliferation and metastasis through JNK signal activation in Drosophila.* EMBO J, 2012. 31(13): p. 2895-907.

[121] De Haro, L. and R. Janknecht, *Functional analysis of the transcription factor ER71 and its activation of the matrix metalloproteinase-1 promoter.* Nucleic Acids Res, 2002. 30(13): p. 2972-9.

[122] Hendrix, M.J., et al., *Expression and functional significance of VE-cadherin in aggressive human melanoma cells: role in vasculogenic mimicry.* Proc Natl Acad Sci U S A, 2001. 98(14): p. 8018-23.

[123] Wallez, Y., I. Vilgrain, and P. Huber, *Angiogenesis: the VE-cadherin switch.* Trends Cardiovasc Med, 2006. 16(2): p. 55-9.

[124] Ostrander, J.H., et al., *Breast tumor kinase (protein tyrosine kinase 6) regulates heregulin-induced activation of ERK5 and p38 MAP kinases in breast cancer cells.* Cancer Res, 2007. 67(9): p. 4199-209.

[125] Hu, W., et al., *Biological roles of the Delta family Notch ligand Dll4 in tumor and endothelial cells in ovarian cancer.* Cancer Res, 2011. 71(18): p. 6030-9.

[126] Hovinga, K.E., et al., *Inhibition of notch signaling in glioblastoma targets cancer stem cells via an endothelial cell intermediate.* Stem Cells, 2010. 28(6): p. 1019-29.

[127] Rapisarda, A. and G. Melillo, *Role of the VEGF/VEGFR axis in cancer biology and therapy.* Adv Cancer Res, 2012. 114: p. 237-67.

[128] Mani, S.A., et al., *Mesenchyme Forkhead 1 (FOXC2) plays a key role in metastasis and is associated with aggressive basal-like breast cancers.* Proc Natl Acad Sci U S A, 2007. 104(24): p. 10069-74.

[129] Sano, H., et al., *The Foxc2 transcription factor regulates tumor angiogenesis.* Biochem Biophys Res Commun, 2010. 392(2): p. 201-6.

[130] Taniwaki, K., et al., *Stroma-derived matrix metalloproteinase (MMP)-2 promotes membrane type 1-MMP-dependent tumor growth in mice.* Cancer Res, 2007. 67(9): p. 4311-9.

[131] Hayashi, H., et al., *The Foxc2 transcription factor regulates angiogenesis via induction of integrin beta3 expression.* J Biol Chem, 2008. 283(35): p. 23791-800.

[132] Zeisberg, E.M., et al., *Discovery of endothelial to mesenchymal transition as a source for carcinoma-associated fibroblasts.* Cancer Res, 2007. 67(21): p. 10123-8.

[133] Crisan, M., et al., *A perivascular origin for mesenchymal stem cells in multiple human organs.* Cell Stem Cell, 2008. 3(3): p. 301-13.

[134] Li, D., et al., *Foxc2 overexpression enhances benefit of endothelial progenitor cells for inhibiting neointimal formation by promoting CXCR4-dependent homing.* J Vasc Surg, 2011. 53(6): p. 1668-78.

[135] Dansen, T.B. and B.M. Burgering, *Unravelling the tumor-suppressive functions of FOXO proteins.* Trends Cell Biol, 2008. 18(9): p. 421-9.

[136] Modur, V., et al., *FOXO proteins regulate tumor necrosis factor-related apoptosis inducing ligand expression. Implications for PTEN mutation in prostate cancer.* J Biol Chem, 2002. 277(49): p. 47928-37.

[137] Paik, J.H., et al., *FoxOs are lineage-restricted redundant tumor suppressors and regulate endothelial cell homeostasis.* Cell, 2007. 128(2): p. 309-23.

[138] Roy, S.K., R.K. Srivastava, and S. Shankar, *Inhibition of PI3K/AKT and MAPK/ERK pathways causes activation of FOXO transcription factor, leading to cell cycle arrest and apoptosis in pancreatic cancer.* J Mol Signal, 2010. 5: p. 10.

[139] Ciechomska, I., et al., *Inhibition of Akt kinase signalling and activation of Forkhead are indispensable for upregulation of FasL expression in apoptosis of glioma cells.* Oncogene, 2003. 22(48): p. 7617-27.

[140] Hu, M.C., et al., *IkappaB kinase promotes tumorigenesis through inhibition of forkhead FOXO3a.* Cell, 2004. 117(2): p. 225-37.

[141] Aoki, M., H. Jiang, and P.K. Vogt, *Proteasomal degradation of the FoxO1 transcriptional regulator in cells transformed by the P3k and Akt oncoproteins.* Proc Natl Acad Sci U S A, 2004. 101(37): p. 13613-7.

[142] Kim, S.Y., et al., *Constitutive phosphorylation of the FOXO1 transcription factor in gastric cancer cells correlates with microvessel area and the expressions of angiogenesis-related molecules.* BMC Cancer, 2011. 11: p. 264.

[143] Lee, B.L., et al., *A hypoxia-independent up-regulation of hypoxia-inducible factor-1 by AKT contributes to angiogenesis in human gastric cancer.* Carcinogenesis, 2008. 29(1): p. 44-51.

[144] Storz, P., et al., *FOXO3a promotes tumor cell invasion through the induction of matrix metalloproteinases.* Mol Cell Biol, 2009. 29(18): p. 4906-17.

[145] Darby, I.A., et al., *Sox18 is transiently expressed during angiogenesis in granulation tissue of skin wounds with an identical expression pattern to Flk-1 mRNA.* Lab Invest, 2001. 81(7): p. 937-43.

[146] Eom, B.W., et al., *The lymphangiogenic factor SOX 18: a key indicator to stage gastric tumor progression.* Int J Cancer, 2012. 131(1): p. 41-8.

[147] Duong, T., et al., *Genetic ablation of SOX18 function suppresses tumor lymphangiogenesis and metastasis of melanoma in mice.* Cancer Res, 2012. 72(12): p. 3105-14.

[148] Azhikina, T., et al., *Heterogeneity and degree of TIMP4, GATA4, SOX18, and EGFL7 gene promoter methylation in non-small cell lung cancer and surrounding tissues.* Cancer Genet, 2011. 204(9): p. 492-500.

Chapter 2

Roles of SRF in Endothelial Cells During Hypoxia

Jianyuan Chai

Additional information is available at the end of the chapter

http://dx.doi.org/10.5772/52182

1. Introduction

Oxygen is a basic need for human life. Maintaining adequate oxygen supply is essential for proper cellular functions. In normal tissue, the oxygen supply usually matches metabolic requirements, and even if there is a brief oxygen shortage, the body can overcome it by an increase in the oxygen extracted from the blood or an increase in local blood flow. In advanced solid tumors, however, due to uncontrolled cell proliferation, the oxygen consumption rate often exceeds the oxygen available around the area, resulting in local hypoxia. The diffusion distance from blood vessels to surrounding tissues is usually no more than 100-200 μm; therefore, the further into the center of the tumors, the lower the oxygen level gets. As measured by Eppendorf probe, pO2 in normal tissue is between 17 and 65 mm Hg, while in wide range of tumors, pO2 can go down to 2 mm or even to zero.

As a result of oxygen deficiency, two things can happen to the suffering cells. Cells can either stop proliferation and die of apoptosis or necrosis, or fight back by taking adaptive processes that lead to increased proliferation, migration and tissue reorganization. While the ultimate fate of the cells varies with tissue type, the severity and duration of hypoxia play critical roles in choosing the direction. In moderate oxygen decline (~ 2-7 mm Hg), the cells in oxygen starvation and the cells carrying oxygen (red blood cells) run towards each other. Cancer cells can move away from their original locations to where oxygen is sufficient, while endothelial cells in the blood vessels can also take an action to move out to form new vessels to bring oxygen towards the center of hypoxia. The former process is known as metastasis, and the latter is angiogenesis. Angiogenesis and metastasis support cancer cells to survive through hypoxic crisis and allow malignant progression. Under severe hypoxic condition (< 1 mm Hg), however, cells are prone to die of apoptosis if glycolytic ATP available, otherwise, die of necrosis.

INTECH
open science | open minds

© 2013 The Author(s). Licensee InTech. This chapter is distributed under the terms of the Creative Commons Attribution License http://creativecommons.org/licenses/by/3.0), which permits unrestricted use, distribution, and reproduction in any medium, provided the original work is properly cited.

Hypoxia-induced apoptosis proceeds through the mitochondrial pathway, as the mitochondria are the primary site of oxygen consumption in a cell. Under normoxic conditions, the mitochondria consume about 90% of available oxygen in the generation of ATP through oxidative phosphorylation in order to meet the metabolic needs of the cell [1, 2]. When there is not sufficient oxygen to support this process, mitochondrial damage occurs, which leads to apoptotic cell death.

To live or to die for a cell under hypoxia is all regulated through different expression and activation of transcription factors. A number of transcription factors have been reported to respond to oxygen deficiency, including AP-1 [3], FOS [4], JUN [4], CREB/ATF [5], DEC1 [6], EGR1 [7], ETS1 [8], GADD153 [9], GATA2 [10], MASH2 [11], NF-IL-6 [12], NFκB [13], RTEF-1 [14], SMADs [15], SP1 [16], STAT5 [17], and of course, the most popular ones, HIF [18] and p53 [19].

2. Hypoxia inducible factor

Hypoxia inducible factor (HIF) is the best studied transcription factor in hypoxia. Whenever there is a discussion about hypoxia, HIF is always an inevitable topic. HIF is composed of two subunits, α and β. While HIFβ is constitutively expressed, HIFα functions more like an oxygen sensor, varying in response to oxygen level [20]. HIFα has an extremely short half-life under normoxic conditions due to ubiquitination by von Hippel-Lindau factor (VHL). Hypoxia does not change HIFα expression per se but stabilizes it by inhibiting hydroxylation at prolines 402 and 564 so that VHL can no longer bind to HIFα to cause proteasomal degradation. Instead, it enables HIFα to bind to HIFβ in the nucleus, generating a functional heterodimeric transcription factor that is able to activate genes that contain hypoxia-response elements (5'-RCGTG-3'), such as genes coding for glucose transporters, vascular endothelial growth factor (VEGF), inducible nitric oxide synthase (iNOS), and erythropoietin (EPO) [21, 22]. In normal tissue, the expression of such genes is to counteract the detrimental impact of hypoxia and to help cells to survive through oxygen crisis. In cancer, however, this role of HIF is abused to support tumor growth and resistance to chemotherapy. Up to date, there are three members in HIF family. HIF-1α is most ubiquitously expressed, while HIF-2α, which shares 48% identity and similar functions with HIF1α, is more restricted to endothelial cells [23]. HIF-3α is the least characterized but may function as a negative regulator of hypoxia, as its dimer with the β subunit has no transcriptional activity [24].

The most prominent role of HIF during hypoxia is to support angiogenesis through transcriptional activation of VEGF. VEGF belongs to a family that contains VEGF-A, VEGF-B, VEGF-C, VEGF-D, VEGF-E and placenta-like growth factor. VEGF-A, the first growth factor that was identified to have special effects on endothelial cells, further splits into five isoforms. VEGF is mainly produced by endothelial cells, macrophages, fibroblasts, and smooth muscle cells. It promotes endothelial cell migration, proliferation and survival through its receptors, VEGFR-1 (Flt-1) and/or VEGFR-2 (Flk-1/KDR), which are predominantly expressed on endothelial cells [25]. In addition, VEGF can also bind to three other transmembrane proteins: VEGFR-3 (Flt-4), which is expressed mainly on lymphatic endothelial cells and only responds to VEGF-C and -D, Neuropilin-1 and Neuropilin-2, which work as co-receptors with VEGFR-2 [26]. Hypoxia-induced VEGF up-regulation is considered to be the major driving force for angiogenesis during tumor progression [27]. Tremendous effort has been made in cancer chemotherapy to inhibit this process and has achieved some significant results, but some expectations have not been met. In addition to VEGF, HIF also regulates several other angiogenic factors such as placenta-like growth factor, platelet-derived growth factor, angiopoietin-1 and -2 [28].

3. p53

Like HIF, p53 is expressed at a low level under normal oxygen conditions and degraded constantly by MDM2 through ubiquitination [29, 30]. Under cellular stress like hypoxia, however, ATM/ATR kinases become active and phosphorylate p53 at its N terminus, which disrupts its interaction with MDM2 and thus, p53 becomes stabilized and moves into the nucleus to activate pro-apoptotic genes [31]. As mentioned above, hypoxia induces apoptosis through mitochondrial damage. The mitochondrial integrity is guarded by Bcl-2 family proteins which include anti-apoptotic members like Bcl-2 and Bcl-X_L, and also pro-apoptotic members, such as Bax and Bak. The balance between these two teams is critical to the fate of a cell. Bcl-2 is an integral membrane protein that targets the outer mitochondrial membrane, and it can form homodimers with each other or heterodimers with Bax. Bax, on the other hand, can do the same. When Bcl-2 predominates, mitochondria stay intact and cells are protected. However, while Bax is in excess, Bax homodimers become dominant, the cells are susceptible to apoptosis. Bax expression is regulated by p53; therefore, p53 activation increases the ratio of Bax to Bacl-2 and reduces the chance of Bcl-2 and Bax association. It has been postulated that 50% reduction in the formation of Bcl-2/Bax complexes can drive the cells toward apoptosis [32]. When Bax inserts into the outer mitochondrial membrane, it opens pores to allow the molecules sequestered in between outer and inner mitochondrial membrane to leak out into the cytosol. One of the released molecules is cytochrome c, which can bind to the apoptotic protease activating factor-1 (APAF-1] and promote it to form an apoptosome. The apoptosome then binds caspase-9 and activates it to cleave two other caspases, caspase-3 and -7. These two caspases orchestrate apoptosis through cleavage of key substrates within the cell, resulting in cell death.

p53 and HIF1α are an odd couple, one supporting cell death and the other supporting cell survival. These two transcription factors can interact with each other directly because HIF1α contains two p53-binding sites within its ODD domain [33]. Unlike HIF, p53 appears to be less sensitive to oxygen level change. Under moderate hypoxic conditions, HIF1α binds to HIF1β to activate genes that promote cell survival, while p53 still remains inactive. Some *in vitro* studies even showed that in such a situation p53 actually promotes HDM2-mediated

HIF1α degradation [34]. Under severe oxygen poverty, however, HIF1α becomes dephosphorylated and may choose to help p53 to induce cell death [35].

4. Hypoxia activates SRF

Although many transcription factors have been studied extensively under hypoxia [36], the reaction of serum response factor (SRF) to oxygen shortage has rarely been discussed.

SRF regulates numerous genes that are involved in cellular responses to mitogenic stimuli as well as cellular stress [37-39]. These genes fall into many diversified categories, including immediate early genes (FOS, EGR1, etc.), cytoskeletal genes (ACTB, CFL1, DES, DSTN, TTN, KRT17, etc.), muscle-related genes (ACTA2, MYH6, MYH11, SM22α, TNNT1, ATP2A1, etc.), growth factors (IGF2, FGF10, FGFR3, TGFB1i1, etc.), extracellular matrix proteins (CCN1, CTGF, etc.), cell adhesion molecules (ITGA1, ITGA5, ITGB1, etc.), intercellular junctional molecules (TJP1, CDH5, CDH11, etc.), neuronal receptors (NR4A1, NR4A2, etc.), and apoptosis regulators (BCL2). This list is still growing. All these genes contain a common DNA sequence, $CC(A/T)_6GG$, so-called CArG box or serum response element (SRE), which SRF recognizes. Some of these genes contain multiple CArG boxes, for example, EGR1 has six and CCN1 has five, and even SRF itself has four SRE sequences [40], indicating a tight regulation by SRF. In addition to the hundreds of genes that SRF directly regulates, a growing number of genes that do not contain SRE have been found to respond to SRF activition [41, 42].

Hypoxia is a form of stress to the cells; therefore, it triggers a response from SRF undoubtedly. As shown in Figure 1, under hypoxic condition, there is not only an increase in the level of SRF expression (Figure 1A), but also an increase in SRF phosphorylation (Figure 1A), which enhances SRF binding activity to SRE (Figure 1B). Moreover, this activation of SRF is independent from either HIF or p53, because neither shut down of HIF with its specific inhibitor Dimethyl Bisphenol A (DBA) (Figure 1C), nor inhibition of p53 with Pifithrin-α (Figure 1D) has impact on hypoxia-induced SRF activation.

5. SRF supports hypoxia-induced angiogenesis

Previously, we have shown that SRF is required for VEGF-induced *in vitro* angiogenesis, and without SRF, VEGF cannot induce endothelial cell proliferation and migration, which are essential for angiogenesis [43]. Our findings were confirmed and extended later by an *in vivo* study on mouse embryonic development, which demonstrated that knockout of SRF in endothelial cells impairs sprouting angiogenesis from arteries to veins [44]. Transcriptional analysis showed that SRF deficiency not only had negative impact on genes responsible for endothelial connection (e.g. VE-cadherin) and adhesion (e.g. integrin $\alpha5$ and $\beta1$), but also suppressed angiogenic factors like VEGF and angiopoietin-1 and -2.

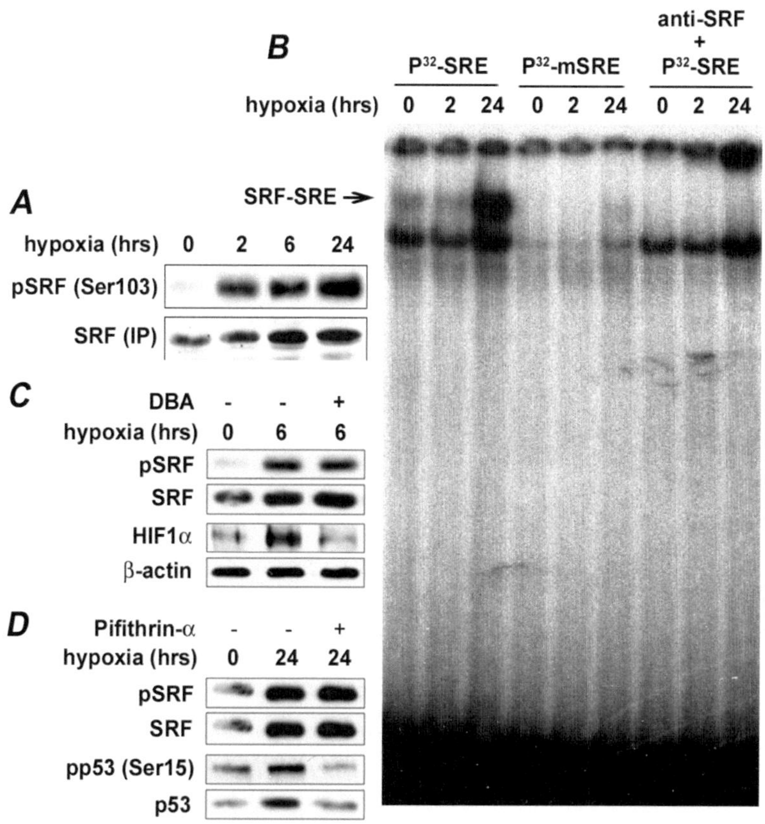

Figure 1. Hypoxia activates SRF in mouse brain endothelial cells (bEND3) regardless HIF and p53 status. A. Cells were cultured in a hypoxic chamber (5% CO_2 : 94% N_2 : 1% O_2) at 37°C for 2, 6 and 24 hours. Total protein was isolated and immune-precipitated with an antibody against SRF. Total and phosphorylated SRF were detected by Western blot analysis. B. SRF protein activity was analyzed by electrophoretic mobility shift assay with P^{32}-labeled consensus SRE (SRE) and mutant SRE (mSRE) oligos. SRF to SRE binding activity was increased by hypoxic treatment. The lack of binding ability to the mutant SRE probe as well as the super shift with the SRF antibody (anti-SRF) confirmed the binding specificity. C. In the presence of Dimethyl Bisphenol A (DBA), a specific inhibitor for HIF, hypoxic treatment failed to stabilize HIF1α, but did not affect SRF activation. D. Incubation with p53 inhibitor Pifithrin-α suppressed p53 activation by hypoxia but did not affect SRF either.

Here we show that hypoxia-induced angiogenic activity in brain endothelial cells is completely lost when SRF is knocked down by RNA interference (Figure 2), indicating that SRF is essential to hypoxia-induced angiogenesis. On the other hand, when extra copies of SRF gene are introduced into these cells, hypoxia-induced angiogenic activity is enhanced. It has been postulated that hypoxia induces angiogenesis through HIF-VEGF-MAPK/Rho-SRF pathway [45]. From our previous study [43], we know that VEGF does activate SRF through MAPK and Rho pathways. However, this is just one side of a coin. As shown above (Figure 1), the increase of VEGF signaling during hypoxia is due to HIF activation, while hypoxia activates SRF independently from HIF and therefore, independently from VEGF as well. SRF responds to hypoxia directly as other transcription factors like HIF and p53. In addition, SRF also serves as a downstream regulator in cell proliferation, adhesion and migration, thus any mitogenic factor that aims to stimulate such cellular activities requires SRF involvement.

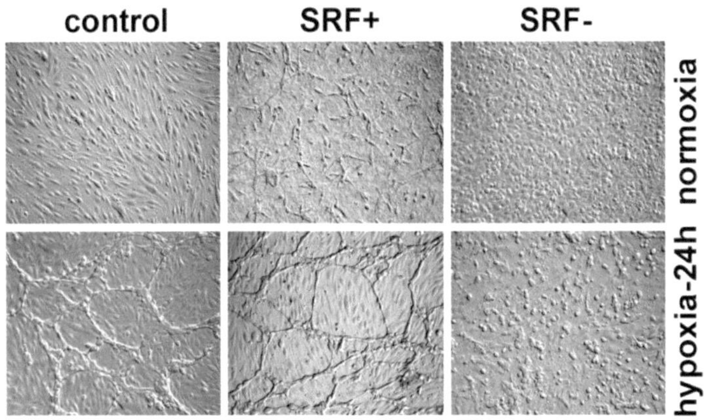

Figure 2. Knockdown of SRF in brain endothelial cells (bEND3) prevents hypoxia-induced angiogenesis. bEND3 cells were cultured in collagen gel matrix under a hypoxic condition. The collagen gel matrix was made of 50% type I collagen in HEPES (pH 8.5) Hanks buffer balanced growth medium. The mixture was solidified in 12-well plates at 37˚C for 20 minutes. Cells were mixed in the liquid gel, plated on top of the solidified gel in the 12-well plates and incubated at 37˚C for additional 20 minutes. More layers of cells were plated in the wells by repeating this step. Eventually, growth medium was added to the top of the solidified gel containing endothelial cells and the plates were incubated at 37˚C for a week. The control cells formed a cobblestone monolayer at the end, while SRF over-expressing cells (SRF+) moved vertically and horizontally within the gel matrix. The cells with SRF knockdown (SRF-), on the other hand, stayed inactively. Under hypoxia, both control and SRF+ cells formed cable-like structure, an indication of angiogenic activity, while the SRF- cells showed sign of death.

6. SRF protects endothelial cells against hypoxia-induced apoptosis

Several studies indicate that hypoxia-induced apoptosis is solely dependent on the mitochondrial pathway [46-48], which is regulated by Bcl-2 family members [49, 50]. Hypoxia induces an increase in the ratio of the pro-apoptotic protein Bax to the anti-apoptotic protein(s) Bcl-2 and/or Bcl-X_L, thereby increases mitochondrial permeability and enables release of cytochrome c to cytoplasm [51]. Cytochrome c released into the cytoplasm forms complexes with Apaf-1 and triggers a caspase cascade to execute apoptotic cell death [52, 53]. It has been demonstrated in neuronal cells that hypoxia-induced Bax expression and DNA fragmentation are mediated through induction of nitric oxide (NO) [54, 55]. NO in endothelial cells is generated by both the endothelial and inducible isoforms of nitric oxide synthase (eNOS and iNOS) via oxidation of the substrate, L-arginine. Hypoxia can induce both iNOS and eNOS expression because the iNOS gene promoter has the hypoxia response element for HIF1 [56, 57] and the eNOS gene promoter has binding sites for HIF2 [58]. NO has a dual action on the vascular endothelium: at low concentrations (nM), as are present under basal conditions, it protects cells against apoptotic stimuli [59]. When its levels become elevated (μM), as in the case of severe ischemia/hypoxia, NO also initiates apoptosis in both endothelial and non-endothelial cells [60, 61].

http://dx.doi.org/10.5772/52182

Activation of eNOS, iNOS and SRF is dependent on Rho GTPase-regulated actin dynamics. Actin de-polymerization activates eNOS [62, 63] and iNOS [64, 65] but suppresses SRF, resulting in apoptosis [66, 67]. Conversely, actin polymerization activates SRF but suppresses eNOS and iNOS, supporting cell survival.

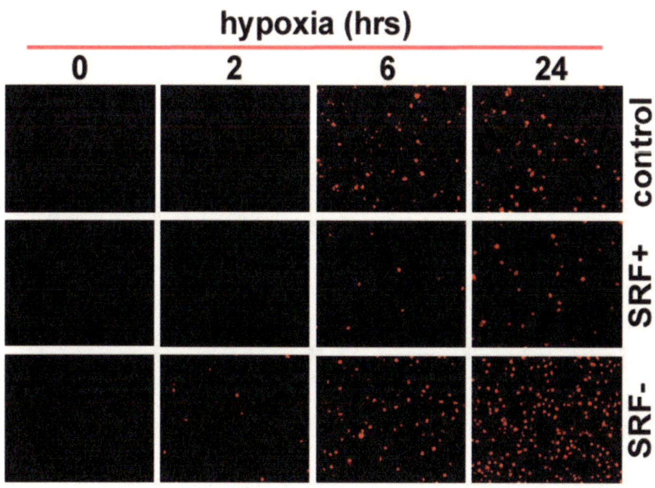

Figure 3. Knockdown of SRF in brain endothelial cells increases hypoxia-induced apoptosis. bEND3 cells were cultured on cover slips under a hypoxic condition for 2, 6 and 24 hours. TUNEL assays were performed to detect apoptosis. Apparently, overexpression of SRF (SRF+) promoted cell survival, while knockdown of SRF (SRF-) made cells more vulnerable to hypoxic damage.

Moderate hypoxia induces cell adaptation but not apoptosis. However, when SRF is insufficient (SRF-), cells become vulnerable to cellular stress and even a brief oxygen shortage can trigger apoptotic cell death (Figure 3). On the other hand, forced overexpression of SRF (SRF +) in these cells can make them more resistant to hypoxic damage and able to survive through even more harsh oxygen crisis. The advantage of SRF over HIF is its broad involvement in the molecular regulation of the cell machinery. Once SRF is activated, it not only promotes cell survival through up-regulation of growth factors and cytoskeletal components, but also protects mitochondrial integrity through up-regulation of anti-apoptotic proteins like Bcl-2 [68]. In another word, SRF supports cell survival at multiple levels. Up-regulation of growth factors stimulates cell proliferation and migration, which require adequate supplies of cytoskeletal proteins, because without cytoskeleton to provide the platform, cells cannot proliferate or migrate, and SRF makes sure these molecules available at the time of need. Finally, SRF also makes sure mitochondria intact so that they can provide the energy that cell proliferation and migration need. Mitochondrial integrity depends on the balance between pro-apoptotic and anti-apoptotic proteins, typically, BAX versus Bcl-2. Severe hypoxia activates p53, which drives up-regulation of BAX, pushing cells toward apoptosis, as BAX gene contains four binding sites for p53. On the other hand, hypoxia also activates SRF (as shown above), which drives up-regulation of Bcl-2, pushing cells toward survival, as Bcl-2 gene contains two SREs in its promoter [68]. The BAX and Bcl-2 fight turns into a wrestle between p53 and SRF. As shown in Figure 4, manipulation of SRF expression can change BAX/Bcl-2 ratio, and ultimately, change the fate of the cells under hypoxia.

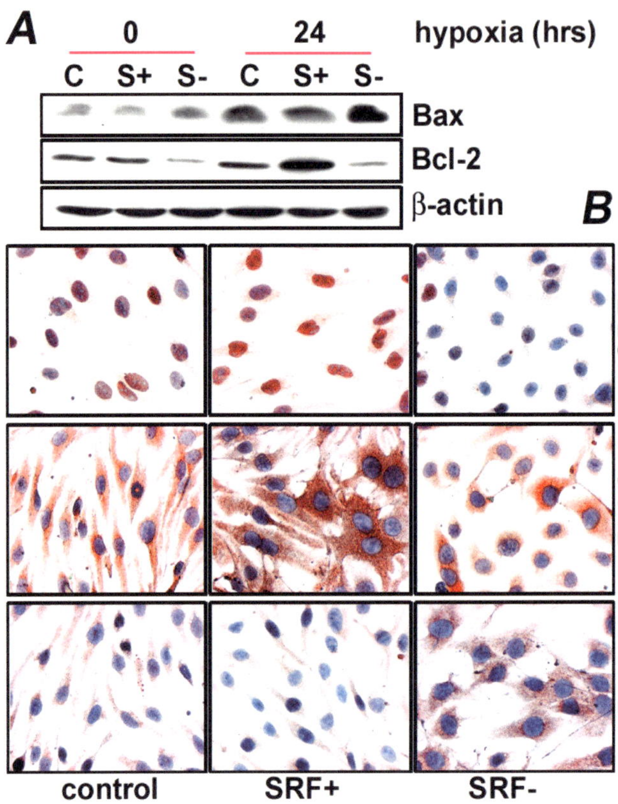

Figure 4. SRF promotes Bcl-2 but suppresses Bax. A. Western blot analysis showed an increase of Bax and a decrease of Bcl-2 in bEND3 cells due to SRF deficiency. B. Immunocytochemistry showed a similar effect.

The impact of SRF on mitochondrial integrity during hypoxia is not only reflected at the molecular level, but it can also be visualized at the subcellular level. As shown in Figure 5, incubation of brain endothelial cells under a hypoxic condition induces mitochondrial leakage, as reflected by the color change of a fluorescent dye. The longer the hypoxic exposure goes, the fewer intact mitochondria exist. However, forced overexpression of SRF in these cells can reverse the effect of hypoxia, protecting mitochondria against hypoxic damage. Conversely, knockdown of SRF can lower the threshold of mitochondrial tolerance to oxygen deprivation, so that a short hypoxic exposure can cause a massive mitochondrial leakage.

http://dx.doi.org/10.5772/52182

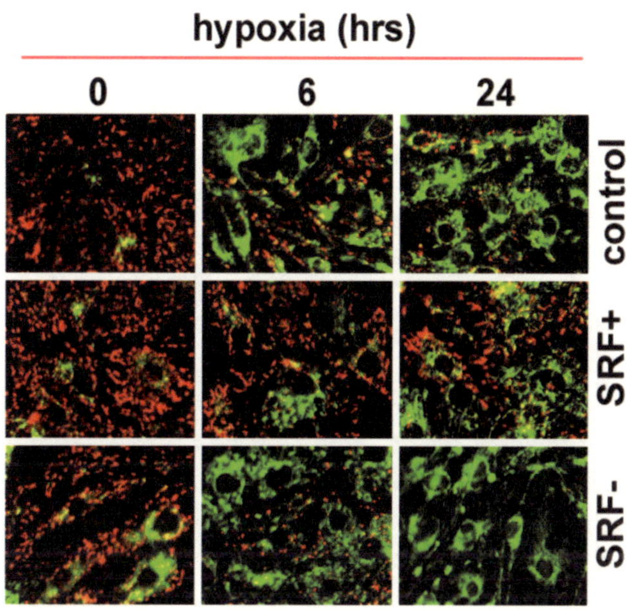

Figure 5. Knockdown of SRF in brain endothelial cells increases mitochondrial permeability during hypoxia. bEND3 cells were cultured on cover slips under a hypoxic condition and stained with a cationic dye. The dye fluoresces differently in healthy vs. apoptotic cells. In healthy cells, the dye accumulates and aggregates in the mitochondria, giving off a bright red fluorescence. While in apoptotic cells, the dye cannot aggregate in the mitochondria due to the altered mitochondrial transmembrane potential, and thus it remains in the cytoplasm in its monomer form, fluorescing green.

Mitochondrial permeability is reflected by the opposite movement of BAX and cytochrome c. Normally, BAX remains in the cytoplasm at a low level, while cytochrome c hides in between the inner and outer membranes of the mitochondria. When cells suffer from an oxygen shortage, BAX jumps, moving toward mitochondria. The insertion of BAX into the outer mitochondrial membrane opens pores to let cytochrome c leak out. Cytoplasmic cytochrome c binds to Apaf-1 and triggers caspase cascade, leading to apoptotic cell death. During this event, the level of SRF is a determining factor for the fate of the cell. As illustrated in Figure 6, as oxygen crisis prolongs the opposite movement of BAX and cytochrome c increases, and cells prone to die. Manipulation of SRF level can either facilitate this process or reverse it, depending on what we desire.

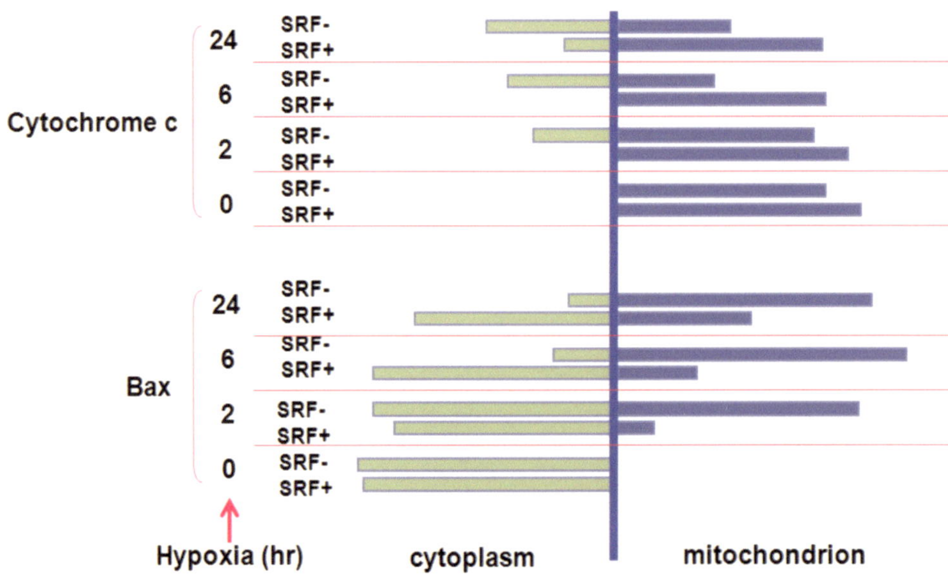

Figure 6. SRF protects mitochondrial integrity. As oxygen deprivation extends, more and Bax binds to mitochondria and opens up channels to allow cytochrome c to escape from mitochondria into cytoplasm, where it forms complexes with Apaf-1 and triggers caspase cascade. With overexpression of SRF, cells can reverse Bcl-2/Bax ratio decrease caused by hypoxia and prevent cytochrome c leakage, while lack of SRF accelerates mitochondrial breakdown.

7. Conclusions

Due to unregulated proliferation of malignant cells, oxygen deficiency is common in tumor development. Cancer cells have learned a few tricks to survive through oxygen crisis, and one of them is to stimulate endothelial cells to build new vessels extending oxygen toward the hypoxic area. However, depending on the severity of hypoxia, endothelial cells may follow the cue to support tumor growth by engaging in angiogenesis, or commit a suicide by engaging in apoptosis and leave the tumor cells to die. It is our interest to guide the endothelial cells to choose the second path. The best known players in the battle against hypoxia are HIF and p53. In general, HIF up-regulates angiogenic factors to promote angiogenesis, while p53 up-regulates pro-apoptotic genes to induce apoptosis. However, the relationship between HIF and p53 is not always a bull-and-bear fight; sometimes they can also join forces to become friends. HIF can bind to MDM2 to stabilize p53 and thereby to promote apoptosis [69]. It has been reported that HIF-deficient embryonic stem cells resist to hypoxia-induced p53 activation and apoptosis [70]. A similar observation was also reported in neuronal cells where HIF helps p53 to endorse cell death [71]. For this reason, treatments targeting HIF do not always achieve inhibition of tumor angiogenesis.

Unlike HIF, SRF promotes cell survival through multi-level and fundamental regulations. Level 1 – growth factors: as discussed above, SRF is not only activated by growth factors, but also turns around to stimulate growth factor expression. This positive feedback reinforces the signal for cell survival. Level 2 – cytoskeletal components: no matter it is for cancer cells to move away from their primary location to look for new places with better oxygen and nutrient supply, or for cancer cells to allure endothelial cells with chemicals to form new vessels to bring oxygen and nutrients to the tumors, cytoskeletal regeneration and rearrangement are essential requirements. The molecules involved in these processes are tightly controlled by SRF. As shown in our previous study [43], without SRF, even the most potent angiogenic factor VEGF cannot stimulate angiogenesis. Level 3 – anti-apoptosis: hypoxia induces apoptosis through disrupting mitochondrial outer membrane, while mitochondrial integrity is guarded by Bcl-2, which is controlled by SRF. Therefore, SRF should be a better candidate for cancer gene therapy, and a treatment targeting SRF, instead of HIF, should achieve better results.

Acknowledgements

This work is supported by the Department of Veterans Affairs of the United States.

Author details

Jianyuan Chai

VA Long Beach Healthcare System, Long Beach and University of California, Irvine, USA

References

[1] Rolfe DF, Brown GC. Cellular energy utilization and molecular origin of standard metabolic rate in mammals. Physiological Reviews. 1997 July 1, 1997;77(3):731-58.

[2] Brown GC, Borutaite V. There is no evidence that mitochondria are the main source of reactive oxygen species in mammalian cells. Mitochondrion. 2012;12(1):1-4.

[3] Yao KS, Xanthoudakis S, Curran T, O'Dwyer PJ. Activation of AP-1 and of a nuclear redox factor, Ref-1, in the response of HT29 colon cancer cells to hypoxia. Molecular and Cellular Biology. 1994 September 1, 1994;14(9):5997-6003.

[4] Webster KA, Discher DJ, Bishopric NH. Induction and nuclear accumulation of fos and jun proto-oncogenes in hypoxic cardiac myocytes. Journal of Biological Chemistry. 1993 August 5, 1993;268(22):16852-8.

[5] Kvietikova I, Wenger RH, Marti HH, Gassmann M. The transcription factors ATF-1 and CREB-1 bind constitutively to the hypoxia-inducible factor-1 (HIF-1)DNA recognition site. Nucleic Acids Research. 1995 January 1, 1995;23(22):4542-50.

[6] Miyazaki K, Kawamoto T, Tanimoto K, Nishiyama M, Honda H, Kato Y. Identification of Functional Hypoxia Response Elements in the Promoter Region of the DEC1 and DEC2 Genes. Journal of Biological Chemistry. 2002 December 6, 2002;277(49): 47014-21.

[7] Yan S-F, Lu J, Zou YS, Soh-Won J, Cohen DM, Buttrick PM, et al. Hypoxia-associated Induction of Early Growth Response-1 Gene Expression. Journal of Biological Chemistry. 1999 May 21, 1999;274(21):15030-40.

[8] Oikawa M, Abe M, Kurosawa H, Hida W, Shirato K, Sato Y. Hypoxia Induces Transcription Factor ETS-1 via the Activity of Hypoxia-Inducible Factor-1. Biochemical and Biophysical Research Communications. 2001;289(1):39-43.

[9] Price BD, Calderwood SK. Gadd45 and Gadd153 Messenger RNA Levels Are Increased during Hypoxia and after Exposure of Cells to Agents Which Elevate the Levels of the Glucose-regulated Proteins. Cancer Research. 1992 July 1, 1992;52(13): 3814-7.

[10] Tabata M, Tarumoto T, Ohmine K, Furukawa Y, Hatake K, Ozawa K, et al. Stimulation of GATA-2 as a mechanism of hydrogen peroxide suppression in hypoxia-induced erythropoietin gene expression. Journal of Cellular Physiology. 2001;186(2): 260-7.

[11] Jiang B, Mendelson CR. USF1 and USF2 Mediate Inhibition of Human Trophoblast Differentiation and CYP19 Gene Expression by Mash-2 and Hypoxia. Molecular and Cellular Biology. 2003 September 1, 2003;23(17):6117-28.

[12] Yan S-F, Zou YS, Mendelsohn M, Gao Y, Naka Y, Yan SD, et al. Nuclear Factor Interleukin 6 Motifs Mediate Tissue-specific Gene Transcription in Hypoxia. Journal of Biological Chemistry. 1997 February 14, 1997;272(7):4287-94.

[13] Royds JA, Dower SK, Qwarnstrom EE, Lewis CE. Response of tumour cells to hypoxia: role of p53 and NFkB. Molecular Pathology. 1998 April 1, 1998;51(2):55-61.

[14] Shie J-L, Wu G, Wu J, Liu F-F, Laham RJ, Oettgen P, et al. RTEF-1, a Novel Transcriptional Stimulator of Vascular Endothelial Growth Factor in Hypoxic Endothelial Cells. Journal of Biological Chemistry. 2004 June 11, 2004;279(24):25010-6.

[15] Zhang H, Akman HO, Smith ELP, Zhao J, Murphy-Ullrich JE, Batuman OA. Cellular response to hypoxia involves signaling via Smad proteins. Blood. 2003 March 15, 2003;101(6):2253-60.

[16] Ryuto M, Ono M, Izumi H, Yoshida S, Weich HA, Kohno K, et al. Induction of Vascular Endothelial Growth Factor by Tumor Necrosis Factor alpha in Human Glioma Cells. Journal of Biological Chemistry. 1996 November 8, 1996;271(45):28220-8.

[17] Dudley AC, Thomas D, Best J, Jenkins A. A VEGF/JAK2/STAT5 axis may partially mediate endothelial cell tolerance to hypoxia. Biochem J. 2005 Sep 1, 2005;390(2): 427-36.

[18] Greer SN, Metcalf JL, Wang Y, Ohh M. The updated biology of hypoxia-inducible factor. EMBO J. 2012;31(11):2448-60.

[19] Hammond EM, Giaccia AJ. The role of p53 in hypoxia-induced apoptosis. Biochemical and Biophysical Research Communications. 2005;331(3):718-25.

[20] Sowter HM, Raval R, Moore J, Ratcliffe PJ, Harris AL. Predominant Role of Hypoxia-Inducible Transcription Factor (Hif)-1alpha versus Hif-2alpha in Regulation of the Transcriptional Response to Hypoxia. Cancer Research. 2003 October 1, 2003;63(19): 6130-4.

[21] Liu Y, Cox SR, Morita T, Kourembanas S. Hypoxia Regulates Vascular Endothelial Growth Factor Gene Expression in Endothelial Cells : Identification of a 5' Enhancer. Circulation Research. 1995 September 1, 1995;77(3):638-43.

[22] Forsythe JA, Jiang BH, Iyer NV, Agani F, Leung SW, Koos RD, et al. Activation of vascular endothelial growth factor gene transcription by hypoxia-inducible factor 1. Molecular and Cellular Biology. 1996 September 1, 1996;16(9):4604-13.

[23] Tian H, McKnight SL, Russell DW. Endothelial PAS domain protein 1 (EPAS1), a transcription factor selectively expressed in endothelial cells. Genes & Development. 1997 January 1, 1997;11(1):72-82.

[24] Hara S, Hamada J, Kobayashi C, Kondo Y, Imura N. Expression and Characterization of Hypoxia-Inducible Factor (HIF)-3alpha in Human Kidney: Suppression of HIF-Mediated Gene Expression by HIF-3alpha. Biochemical and Biophysical Research Communications. 2001;287(4):808-13.

[25] Ferrara N. Vascular Endothelial Growth Factor: Basic Science and Clinical Progress. Endocrine Reviews. 2004 August 1, 2004;25(4):581-611.

[26] Stuttfeld E, Ballmer-Hofer K. Structure and function of VEGF receptors. IUBMB Life. 2009;61(9):915-22.

[27] Carmeliet P. VEGF as a Key Mediator of Angiogenesis in Cancer. Oncology. 2005;69(Suppl. 3):4-10.

[28] Yamakawa M, Liu LX, Date T, Belanger AJ, Vincent KA, Akita GY, et al. Hypoxia-Inducible Factor-1 Mediates Activation of Cultured Vascular Endothelial Cells by Inducing Multiple Angiogenic Factors. Circulation Research. 2003 October 3, 2003;93(7):664-73.

[29] Haupt Y, Maya R, Kazaz A, Oren M. Mdm2 promotes the rapid degradation of p53. Nature. 1997;387(6630):296-9.

[30] Yang Y, Li C-CH, Weissman AM. Regulating the p53 system through ubiquitination. Oncogene. 2004;23(11):2096-106.

[31] Slee EA, O'Connor DJ, Lu X. To die or not to die: how does p53 decide? Oncogene. 2004;23(16):2809-18.

[32] Yang E, Zha J, Jockel J, Boise LH, Thompson CB, Korsmeyer SJ. Bad, a heterodimeric partner for Bcl-xL and Bcl-2, displaces bax and promotes cell death. Cell. 1995;80(2): 285-91.

[33] Hansson LO, Friedler A, Freund S, Rudiger S, Fersht AR. Two sequence motifs from HIF-1alpha bind to the DNA-binding site of p53. Proceedings of the National Academy of Sciences. 2002 August 6, 2002;99(16):10305-9.

[34] Ravi R, Mookerjee B, Bhujwalla ZM, Sutter CH, Artemov D, Zeng Q, et al. Regulation of tumor angiogenesis by p53-induced degradation of hypoxia-inducible factor 1alpha. Genes & Development. 2000 January 1, 2000;14(1):34-44.

[35] Suzuki H, Tomida A, Tsuruo T. Dephosphorylated hypoxia-inducible factor 1alpha as a mediator of p53-dependent apoptosis during hypoxia. Oncogene. 2001;20(41): 5779-88.

[36] Cummins E, Taylor C. Hypoxia-responsive transcription factors. Pflügers Archiv European Journal of Physiology. 2005;450(6):363-71.

[37] Chai J. Gastric ulcer healing - Role of serum response factor. In: Chai J, editor. Peptic Ulcer Disease. Rijeka, Croatia: InTech; 2011. p. 143-64.

[38] Chai J, Tarnawski A. Serum response factor: discovery, biochemistry, biological roles and implications for tissue injury healing. Journal of Physiology and Pharmacology. 2002;53(2):147-57.

[39] Modak C, Chai J. Serum response factor: Look into the gut. . World Journal of Gastroenterology. 2010;16:2195-201.

[40] Sun Q, Chen G, Streb JW, Long X, Yang Y, Stoeckert CJ, et al. Defining the mammalian CArGome. Genome Research. 2006 February 1, 2006;16(2):197-207.

[41] Khachigian LM, Collins T. Inducible Expression of Egr-1–Dependent Genes : A Paradigm of Transcriptional Activation in Vascular Endothelium. Circulation Research. 1997 October 19, 1997;81(4):457-61.

[42] Miano JM, Long X, Fujiwara K. Serum response factor: master regulator of the actin cytoskeleton and contractile apparatus. American Journal of Physiology - Cell Physiology. 2007 January 2007;292(1):C70-C81.

[43] Chai J, Jones MK, Tarnawski AS. Serum response factor is a critical requirement for VEGF signaling in endothelial cells and VEGF-induced angiogenesis. The FASEB Journal. 2004 June 4, 2004;18(11):1264-6.

[44] Franco CA, Mericskay M, Parlakian A, Gary-Bobo G, Gao-Li J, Paulin D, et al. Serum Response Factor Is Required for Sprouting Angiogenesis and Vascular Integrity. Developmental Cell. 2008;15(3):448-61.

[45] Franco CA, Li Z. SRF in angiogenesis: Branching the vascular system. Cell Adhesion & Migration. 2009;3(3):264-7.

[46] McClintock DS, Santore MT, Lee VY, Brunelle J, Budinger GRS, Zong W-X, et al. Bcl-2 Family Members and Functional Electron Transport Chain Regulate Oxygen Deprivation-Induced Cell Death. Molecular and Cellular Biology. 2002 January 1, 2002;22(1):94-104.

[47] Matsushita H, Morishita R, Nata T, Aoki M, Nakagami H, Taniyama Y, et al. Hypoxia-Induced Endothelial Apoptosis Through Nuclear Factor-kB (NF-kB)–Mediated bcl-2 Suppression : In Vivo Evidence of the Importance of NF-kB in Endothelial Cell Regulation. Circulation Research. 2000 May 12, 2000;86(9):974-81.

[48] Shimizu S, Eguchi Y, Kosaka H, Kamiike W, Matsuda H, Tsujimoto Y. Prevention of hypoxia-induced cell death by Bcl-2 and Bcl-xL. Nature. 1995;374(6525):811-3.

[49] Vander Heiden MG, Thompson CB. Bcl-2 proteins: regulators of apoptosis or of mitochondrial homeostasis? Nat Cell Biol. 1999;1(8):E209-E16.

[50] Martinou J-C, Youle RichardÂ J. Mitochondria in Apoptosis: Bcl-2 Family Members and Mitochondrial Dynamics. Developmental Cell. 2011;21(1):92-101.

[51] Kaufmann SH, Hengartner MO. Programmed cell death: alive and well in the new millennium. Trends in Cell Biology. 2001;11(12):526-34.

[52] Riedl SJ, Salvesen GS. The apoptosome: signalling platform of cell death. Nat Rev Mol Cell Biol. 2007;8(5):405-13.

[53] Pop C, Salvesen GS. Human Caspases: Activation, Specificity, and Regulation. Journal of Biological Chemistry. 2009 August 14, 2009;284(33):21777-81.

[54] Zubrow AB, Delivoria-Papadopoulos M, Ashraf QM, Ballesteros JR, Fritz KI, Mishra OP. Nitric oxide-mediated expression of Bax protein and DNA fragmentation during hypoxia in neuronal nuclei from newborn piglets. Brain Research. 2002;954(1):60-7.

[55] Kindler DD, Thiffault C, Solenski NJ, Dennis J, Kostecki V, Jenkins R, et al. Neurotoxic nitric oxide rapidly depolarizes and permeabilizes mitochondria by dynamically opening the mitochondrial transition pore. Molecular and Cellular Neuroscience. 2003;23(4):559-73.

[56] Melillo G, Taylor LS, Brooks A, Musso T, Cox GW, Varesio L. Functional Requirement of the Hypoxia-responsive Element in the Activation of the Inducible Nitric Ox-

ide Synthase Promoter by the Iron Chelator Desferrioxamine. Journal of Biological Chemistry. 1997 May 2, 1997;272(18):12236-43.

[57] Jung F, Palmer LA, Zhou N, Johns RA. Hypoxic Regulation of Inducible Nitric Oxide Synthase via Hypoxia Inducible Factor-1 in Cardiac Myocytes. Circulation Research. 2000 February 18, 2000;86(3):319-25.

[58] Coulet F, Nadaud S, Agrapart M, Soubrier F. Identification of Hypoxia-response Element in the Human Endothelial Nitric-oxide Synthase Gene Promoter. Journal of Biological Chemistry. 2003 November 21, 2003;278(47):46230-40.

[59] Shen YH, Wang XL, Wilcken DEL. Nitric oxide induces and inhibits apoptosis through different pathways. FEBS Letters. 1998;433(1-2):125-31.

[60] Lee VY, McClintock DS, Santore MT, Budinger GRS, Chandel NS. Hypoxia Sensitizes Cells to Nitric Oxide-induced Apoptosis. Journal of Biological Chemistry. 2002 May 3, 2002;277(18):16067-74.

[61] Walford GA, Moussignac R-L, Scribner AW, Loscalzo J, Leopold JA. Hypoxia Potentiates Nitric Oxide-mediated Apoptosis in Endothelial Cells via Peroxynitrite-induced Activation of Mitochondria-dependent and -independent Pathways. Journal of Biological Chemistry. 2004 February 6, 2004;279(6):4425-32.

[62] Su Y, Edwards-Bennett S, Bubb MR, Block ER. Regulation of endothelial nitric oxide synthase by the actin cytoskeleton. American Journal of Physiology - Cell Physiology. 2003 June 1, 2003;284(6):C1542-C9.

[63] Kook H, Ahn KY, Lee SE, Na HS, Kim KK. Nitric oxide-dependent cytoskeletal changes and inhibition of endothelial cell migration contribute to the suppression of angiogenesis by RAD50 gene transfer. FEBS Letters. 2003;553(1â€"2):56-62.

[64] Witteck A, Yao Y, Fechir M, Forstermann U, Kleinert H. Rho protein-mediated changes in the structure of the actin cytoskeleton regulate human inducible NO synthase gene expression. Experimental Cell Research. 2003;287(1):106-15.

[65] Zeng C, Morrison AR. Disruption of the actin cytoskeleton regulates cytokine-induced iNOS expression. American Journal of Physiology - Cell Physiology. 2001 September 1, 2001;281(3):C932-C40.

[66] Kim S-J, Hwang S-G, Kim I-C, Chun J-S. Actin Cytoskeletal Architecture Regulates Nitric Oxide-induced Apoptosis, Dedifferentiation, and Cyclooxygenase-2 Expression in Articular Chondrocytes via Mitogen-activated Protein Kinase and Protein Kinase C Pathways. Journal of Biological Chemistry. 2003 October 24, 2003;278(43): 42448-56.

[67] Hippenstiel S, Schmeck B, N'Guessan PD, Seybold J, Krull M, Preissner K, et al. Rho protein inactivation induced apoptosis of cultured human endothelial cells. American Journal of Physiology - Lung Cellular and Molecular Physiology. 2002 October 1, 2002;283(4):L830-L8.

[68] Schratt G, Philippar U, Hockemeyer D, Schwarz H, Alberti S, Nordheim A. SRF regulates Bcl-2 expression and promotes cell survival during murine embryonic development. EMBO J. 2004;23(8):1834-44.

[69] Chen D, Li M, Luo J, Gu W. Direct Interactions between HIF-1alpha and Mdm2 Modulate p53 Function. Journal of Biological Chemistry. 2003 April 18, 2003;278(16): 13595-8.

[70] Carmeliet P, Dor Y, Herbert J-M, Fukumura D, Brusselmans K, Dewerchin M, et al. Role of HIF-1[alpha] in hypoxia-mediated apoptosis, cell proliferation and tumour angiogenesis. Nature. 1998;394(6692):485-90.

[71] Halterman MW, Miller CC, Federoff HJ. Hypoxia-Inducible Factor-1alpha Mediates Hypoxia-Induced Delayed Neuronal Death That Involves p53. The Journal of Neuroscience. 1999 August 15, 1999;19(16):6818-24.

Chapter 3

Manipulating Redox Signaling to Block Tumor Angiogenesis

Vera Mugoni and Massimo Mattia Santoro

Additional information is available at the end of the chapter

http://dx.doi.org/10.5772/54593

1. Introduction

A tumor consists of a population of rapidly dividing and growing cancer cells. Cancer cells have lost their ability to divide in a controlled fashion and as a consequence they rapidly accumulate mutations. In such way cancer cells (or sub-populations of cancer cells within a tumor) will acquire stronger proliferative capacity [1]. Tumors cannot grow beyond a certain size due to a lack of oxygen and other essential nutrients. Tumors cells have then acquired a specific feature that is to induce blood vessel growth, a process called tumor angiogenesis. Tumor angiogenesis is a necessary and required step for transition from a small harmless cluster of cells to a large tumor [2]. The early induction of tumor vasculature is termed "angiogenic switch", that occurs when a tumor mass reaches about dimensions of 2 mm^2 and moves towards progression. The "angiogenic switch" is a rate-limiting step for tumor growth that is not limited at earliest stages, but occurs also at different stages of tumor-progression. The angiogenic switch induces angiogenic sprouting and new vessels formation and maturation. Activation of angiogenesis in premalignant lesions and dormant metastasis is mandatory for tumor survival. The fact that tumor mass is depending on angiogenesis has driven the medical research towards the characterization of molecular pathways and cellular dynamics for the induction and regulation of angiogenesis.

Tumor angiogenesis is regulated by several growth factors (EGF, TGFα, bFGF, VEGF). Induction of these angiogenic factors is triggered by various stresses [3]. For instance, tissue hypoxia exerts its pro-angiogenic action through various angiogenic factors, the most notable is VEGF (vascular endothelial growth factor), which has been mainly associated with initiating the process of angiogenesis through the recruitment and proliferation of endothelial cells [4]. Recently, reactive oxygen species (ROS) have been found to stimulate angiogenic response in the normal and pathological angiogenesis. ROS can cause tissue injury in one hand and

INTECH
open science | open minds

© 2013 The Author(s). Licensee InTech. This chapter is distributed under the terms of the Creative Commons Attribution License http://creativecommons.org/licenses/by/3.0), which permits unrestricted use, distribution, and reproduction in any medium, provided the original work is properly cited.

promote tissue repair in another hand by promoting angiogenesis. It thus appears that after causing injury to the cells, ROS promptly initiate the tissue repair process by triggering angiogenic response. Recently, it has been reported that redox signaling may influence pathological angiogenesis as well [5,6].

2. Redox signaling in normal and pathological angiogenesis

Redox signaling is a biochemical communication by free radicals, reactive oxygen species (ROS), and other electronically activated species such as nitric oxide and other oxides of nitrogen acting as biological messengers [7]. Pro- and anti-oxidative species act as second messengers. Pro-oxidative species are physiologically produced by cells and tightly regulated with antioxidant systems. Down-regulation of antioxidant system or up-regulation in production of pro-oxidative species leads to oxidative stress state. This condition is reported as dangerous for cells since it conveys macromolecules damage. Importantly, it has been reported that oxidative stress plays a key role in the regulation of tumor angiogenesis [8]. The complex molecular network that regulates endothelial cells homeostasis during angiogenesis includes molecules sensitive to redox state of biological environment. The redox state is determined by the relative abundance of highly chemically reactive species derived from oxygen (ROS: Reactive Oxygen Species) or nitrogen (RNS: Reactive Nitrogen Species) (Table 1).

ReactiveOxygen Species (ROS)	Symbol	ReactiveNitrogen Species (RNS)	Symbol
Hydroxyl	$OH^{\cdot}$	Nitrous oxide	$NO^{\cdot}$
Superoxyde	$O_2^{\cdot -}$	Peroxynitrate	$OONO^-$
Nitric Oxide	$NO^{\cdot}$	Peroxynitrous acid	ONOOH
Peroxyl	$RO_2^{\cdot}$	Nitroxyl anion	NO^-
Lipid peroxyl	$LOO^{\cdot}$	Nitrogen dioxide	$NO^{\cdot}_2$
Peroxynitrate	$ONOO^-$	Dinitrogen trioxide	N_2O_3
Hydrogen Peroxide	H_2O_2	Nitrous acid	HNO_2
Singlet Oxygen	$^{\cdot 1}O_2$	Nitryl chloride	NO_2Cl
Hypochloric acid	HOCl	Nitrosyl cation	NO^+

Table 1. List of oxygen (ROS) and nitrogen (RNS) reactive species commonly found in normal and pathological tissues.

Reactive oxygen species (ROS) and reactive nitrogen species (RNS) are important in regulation of cell survival. In general, moderate levels of ROS/RNS functions as signals to promote cell proliferation and survival, whereas severe increase of ROS/RNS can induce cell death. Under physiologic conditions, the balance between generation and elimination of ROS/RNS maintains the proper function of redox-sensitive signaling proteins. Normally, the redox homeostasis ensures that cells respond properly to endogenous and exogenous stimuli. However, when the redox homeostasis is disturbed, oxidative stress may lead to aberrant cell death and contribute to disease development [9].

Reactive species are highly reactive chemical molecules or ions, characterized by unpaired electrons that react with other molecules in order to stabilize their electron configuration and gain a more stable state. Consequently, the reaction of ROS/RNS with cellular molecules is a damaging reaction of oxidation. Oxidized molecules are dysfunctional and may induce cell death. Initially, the presence of ROS/RNS was linked only to cellular damage and cell degenerative processes. However, accumulating evidences derived from the characterization of mechanisms for buffering and regulating reactive species opened the possibility that oxidative species are important for cellular homeostasis. Reactive species had been also described as second messenger molecules and their interaction with molecules is identified as a post-translational modification (i.e. S- nitrosylation of proteins) that can trigger a specific intracellular signal. At the present, the evidence is that a tight regulation of pro-oxidative species levels is essential for cellular homeostasis and that such regulatory mechanism is fundamental to maintain a safe redox state and activate related redox signaling pathways [10].

In vascular beds, the redox state is mainly modulated by oxygen concentration and by mechanical forces (i.e. shear stress caused by blood flow) [11]. In normal conditions oxygen levels are constant and essential to guarantee sufficient provision for tissues oxygenation. Mechanisms for sensing oxygen tension are based on redox-mediated signaling. During normoxic conditions the transcription factor HIF1α (hypoxia inducible factor) is degraded in a ROS-dependent manner, while during hypoxia the concentration of oxygen is lower and ROS levels are differentially modulated. Consequently, HIF1α couples with HIF1β and activates transcription of genes involved in angiogenesis, vascular remodeling and cell proliferation [12].

Redox signaling events are also activated in endothelial cells during normal angiogenesis for sensing mechanical forces. Shear forces are constantly present on endothelial cells where regulate cell proliferation, survival and migration. Vascular forces exercise a mechanical stimulus that is perceived by endothelial cells and translated into intracellular molecular pathways. Therefore, concomitant to shear forces there is an upregulation in production of RNS and ROS. In adult ECs, the mechanical oscillatory shear stress induces the activation of specific antioxidant enzymes or proteins like peroxiredoxins (Prx) that act as "mechano-sensitive antioxidants" [13]. Moreover, specific antioxidant and protective genes are induced. Shear stress causes upregulation of specific "antioxidant transcriptional factors" Nrf2 and ATF in developing embryonic vasculature as well as in adult ECs [14]. Most of the molecules with oxidative properties that modulate endothelial cell homeostasis in normal conditions are included in redox molecular pathways that are altered in pathogenic angiogenesis [15]. There are specific oxidized products or redox sensitive proteins that behave differentially. ROS-activated factors play different role in context of pathologic angiogenesis or normal angiogenesis. The ATM kinase protein, which is involved in regulation of endothelial cells survival and proliferation is activated in tumor condition under upregulation of ROS and promotes new vessel formation, while it is not activated in normal vasculature [16]. Oxidative stress triggered by inflammation in tumor conditions (i.e. human melanoma) causes lipid peroxidation with consequent accumulation of an oxidized compound: ω-(2-carboxyethyl)-pyrrole (CEP). The CEP acts as a ligand for Toll-like receptor 2 (TLR2) and induces angiogenesis independently from VEGF [17]. Similarly, oxidized lipid (carboxyalkyl pyrroles, CAPs) molecules bind to their TLRs receptors and activate angiogenesis in some specific pathological conditions such us age related macular degeneration [18].

In the following three different paragraphs we will define the cellular systems regulating redox signaling and how they control molecules and factors clearly involved in angiogenesis. In addition, here we plan to present paragraphs about main sources for production of oxidative species and systems for counteract their products and maintenance of an equilibrated cell redox state. Finally, we will describe molecules sensitive to redox signaling that are known for being part of established pathway for tumor angiogenesis signaling.

3. Molecules generating oxidative species in endothelial cells

In endothelial cells the endogenous production of pro-oxidative species is mainly generated by four different enzymes: NADPH oxidases (NOX), Cyclooxygenases (COX), Xanthine oxidoreductase (XOR), and dysfunctional endothelial NOS (eNOS).

NADPH oxidases (NOX). NADPH oxidases are a family of enzymes composed by seven members: NOX1, NOX2, NOX3, NOX4, NOX5 and two homologues DUOX1, DUOX2. All of them are transmembrane proteins containing a NADPH-binding site, a FAD binding region, heme-binding sites and several subunits that function in the regulation and maturation of enzymes. $p22^{phox}$, DUOX activator 1 (DUAX1) and DUOX activator 2 (DUOX2) are important factors for NOX and DUOX maturation. Among factors important for NOX and DUOX enzyme activation we found $p67^{phox}$, NOX activator1 (NOXA1), small GTPase (RAC1 and RAC2). On the contrary specific regulator of NOX4 is polymerase δ-interacting protein 2 (POLDIP2) and Ca^{2+} ions are specific activators of NOX5 and DUOX1/DUOX2 isoforms. These enzymes are also associated to spatial regulator subunits $p40^{phox}$, $p47^{phox}$ and NOX organizer1 (NOXO1) that are important for the enzyme complex structure [19]. NADPH oxidase catalytic activity consists in the generation of superoxide anions (O_2^-) through an electrons transfer cycle from an electron donor (NADPH) to FAD subunit, heme groups and to a final electron acceptor that is a molecule of oxygen. Activation of NOX4, DUOX1 and DUOX2 results mainly in the release of hydrogen peroxide instead of superoxide anions. The specific role of this enzyme family consists in the production and release of pro-oxidative species. Such class of enzymes is considered one of the main player in the redox signaling in cardiovascular system [20]. NADPH oxidases are expressed in various types of cells along the vascular wall, including vascular smooth muscle cells, monocytes and macrophages. NOX1, NOX2, NOX4 and NOX5 are constitutively expressed in the endothelial cells and their functionality is regulated by several vascular conditions like shear stress, hypoxia or stimuli as hormones, cytokines, pro-angiogenic factors [21]. It has been demonstrated that NADPH oxidase are sensitive to pro-angiogenic vascular endothelial growth factor (VEGF) activation and it seems probable that reactive oxygen species derived from their oxidase activity may sustain activated VEGFR2 and promote endothelial cells migration and proliferation [22]. In endothelium the regulation of NOX activity is tightly associated with redox balance, since it has been demonstrated that NOX are involved with a series of cardiovascular disease like hypertension, atherosclerosis or ischemia/reperfusion injury [23]. A specific role of NADPH oxidase activity is also reported during the angiogenesis process [24]. NOX1 activity mediates the interaction between leukocyte cells and endothelium and is involved in the initiation of cell migration. NOX1 levels are sensitive to oscillatory shear stress conditions and are positively regulated by HIF-1 and PDGF. Also NOX1 is involved in angiogenic switch by sustaining VEGF signaling and upregulation of matrix metalloproteinase production [25]. NOX2 is also sensitive to vascular pro-angiogenic factors and is reported to be involved in the regulation of ROS signaling for cytoskeleton organization in ECs migration [26]. NOX4 is the most abundant isoform in endothelial tissues and is responsible for basal superoxide production. As a matter of fact the role of NOX4 in vascular tissues is still far from been understood [27]. NOX5 isoform is present in mammalian cells, but its function can be substituted by other isoforms (i.e. DUOX in rodents). In vitro studies report upregulation of NOX5 stimulates endothelial cells proliferation and organization in microvascular tubules. Also NOX5 is sensitive to pro-angiogenic stimuli like angiopoietins [28]. Considering vascular pro-angiogenic factors tightly regulate by NADPH oxidases several inhibitors have been developed as possible approach to modulate redox signaling in tumor angiogenesis. The most studied NADPH oxidase inhibitors are apocyanin and diphenyleneiodonium (DPI). They are quite non-specific inhibitors since they block assembly of enzyme or electron flow. Emerging new inhibitors for endothelial NOX isoforms are triazolopyrimidines inhibitors such as VAS2870 and VAS3947, whose preliminary in vitro and in vivo studies have been reported beneficial for endothelium dysfunctions under oxidative stress [29].

Cyclooxygenases (COX). Cyclooxygenases act in the rate-limiting step of prostanoids biosynthesis. There are two kinds of enzymes: cyclooxygenase-1 (COX-1) and cyclooxygenase-2, also known as prostaglandin endoperoxide H synthase -1 and -2 (PGHS-1 and PGHS-2). Recently, a cyclooxygenase-1 isoenzyme was identified as COX-3 [30]. Prostanoids are lipid molecules that are produced from all animal cells in response to specific stimuli, like hormones. After activation COX produce prostanoids from free fatty acids, typically from arachidonic acid (AA). In particular COX catalyze the bis-oxygenation of AA into the prostaglandin endoperoxide PGG_2, an intermediate molecule that is subsequently converted into different kinds of prostanoids by specific enzymes that are downstream COX. There are five main categories of prostanoid molecules and their specific receptors: 1) prostaglandin D_2 (PGD_2) whose receptors are named DP1-DP-2; 2) prostaglandin E_2 (PGE_2) whose receptors are named EP1-EP4, 3) prostaglandin $F_{2\alpha}$ ($PGF_{2\alpha}$) whose receptors are named FP, 4) prostaglandin I_2

(PGI_2) whose receptors are named IP and 5) thromboxane A_2 (TXA_2) whose receptors are named TP. It is also been reported that some categories of prostanoids can bind peroxisome proliferator-activated receptors (PPARs). PPARs are key activators of prostanoids signaling, the binding to their specific G-protein linked receptor activates an intracellular second messenger (i.e. IP_3/cAMP/DAG/Ca^{2+}) that starts a molecular pathway, which is characteristic for each kind of ligand-receptor. Prostanoids are a class of short-life molecules: immediately after their production they are released outside from cells by specific receptors (prostaglandin transporters, PTG), allowing them to act in a paracrine or autocrine way. Prostanoids are implicated in the regulation of several physiological states (i.e. renal system, kidney functions) such us pathological states (i.e. inflammation, cancer). In the cardiovascular system this class of molecules is relevant for the homeostasis of the vasculature. Prostanoids differentially modulate vascular remodeling by direct action on endothelial cells and their progenitors (endothelial progenitor cells, EPCs) as well as on platelets and smooth muscle cells. Mainly prostacyclin PGI_2 and thromboxane (TXA_2) are involved in the regulation of cardiovascular system homeostasis, even though they act in a different way. PGI_2 is synthetized from COX-2 and is a local vasodilator. It also regulates vascular relation by modulation of smooth muscle cells. Moreover PGI_2 limits the aggregation of platelets and favorites angiogenesis by exerting a direct effect on cellular pathways of EPCs [31,32]. There are contradictory studies on PGI_2 action during tumor angiogenesis, it is reported PGI_2 induces tumor angiogenesis by binding to peroxisomes proliferator-activated receptor – δ (PPAR- δ)[33], on the other hand it is also been reported that healthy tissues have higher levels of PGI synthases than tumor cells. So, it has been speculated that tumor cells might induce PGI_2 in neighboring endothelial cells and so they take advantage of its angiogenic property for growth. On the contrary, TXA_2 is synthetized from COX-1 in platelets and promotes vasoconstriction and platelets aggregates. TXA_2 plays an important role in tissue repair as well as on pathological conditions by favouring atherogenesis. Consequently, the ratio between TXA_2 and PGI_2 is fundamental for the maintenance of physiological homeostasis [34]. In tumor conditions there are also prostanoids PGE_2 and $PGF_{2\alpha}$, PGD_2. Signaling of PGE_2 and its receptor is involved in tumor angiogenesis. PGE_2 induces upregulation of metallopeptidase 9 and activates the fibroblast factor receptor type 1 (FGFR1) [35]. Also $PGF_{2\alpha}$ is considered a prostanoids molecule that sustains tumor angiogenesis by inducing activation of EGR-1, HIF-1a and VEGF. Regarding PGD_2 and its receptor DP1 there are evidences for their signaling implication in vessels homeostasis, but there are opposing reports about the role of PGD_2 for normal and tumor angiogenesis [36]. While molecular pathways regarding prostanoids signaling in the regulation of vessels proliferation are not fully described, their metabolism is considered of significant importance for development of anti-angiogenic drugs. Drugs for modulation of prostanoids levels are divided into two classes of molecules: 1) inhibitors of prostanoids biosynthetic enzymes (e.g. limiting prostanoids biosynthesis) and 2) antagonists of prostanoids receptors (e.g. blocking prostanoids 'cellular signaling). The most important drugs of the first class molecules are COX inhibitors like NSAIDs (aspirin, non-selective COX inhibitor) and COXIBs (selective COX-2 inhibitor) whose evidence as chemo preventive agents is yet reported in preclinical studies. Among inhibitor molecules, there are also available inhibitors of terminal prostaglandin synthetize (tPGSs), and in particular for mPGES-1 (microsomal prostaglandin E synthetize -1). Inhibitors of mPGES-1, like AF3442e, are now at the beginning of clinical trials. Regarding the second class of drugs, there are many selective and isoform specific molecules. In particular EP antagonists have been successfully tested for limiting angiogenesis in different kinds of pathologies: the ONO8711 (EP1 antagonist) has been tested for inhibitory effects on metastasis and invasion in hepatocellular carcinoma, the EP3 antagonist ONOA23240 has been tested for limiting metastasis in Lewis lung carcinoma, the EP4 antagonists ONOA23208 and AH23848 have been tested for limiting angiogenesis and metastasis in skin melanoma, colorectal adenomas, lung carcinoma and ovarian carcinoma. The limits in application of EP antagonists is the high level of specificity of action: EP isoform antagonists effects are mediated by signaling related to a specific EP isoform relative expression in a tumor, that is always tissue and tumor dependent [37]. An alternative approach that is still needs to be validated is the application of drugs that modulate the activation of PPAR. Even though prostanoids are a heterogeneous class of molecules whose metabolism and signaling still needs to be largely characterized in tumors, they are involved in angiogenesis processes and targetable from drugs.

Xanthine oxidoreductase (XOR). Xanthine oxidoreductase is molybdenum-iron-sulfur flavin hydrolase and, consequently, its essential cofactors are molybdopterin (Mo-Co), two iron-sulfur centers (Fe_2-S_2) and flavin adenine dinucleotide (FAD). XOR shifts between two inter-convertible forms: Xanthine oxidase (XO; EC 1.1.3.22) and Xanthine Dehydrogenase (XDH; EC 1.17.14). XOR enzyme works in the purine degradation pathway where it converts hypoxanthine and xanthine to uric acid. The catalytic reaction consists of an electron flow from precursor molecules to electron acceptors (cofactors). In the first part of reaction xanthine reduces XOR at the Mo-Co core and subsequently the Fe_2-S_2 coordination core mediates the re-oxidation of XOR by reducing FAD into $FADH_2$. In order to restore FAD+, electrons are shifted to NAD+ and in turns directly to oxygen. Consequently, the re-oxidation reaction of XOR yields to two molecules of hydrogen peroxide (H_2O_2) and two molecules of superoxide anion (O_2^-) [38]. XOR enzyme is expressed at highest levels in the gut and in the liver. However, it has been also detected in the heart and in endothelial cells [39]. Behind purine metabolism, XOR is reported to be important for redox signaling since superoxide radicals generated as side products have shown in pathological conditions of cardiovascular system. In vitro overexpression of XOR in cultured endothelial cells reduces cell viability, proliferation and ability to generate vascular tubes due to upregulation of ROS levels [40]. It has also been described that XOR-generated ROS affect heart cardiac contractility by reacting with nitric oxide and generation of $ONOO^-$ species [41] or by regulating myofilaments sensitivity to Ca^{2+} [42]. Moreover XOR activity seems to play a role in oxidative state of infusion/reperfusion injury as well as in myocardial infarction. Treatments with inhibitors of XOR as allopurinol and oxypurinol are reported as benefic for cardiovascular pathologies related to XOR-generated ROS overload. Clinical studies have demonstrated that XOR-inhibition diminishes endothelium dysfunctions by limiting oxidation of molecules and in particular of lipids by favoring vaso-relaxation. In particular allopurinol treatment improves endothelium functions in patients with congestive heart failure by reducing plasma levels of malondyaldehyde (i.e. lipid peroxidation) and improving NO bioavailability [43].

Endothelial Nitric Oxide Synthase (eNOS). eNOS is one of the three isoform of nitric oxide synthase family and it is constitutively expressed in endothelial cells. eNOS is important since it is the major source of endothelial nitric oxide (NO). NOS enzymes work as homodimers with support of several cofactors. One monomer is linked to flavin adenine dinucleotide (FAD), nicotinamide adenine dinucleotide phosphate (NADPH), flavin mononucleotide (FMN) and binds the second monomer at the oxygenase domain that contains a prosthetic heme group. The second monomer is also linked to cofactors: tetrahydrobiopterin (BH_4) and molecular oxygen. The catalytic activity consists in an electron flow between NOS cofactors where the substrate: L-arginine is oxidized to L-citrulline with concomitant production of NO. Moreover calmodulin (CaM) and Ca^{2+} are essential for functional enzyme [44]. When eNOS is not able to produce NO due the absence of specific cofactors the reduction of oxygen and concomitant production of NO are uncoupled. As consequence of uncoupled eNOS the superoxide anion is produced instead of NO [45]. The importance of eNOS for endothelium homeostasis is related to NO as well as to its side product O_2^-. In physiological conditions NO function is widely characterized as regulator molecule for vasorelaxation and maintenance of healthy vascular beds. However the level of NO is critical for vascular homeostasis. Low and medium NO levels are involved in cellular signaling, while high NO levels are related to apoptosis and cell damage. NO is a gas that diffuse among tissues. NO is a very reactive molecule that spontaneously reacts with free radicals (i.e. superoxide anions) generating reactive nitrogen species (RNS) among which the most common is peroxynitrate (ONOO-). Peroxynitrate is a potent pro-oxidative radical that cause intracellular damage by nitration and S-nitrosylation of proteins, lipid and DNA [46]. Excessive cellular damage causes severe endothelium dysfunctions as reported in multiple cases of cardiovascular disease as diabetes and hypertensions or inflammation [47,48]. eNOS expression and NO are important players for angiogenesis not only in physiological conditions, but also in tumor conditions. NO contributes to angiogenesis by activating intracellular molecular pathway such as the mitogen activated kinases (MAPK), cyclic GMP (cGMP), and by regulating expression of fibroblast growth factor (FGF-2) and controlling the balance between metalloprotease (MMP) and their inhibitors in surrounding tissues. In tumor conditions it has been reported that tumor cells can upregulate NO levels by induction of specific intracellular NOS isoforms (iNOS and nNOS) in order to activate NO-dependent angiogenic signaling. Also eNOS is normally expressed by endothelial tumor cells and is sensitive to multiple factors present in the tumor microenvironment. Pro-angiogenic factors such as vascular endothelial growth factor (VEGF), sex hormones or angiopoietins activate eNOS and positively regulate eNOS in endothelial cells through specific molecular pathways such as 1) Akt-phosphoinositide3 (PI3K) pathway, 2) phospholipase Cγ (PLCγ)-diacylglicerol (DAG)/Ca^{2+} 3) adenilate cyclase (AC) -protein kinase A (PKA). Upregulation of eNOS triggers NO-specific intracellular signaling not only through cGMP, but also leading to post-translational modifications of proteins to form S-nitrosothiol and, thus, generating a specific oxidative signaling mediated by S-nitrosylation. An example of such mechanism is the nitrosylation of caspase 3 that inhibits apoptosis or the nitrosylation of p21Ras that enforces cGMP signaling by increasing endothelial cell proliferation [49,50]. Supporting evidences for NO involvement in tumor progression come from in vivo studies

http://dx.doi.org/10.5772/54593

with NOS inhibitors that have demonstrated a peculiar role for NO in sustaining tumor growth. Anti-metastatic effects have been reported in several kinds of tumors under treatment with NOS inhibitors N^G-methyl-L-arginine (NMMA) and N^G – Nitro-L-arginine methyl ester (L-NAME) [51,52].

Together with these enzymes the mitochondrial electron transport chain (ETC) has been recognized as responsible for pro-oxidative species production. The mitochondrial respiratory chain is one of the first sources of pro-oxidative species to have been characterized in cells. Mechanism through witch oxidative species are produced in mitochondria are widely described as side products of ETC [53,54]. As it has been described ETC consists in an electron flow among different protein complexes in the inner mitochondria membranes. Electrons from NADPH are transferred NADPH-ubiquinone oxidoreductase complex I which consequently transfer electrons downstream to complex II. Then, electrons according to electrochemical gradients flow to complexes III and IV. The final step of the chain is the reduction of oxygen to water, however it has been quantified that about 1-4% of oxygen fails to be properly reduced and superoxide is produced as consequence. Dysfunctional ETC leads to high levels of ROS in mitochondria that are reported as cytotoxic, however this condition has been also associated with induction of pro-angiogenic signaling [55]. In vitro and in vivo treatments with inhibitors of ETC (i.e. rotenone) inhibits VEGF -induced signaling and vascular walls remodeling [56] suggesting that ETC may play a role in redox signaling in normal and pathological angiogenesis.

4. Cellular systems for counterbalance oxidative species in angiogenesis: Natural antioxidants and scavenging systems

4.1. Antioxidant enzymes

In order to limit oxidative stress levels cells are armed with a series of enzymes and molecules. Important enzymes for degradation of hydrogen peroxide and superoxide are family of superoxide dismutase (SOD), catalase (CAT), peroxiredoxins (PRX), thioredoxin (TRX) and gluthatione peroxidase (GPx). All these enzymes play a critical role in modulation redox signaling.

Superoxide dismutase (SOD) is the most important cellular mechanism of protection against superoxide anion (O_2^-). SOD catalyzes the dismutation of O_2^- into hydrogen peroxide (H_2O_2). The catalytic reaction of SOD involves metal cations (i.e. Cu, Zn, Mn) as cofactors that continuously shift between reduced and oxidized forms in the active site of the enzymes. In humans there are three isoforms of superoxide dismutase enzymes that are distinguished for their cellular localization: SOD1 (CuZn-SOD) which is localized essentially in the cytosol, SOD2 (Mn-SOD) which is localized in the mitochondria and SOD3 (CuZn-SOD, also known as ec-SOD) which is localized in the extracellular matrix. All three isoforms catalyze the same reaction, which is important, not only to scavenge the cytotoxic effects of superoxide anion accumulation (i.e. oxidation and inactivation of proteins), but also to prevent the reaction of

O_2^- with nitric oxide (NO) to generate peroxynitrate. In this way these enzymes guarantee the metabolism of H_2O_2, important for redox signaling [57]. In the vasculature the signaling of H_2O_2 produced by SODs activates multiple pathways important for angiogenesis. The H_2O_2 generated by SOD3 in the extracellular space favorites VEGFR2 signaling and consequently modulates angiogenesis. H_2O_2 produced by SOD3 under conditions of ischemic injury, protects tissues and promotes neovascularization by enhancing Ras-ERK, PI3kinase-Akt pathways and VEGF expression [58].

The H_2O_2 generated by SOD1 is actively produced in endosomes under inflammation signals and activates NF-kB. Moreover such H_2O_2 generated by SOD1 is particularly important in endothelial cells where acts as endothelium–derived hyperpolarization factor (EDHF). It has been demonstrated that in the tumorigenic context, SOD1 overexpression promotes angiogenesis and tumor growth. Also the H_2O_2 generated by SOD2 is important for endothelium. It has been demonstrated that SOD2 overexpression favorites Akt pathway activation and enhances vessels formations *in vivo* by favoring endothelial cells sprouting. On the contrary, SOD2 deficiency causes increased mitochondrial O_2^- that results in mitochondria damage (i.e. mtDNA and mitochondrial proteins oxidation) and endothelial dysfunctions [59,60]. Additionally, all SODs enzymes modulate vessels homeostasis by influencing EPCs. $SOD3^{-/-}$ mice show EPCs failure in physiological processes of migration and differentiation. A recent report indicate that SOD1-deficient EPCs show shortages in migration and ability to generate small vessels networks [61]. Thus, SODs enzymes play their role in redox signaling by regulating angiogenesis through H_2O_2 and protecting EPCs from excess of O_2^-.

Catalase (CAT) catalyzes the decomposition of hydrogen peroxide (H_2O_2) into water and oxygen by helping the antioxidant machinery in cells. The active site of the enzyme is made by four porphyry heme groups, that are essential to catalyze the flow of electrons between atoms. The mechanism of reaction is not jet fully characterized however it is supposed to occur into two steps: in the first step the iron is reduced with concomitant production of water, in the second step another molecule of hydrogen peroxide enters into the active site and allows the re-oxidation of iron with contemporary production of water and oxygen [62]. The balance of the reaction consists of two molecules of H_2O_2 that are decomposed into two molecules of water and one molecule of oxygen. Catalase is intracellular localized, mainly in peroxisomes of animal and vegetal cells. In addition, there are also data supporting its localization in the mitochondria and cytosol. Catalase is an enzyme shared between all organisms. All cells contain catalase, however knock-out animal models do not display severe phenotypes. Also human patients showing reduced levels of catalase enzymes do not display severe health disorder [63]. It is supposed that the lack of catalytic activity of catalase may be replaced by multiple alternative antioxidant systems. The catalase plays an important role in the redox signaling since it regulates H_2O_2 levels, which is important for homeostasis of vascular beds. Catalase of endothelial cells protects smooth muscle cells from oxidative damage of luminal peroxide [64] and is involved in mechanisms of vessels relaxation [65]. Moreover, it has been also reported that catalase in combination with SOD play a synergistic role in the regulation of endothelium permeability. Overexpression of catalase was also applied to breast cancer cells in order to down-regulate intracellular ROS levels and make tumor cells more sensitive to therapy (paclitaxel, etoposide and arsenic triosside) [66].

Peroxiredoxins (PRX) are a family of ubiquitous antioxidant enzymes constituted by several isoforms. PRX catalytic activity consists in the reduction of cellular hydrogen peroxide and for some aspects it overlaps with enzyme activity of other antioxidant enzymes (i.e. catalase and GPx) [67]. However, PRXs differentiate from other antioxidant enzymes for their mechanism of activity. Their enzymatic active site is constituted by cysteine amminoacids that metabolize H_2O_2 by cycling between oxidation and reduction reactions. When a molecule of hydrogen peroxide enters, the active Cys-SH oxides into Cys-SOH. This intermediate form can be further oxidized to Cys-SO_2H. The recycling of cysteine is mediated by glutathione, ascorbic acid or sulfiredoxins. According with the setting of the active site PRX are divided into three groups. The first two groups are Typical 2-Cys-PRX and Atypical 2-Cys-PRX, according with folding structure, and both contains two residues of Cys in their active site are. The third class, 1-Cys-PRX contains only one Cys in the active site. Besides the difference in the number of active cysteine, all PRXs act as intracellular H_2O_2 scavengers. PRXs are localized primarily in the cytosol, but they are localized also in intracellular organelles (peroxisomes, mitochondria) where they take part to regulation of H_2O_2 levels and redox signaling [68,69]. In vivo knockout mice for PRX-VI are more sensitive to oxidative stress under hyperoxia exposure, while knockout mice for PRX-I and PRX-II develop severe blood cells disease (hemolytic anemia and hematopoietic cancer) [70,71]. The role of PRXs in redox signaling in cardiovascular system is still not clear.

Thioredoxins (TRX) are a small class of antioxidant enzymes composed of two isoforms: TRX1, which is primarily localized in the cytosol and nucleus, and TRX, which is found in mitochondria. All TRX enzymes are ubiquitously expressed and are characterized by a dithiol-disulfide site. The active site of TRX contains a specific and highly conserved motif with two residues of Cysteine that are essentials to reduce oxidized proteins and buffer ROS. TRX can be continuously reconverted from oxidized form into reduced form thanks to thioredoxin reductase enzymes activity. The TRX system is modulated by an endogenous inhibitor protein, called TXNIP (TRX-interacting protein), that prevents TRX to form disulfides [72]. The TRX system has been shown to be essential for life since the knockout mice of either isoform is lethal for embryo development [73,74]. Moreover endothelium specific *Trx2* transgenic mice as well as mice overexpressing *Trx1* demonstrate a crucial role of this class of enzymes in buffering oxidative stress in endothelial cells. TRX1 can modulate different cellular processes involved with endothelial cell homeostasis and angiogenesis. In endothelial cells TRX1 prevents degradation of HIF1α and consequently modulate VEGF expression facilitating pro-angiogenic processes. Moreover, TRX1 can regulate proliferation and migration of endothelial cells by modulation of NF-kB activity and upregulation of matrix metalloproteases (MMPs). TRX2 have been demonstrated to play also a specific role in endothelial cells by inducing angiogenesis and arteriogenesis in pathological conditions (i.e. murine model of ischemia) [75]. The importance of this antioxidant system for promoting angiogenesis has been considered for development of anticancer drugs. In vitro studies performed with TRX inhibitors (i.e. PMX464, AJM290) confirm the pivotal role of this class of enzymes in preventing endothelial cell proliferation and differentiation [76].

Glutathione peroxidases (GPx) are a family of enzymes that catalyze the reduction of hydrogen peroxide and organic hydroperoxides to water. The reaction consists in the oxidation of monomeric glutathione to glutathione disulfide with the involvement of a selenic acid group. Oxidized glutathione molecules are then reduced by a specific glutathione reductase [77]. In humans there are eight isoforms of glutathione peroxidases with different intracellular localizations and different relative abundance in tissues. Human GPx1, GPx2, GPx3, GPx4 and Gpx6 are different from other isoforms for containing seleno-cysteines in their catalytic sites, which identifies them as seleno-proteins. All GPxs play a fundamental role in the antioxidant molecular network as peroxide scavenging enzymes, however specific notes are reported for different isoforms. GPx4 has been identified mainly as phospholipid hydroperoxidase since it not only reduces peroxides but it is also efficient in reducing phospholipids, cholesterol and lipoproteins hydroperoxide [78]. In pig livers GPx4 activity was reported for inhibition of lipid peroxidation [79] and curiously crucial for sperm maturation [80]. GPx3 is produced in the tubules of kidney and secreted in extracellular fluids as well as in the plasma, but its antioxidant activity does not seem to be essential since GPx3$^{-/-}$ mice do not show abnormal phenotype [81]. Recent studies on GPx3 promoter regulation suggest that its expressivity is implicated in epithelial tumor development but a specific role needs to be addressed [82]. GPx2 is expressed in the gastrointestinal system and is supposed to play a key role as antioxidant enzyme in the gut. Also, GPx2$^{-/-}$ mice do not show abnormal phenotype [83] but in vitro and in vivo data regarding loss of GPx2 expression report a role for GPx2 in regulation of inflammation-mediated carcinogenesis and for supporting growth of established tumors. Among the GPxs isoforms the most studied and characterized is GPx1, which is also the most abundant one. It is ubiquitously expressed and it is localized mainly in the cytosol and in mitochondria. GPx1 is believed to be the most important peroxide scavenger in the family [84], even tough also GPx1$^{-/-}$ mice are not lethal and develop normally [85]. In vivo data indicate that the loss of this enzyme is correlated with high oxidative damage condition. Loss of GPx1 in condition of cerebral inflammation increases pro-oxidative species level and favors interactions between leukocytes and endothelial cells of cerebral microvasculature [86]. Loss of GPx1 in human microvascular cells as well as in GPx1$^{-/-}$ mice favors endothelium response to lipo-polisaccaride pro-oxidant stimuli favoring intracellular reactive oxygen species accumulation and altering expression of adhesion molecules. Levels of GPx1 are also reported to modulate angiogenic endothelial progenitor cells (EPCs) in correlation with aging. EPCs of old subjects, that have impaired GPx1 levels, are more sensitive to oxidative damage [87].

4.2. Antioxidant molecules

Recent evidence suggests that many natural **antioxidant molecules** contained in foods or plants have beneficial effects against tumor progression. Polyphenols as well as terpenoids act on overall oxidative stress levels. By modulation of cytokines, metabolizing enzymes, growth factors and various molecules in redox signaling, antioxidants regulate pathways for tumor angiogenesis. Natural **polyphenols** are a class of compounds constituted by molecules containing repetitive units of phenols that characterize them with antioxidant properties. Polyphenols are naturally present in vegetal derived foods (i.e. fruits, tea, red wine, honey, olive oil) and can be assumed directly with the diet [88]. Data regarding alimentary habits correlate black tea assumption with beneficial effects on endothelium dysfunctions in individuals with chronic heart disease and hypercholesterolemia [89]. In vitro studies on endothelial cells demonstrate polyphenols modulate redox signaling by regulation of arachidonic acid cascade. In particular, it has been reported that polyphenols from virgin olive oil and red wine reduce significantly angiogenesis by inhibition of cyclooxigenase2 (COX2) and activation of redox sensitive NF-kB pathway [90]. Microarray data and RT-PCR analyses show that treatment of endothelial cells (HUVEC) with resveratrol (contained in red wine) can upregulate eNOS and decrease the levels of endothelin-1, suggesting a protective role against endothelium contractions. Moreover, resveratrol exerts a protective effects on endothelium as assed also under pro-oxidative state (in presence of H_2O_2). Together with anthocyanin, also polyphenols (contained in berries that have red pigments) are reported to have an antioxidant positive effect for cardiovascular system. Recently, anthocyanins from six berries extracts have been mixed in a formula (OptiBerry), which in vitro exhibits anti-angiogenic properties on human microvascular endothelial cells and also in vivo impairs endothelioma cells for tumor growth [91].

Among **lipids** there are also very important antioxidant molecules. They are naturally present in plants like carotenes (retinol and b-carotene), alpha-tocopherol (also known as Vitamin E) or synthetized by animal cells, like CoenzymeQ10. The characteristic lipid character of these molecules allows them to localize in cell membranes (intracellular organelles and plasma membrane) where they can buffer lipid radicals and prevent reactions of peroxidation. Antioxidant Vitamin E properties for lipid peroxidation were efficiently assayed in $GPx4^{-/-}$ mice [92]. Carotenoids are tetraterpenoid pigments contained exclusively in plant cells that can be assumed with diet and act as terminal antioxidant molecules, once oxidized they can not be "re-used" from cells [93]. CoenzymeQ10 (CoQ10) is a terpenoid molecule whose antioxidant activity has been reported for maintenance of healthy cardiovascular system. Recent clinical trials have also show the use of CoQ10 for lowering blood pressure. At the present there are not evidences regarding the involvement of lipid antioxidant molecules in conditions of tumor angiogenesis [94].

Several other **antioxidant genes** are normally induced in cells to shield against dangerous deregulation of redox balance. Among those which play a key role in angiogenesis we can find heme-oxygenase-1 (HMOX-1) and nuclear factor erythroid 2 (NRF2) [95]. Upregulation of these genes are correlates to tumor metastasis and progression suggesting how oxidative stress is a condition implicated in tumor angiogenesis [96].

5. Angiogenic molecules regulated by redox signaling

Vascular Endothelial Growth Factor (VEGF) family encloses six glycoproteins: VEGF-A, VEGF-B, VEGF-C, VEGF-D AND VEGF-E, all of them belong to a superfamily of growth factors. Endothelial cells have three types of specific VEGF receptors: VEGFR-1 (Flt-1), VEGFR-2 (KDR, Flk-1), VEGFR-3 (Flt-4). Signaling mediated by VEGF and respective receptors has been characterized as one of the most powerful factors for induction and maintenance of angiogenesis in a series of physiological as well as pathological (i.e. tumor) angiogenesis [97,98]. Among the multiple mechanisms of VEGF signaling regulation we can also found its redox state. Modulators of redox state as the concentration of oxygen directly regulates VEGF levels. VEGF promoter contains a hypoxia responsive element that can be bound by transcription factors HIF-1α- HIF1β under conditions of low oxygen concentration in vascular vessels (hypoxia). In vitro studies by using human genome array on pulmonary artery endothelial cells maintained in hypoxia for 24hours report up-regulation of expression of VEGF genes. Accordingly, in vivo hypoxia conditions induce VEGF and VEGFR-1/2 expression [99,100]. It has been also reported that modulation of redox state by NO levels regulates angiogenesis and tumor progression through modulation of VEGF–VEGFR signaling. In vitro treatments of human tumor cells with NO-donor (i.e. SNAP) or NO-generating compounds upregulate VEGF expression and stimulate angiogenesis [101]. Further specifications about VEGF modulation by NO are related to endothelial NOS activity.

Angiopoietins (Ang) are a group of four growth factors (Ang-1, Ang-2, Ang-3, Ang-4) involved in blood vessels formation. Signaling mediated by angiopoietins and their specific receptors (TIE, tyrosine kinases receptor) has been characterized as key factors in angiogenesis [102]. They are particularly sensitive to endothelium environment since angiopoietins are modulated by pro-oxidative species. In vitro and in vivo studies in endothelial cells report Ang1 is induced by hydrogen peroxide and abrogation of catalase activity relates to low ability in cell migration and vessels formation [103]. Also, angiopoietin-like proteins (ANGPTL) are involved in redox signaling in tumor conditions. Up-regulation of expression of ANGPL4 promotes NADPH oxidases activity causing an alteration in relative abundance of superoxide anion over hydrogen peroxide. Finally, such redox alteration induces tumor cells escape from anoikis and promotes survival via specific activation of PI3K/PKBα/ERK pathway [104].

Vascular Endothelial (VE)-Cadherin is an adhesion protein in the adherent junction complexes of endothelial cells and has been characterized as the major system for controlling endothelial cells junctions [105]. VE-Cadherin controls vascular permeability and remodeling of blood vessels also under mechanical stimuli (shear forces) [106]. VE-Cadherin regulation is sensitive to pro-angiogenic factors, in particular to VEGF [107]. VE-Cadherin is also directly regulated by redox signaling pathway. In vitro assays showed that resveratrol promotes proliferation and migration of cerebral endothelial cells by modulation of VE-cadherin as result of activation of MAPK/ERK pathway and NO upregulation [108]. It has also been demonstrated that resveratrol control initiation of arteriogenesis by blocking oxidative stress dependent phosphorylation of VE-Cadherin [109]. Interestingly, it is also reported that nitrate concentration contributes to control VE-Cadherin stability in adherent junction of human primary endothelial cells (HUVEC) and prevents blood vessel leakage [110].

Nuclear factor-kB (NF-kB) is a transcriptional factor that promotes tumor growth and invasiveness by activation of angiogenic molecules in endothelial cells [111]. Using a zebrafish animal model it has been shown that in vivo NF-kB inhibition causes loss of vascular integrity and interferes with physiologic vessels morphology [112]. Inhibition or negative modulation of NF-kB is considered an alternative approach to block pathological angiogenesis. Among inhibitors of NF-kB it has been reported evidence for antioxidant molecules. In vitro treatments of cells with pro-oxidative species (hydrogen peroxide, LPS, TNF-α) activates NF-kB, while contemporary antioxidants addiction inhibit its response [113,114]. NF-kB activation can also be impaired by N-acetylcysteine (that acts in the NO pathway), terpenoids (vitamin E) and mitochondria-specific antioxidant (rotenone) [115,116]. At the present it is not fully clarified as antioxidants interact with NF-kB and inactivate it. It is supposed they can act indirectly by altering different molecules that interact with NF-kB on redox pathways or directly by inhibition of IKK kinase activity [117].

6. Conclusion: Manipulating redox signaling as anti-tumor angiogenesis therapy

Increased generation of reactive oxygen species (ROS) and an altered redox status have long been observed in cancer cells, and recent studies suggest that this biochemical property of cancer cells can be exploited for therapeutic benefits. Cancer cells in advanced stage tumors frequently exhibit multiple genetic alterations and high oxidative stress, suggesting that it might be possible to preferentially eliminate these cells by pharmacological ROS insults [118].

Reactive oxygen species (ROS) might function as a double-edged sword in endothelial cells. A moderate increase of ROS may promote cell proliferation and survival. However, when the increase of ROS reaches a certain level (the toxic threshold), it may overwhelm the antioxidant capacity of the cell and trigger cell death. Under physiological conditions, normal endothelial cells maintain redox homeostasis with a low level of basal ROS by controlling the balance between ROS generation (pro-oxidants) and elimination (antioxidant capacity). Endothelial cells in normal vessels can tolerate a certain level of exogenous oxidative stress owing to their 'reserve' antioxidant capacity, which can be mobilized to prevent the ROS level from reaching the cell-death threshold. In In endothelial cells of tumor vessels the increase in ROS generation from metabolic abnormalities and oncogenic signaling may trigger a redox adaption response. This response leads to an upregulation of antioxidant capacity and a shift of redox dynamics that maintain the ROS levels below the toxic threshold. As such, tumor angiogenic cells would be more dependent on the antioxidant system and more vulnerable to further oxidative stress induced by exogenous ROS-generating agents or compounds that inhibit the antioxidant system. A further increase of ROS stress in these cancer cells using exogenous ROS-modulating agents is likely to cause elevation of ROS above the threshold level, leading to cell death. This might constitute a biochemical basis to design therapeutic strategies to selectively kill tumor angiogenic cells using ROS-mediated mechanisms [119-121].

The role of redox signaling in tumor angiogenesis is not yet completely characterized. Although converse mechanisms are postulated about how oxidative species recruit new blood vessels for tumor progression, it is well established redox signaling modulates angiogenesis. Analysis and characterization of molecules that sustain redox signaling is a new opportunity for set up innovative strategies of anti-cancer therapy (Figure 1).

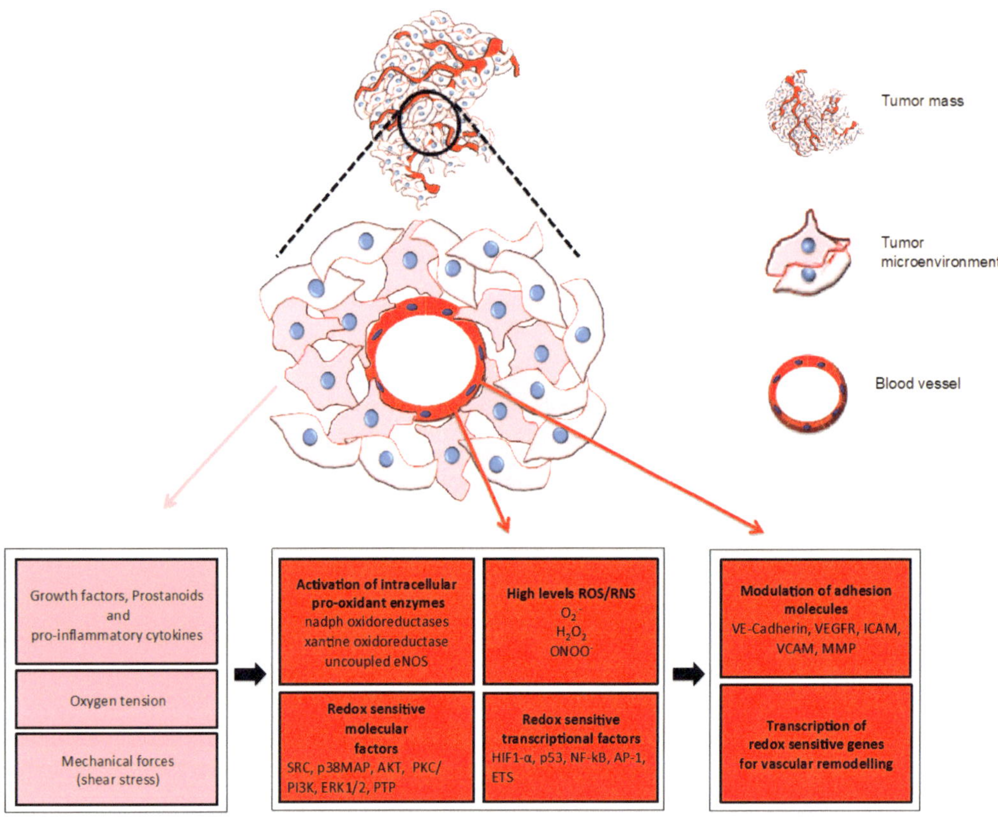

Figure 1. Schematic representation of redox mechanisms in tumor angiogenesis. Multiple stimuli coming from tumor microenvironment (growth factor, prostanoids, oxygen tension, mechanical forces) induce specific activation of intracellular pro-oxidant enzymes (NADPH oxidase, xantine oxidoreductase, uncoupled eNOS). Consequently, raising levels of oxygen and nitrogen pro-oxidant species (ROS/RNS) modulate the activation of multiple cellular pathways by acting on molecular and transcriptional factors. Signaling induced by oxidative species results mainly in endothelial cells motility and proliferation towards vascular remodeling and formation of new blood vessels. HIF-1α hypoxia-inducible transcription factor; ETS E-twenty six family transcription factor; AP-I activator protein 1; p53 tumor suppressor protein; NF-kB nuclear factor – kB. PKC protein kinase C; PI3K phosphatidylinositol3-OH kinase; PTP protein tyrosine phosphatase; SRC tyrosine protein kinase; p38MAPK p38 mitogen-activated protein kinase; Akt serine/threonine-specific protein kinase; ERK1/2 extracellular signal-regulated kinases; MMP matrix metalloproteinase; VE–Cadherin: vascular endothelial-cadherin; VEGFR vascular endothelial growth factor receptor; ICAM intracellular adhesion molecule 1; VACAM vascular cell adhesion molecule 1.

Acknowledgements

We apologize to the many researchers whose work was not cited in this review due to space limitations. We would like to thank all members of Santoro lab for support and discussion. MMS is supported by grants from HFSP, Marie Curie IRG, Telethon and AIRC.

Author details

Vera Mugoni and Massimo Mattia Santoro*

*Address all correspondence to: massimo.santoro@unito.it

Department of Molecular Biotechnology and Health Sciencesm, Molecular Biotechnology Center, University of Torino, Italy

References

[1] Holland AJ, Cleveland DW.Boveri revisited: chromosomal instability, aneuploidy and tumorigenesis. Nat Rev Mol Cell Biol 2009; 10(7): 478-87

[2] Albini A, Tosetti F, Li VW, Noonan DM, Li WW. Cancer prevention by targeting angiogenesis. Nat . Rev Clin Oncol 2012; 9(9):498-509. http://www.ncbi.nlm.nih.gov/pubmed/22850752

[3] Carmeliet P, Jain RK. Angiogenesis in cancer and other diseases. Nature 2000; 407(6801):249– 257.

[4] Fraisl P, Mazzone M, Schmidt T, Carmeliet P. Regulation of angiogenesis by oxygen and metabolism. Dev Cell. 2009; 16(2):167-79. http://www.ncbi.nlm.nih.gov/pubmed/19217420

[5] Wu WS. The signaling mechanism of ROS in tumor progression. Cancer Metastasis Rev. 2006 Dec; 25(4):695-705. http://www.ncbi.nlm.nih.gov/pubmed/17160708

[6] Blanchetot C, Boonstra J. The ROS-NOX connection in cancer and angiogenesis. Crit Rev Eukaryot Gene Expr 2008; 18(1):35-45.

[7] Fridovich I. The biology of oxygen radicals. Science 1978; 201(4359):875–80.

[8] Xia C, Meng Q, Liu LZ, Rojanasakul Y, Wang XR, Jiang BH. Reactive oxygen species regulate angiogenesis and tumor growth through vascular endothelial growth factor. Cancer Res 2007; 67(22):10823-30. http://www.ncbi.nlm.nih.gov/pubmed/18006827

[9] Trachootham D, Lu W, Ogasawara MA, Nilsa RD, Huang P. Redox regulation of cell survival. Antioxid Redox Signal 2008;10(8):1343-74. http://www.ncbi.nlm.nih.gov/pubmed/18522489

[10] Cai H, Garrison DG. Endothelial dysfunction in cardiovascular diseases. The role of oxidant stress. Circ. Res 2000. 87: 840–4.

[11] Noguchi N, Jo H. Redox going with vascular shear stress. Antioxid Redox Signal 2011; 15(5):1367-8.

[12] Hirota K, Semenza GL. Regulation of angiogenesis by hypoxia-inducible factor 1. Crit Rev Oncol Hematol 2006; 59(1):15-26.

[13] Mowbray AL, Kang DH, Rhee SG, Kang SW, Jo H. Laminar shear stress up-regulates peroxiredoxins (PRX) in endothelial cells: PRX 1 as a mechanosensitive antioxidant. J Biol Chem 2008; 283(3):1622-7.

[14] He CH, Gong P, Hu B, Stewart D, Choi ME, Choi AM, Alam J. Identification of activating transcription factor 4 (ATF4) as an Nrf2-interacting protein. Implication for heme oxygenase-1 gene regulation. J Biol Chem 2001; 276(24):20858-65.

[15] Vurusaner B, Poli G, Basaga H. Tumor suppressor genes and ROS: complex networks of interactions.Free Radic Biol Med 2012; 52(1):7-18. http://www.ncbi.nlm.nih.gov/pubmed/22019631

[16] Okuno Y, Nakamura-Ishizu A, Otsu K, Suda T, Kubota Y. Pathological neoangiogenesis depends on oxidative stress regulation by ATM. Nat Med. 2012. doi: 10.1038/nm.2846.

[17] West XZ, Malinin NL, Merkulova AA, Tischenko M, Kerr BA, Borden EC, Podrez EA, Salomon RG, Byzova TV. Oxidative stress induces angiogenesis by activating TLR2 with novel endogenous ligands. Nature 2010; 467(7318):972-6.

[18] Ebrahem Q, Renganathan K, Sears J, Vasanji A, Gu X, Lu L, Salomon RG, Crabb JW, Anand-Apte B. Carboxyethylpyrrole oxidative protein modifications stimulate neovascularization: Implications for age-related macular degeneration. Proc Natl Acad Sci USA 2006; 103(36):13480-4. Erratum in: Proc Natl Acad Sci USA 2006; 103(42): 15722.http://www.ncbi.nlm.nih.gov/pubmed/16938854

[19] Lambeth JD . NOX enzymes and the biology of reactive oxygen. Nat Rev Immunol 2004; 4: 181–9.

[20] Ushio-Fukai M, Alexander RW. Reactive oxygen species as mediators of angiogenesis signaling: role of NAD(P)H oxidase. Mol Cell Biochem 2004; 264 (1–2):85–97.

[21] Lambeth JD, Kawahara T, and Diebold B. Regulation of Nox and Duox enzymatic activity and expression. Free Radic Biol Med 2007;43: 319–31.

[22] Ushio-Fukai M. VEGF signaling through NADPH oxidase-derived ROS.Antioxid Redox Signal 2007;9(6):731-9. http://www.ncbi.nlm.nih.gov/pubmed/17511588

[23] Lassègue B, San Martín A, Griendling KK. Biochemistry, physiology, and pathophysiology of NADPH oxidases in the cardiovascular system. Circ Res 2012;110(10): 1364-90. http://www.ncbi.nlm.nih.gov/pubmed/22581922

[24] Ushio-Fukai M. Redox signaling in angiogenesis: role of NADPH oxidase.Cardiovasc Res 2006; 71(2):226-35. http://www.ncbi.nlm.nih.gov/pubmed/16781692

[25] Arbiser JL, Petros J, Klafter R, Govindajaran B, McLaughlin ER, Brown LF, Cohen C, Moses M, Kilroy S, Arnold RS, Lambeth JD. Reactive oxygen generated by Nox1 triggers the angiogenic switch. Proc Natl Acad Sci USA 2002;99(2):715–20.

[26] Ushio-Fukai M, Tang Y, Fukai T, Dikalov S, Ma Y, Fujimoto M, Quinn MT, Pagano PJ, Johnson C, Alexander RW. Novel role of gp91phox-containing NAD(P)H oxidase in vascular endothelial growth factor-induced signaling and angiogenesis. Circ Res 2002;91:1160–7.

[27] Datla SR, Peshavariya H, Dusting GJ, Jiang F. Important Role of Nox4 Type NADPH Oxidase in Angiogenic Responses in Human Microvascular Endothelial Cells In Vitro. Arterioscler Thromb Vasc Biol 2007; 27(11):2319-24.

[28] BelAiba RS, Djordjevic T, Petry A, Diemer K, Bonello S, Banfi B, Hess J, Pogrebniak A, Bickel C, Gorlach A. NOX5 variants are functionally active in endothelial cells. Free Radic Biol Med 2007; 42(4):446–59.

[29] Ushio-Fukai M, Nakamura Y. Reactive oxygen species and angiogenesis: NADPH oxidase as target for cancer therapy. Cancer Lett 2008; 266(1):37-52. http://www.ncbi.nlm.nih.gov/pubmed/18406051

[30] The lipid library. Lipid Chemistry, Biology, Technology & Analysis. AOCS. http://lipidlibrary.aocs.org/index.html (accessed 28 September 2012).

[31] He T, Lu T, d'Uscio LV, Lam CF, Lee HC, Katusic ZS. Angiogenic function of prostacyclin biosynthesis in human endothelial progenitor cells. Circ Res. 2008;103(1):80-8.

[32] Kawabe J, Yuhki K, Okada M, Kanno T, Yamauchi A, Tashiro N, Sasaki T, Okumura S, Nakagawa N, Aburakawa Y, Takehara N, Fujino T, Hasebe N, Narumiya S, Ushikubi F. Prostaglandin I2 promotes recruitment of endothelial progenitor cells and limits vascular remodeling. Arterioscler Thromb Vasc Biol 2010; 30(3):464-70.

[33] Gupta RA, Tan J, Krause WF, Geraci MW, Willson TM, Dey SK, DuBois RN. Prostacyclin-mediated activation of peroxisome proliferator-activated receptor delta in colorectal cancer. Proc Natl Acad Sci USA 2000;97(24):13275-80.

[34] Cathcart, M.C. et al. (2010) The role of prostacyclin synthase and thromboxane synthase signaling in the development and progression of cancer. Biochim. Biophys. Acta 1805, 153–166

[35] Greenhough A, Smartt HJ, Moore AE, Roberts HR, Williams AC, Paraskeva C, Kaidi A. The COX-2/PGE2 pathway: key roles in the hallmarks of cancer and adaptation to the tumour microenvironment. Carcinogenesis 2009;30(3):377-86.

[36] Murata T, Lin MI, Aritake K, Matsumoto S, Narumiya S, Ozaki H, Urade Y, Hori M, Sessa WC. Role of prostaglandin D2 receptor DP as a suppressor of tumor hyperpermeability and angiogenesis in vivo. Proc Natl Acad Sci USA 2008;105(50):20009-14.

[37] Salvado MD, Alfranca A, Haeggström JZ, Redondo JM. Prostanoids in tumor angiogenesis: therapeutic intervention beyond COX-2. Trends Mol Med 2012; 18(4):233-43.

[38] Olson JS, Ballou DP, Palmer G, Massey V. The mechanism of action of xanthine oxidase. J Biol Chem 1974; 249(14):4363-82. http://www.ncbi.nlm.nih.gov/pubmed/4367215

[39] Parks DA, Granger DN. Xanthine oxidase: biochemistry, distribution and physiology. Acta Physiol Scand Suppl 1986;548:87–99.

[40] Kou B, Ni J, Vatish M, Singer DR. Xanthine oxidase interaction with vascular endothelial growth factor in human endothelial cell angiogenesis Microcirculation 2008;15(3):251-67.

[41] Ferdinandy P, Panas D, Schulz R. Peroxynitrite contributes to spontaneous loss of cardiac efficiency in isolated working rat hearts. Am J Physiol 1999; 276(6 Pt 2):H1861-7. http://www.ncbi.nlm.nih.gov/pubmed/10362664

[42] Pérez NG, Gao WD, Marbán E. Novel myofilament Ca2+-sensitizing property of xanthine oxidase inhibitors. Circ Res 1998;83(4):423-30.http://www.ncbi.nlm.nih.gov/pubmed/9721699

[43] Miyamoto Y, Akaike T, Yoshida M, Goto S, Horie H, Maeda H. Potentiation of nitric oxide-mediated vasorelaxation by xanthine oxidase inhibitors.Proc Soc Exp Biol Med 1996; 211(4):366-73.

[44] Nathan C, Xie QW. Nitric oxide synthases: roles, tolls, and controls. Cell 1994;78(6): 915-8. http://www.ncbi.nlm.nih.gov/pubmed/7522969

[45] Förstermann U, Sessa WC. Nitric oxide synthases: regulation and function. Eur Heart J 2012;33(7):829-37, 837a-837d. http://www.ncbi.nlm.nih.gov/pubmed/21890489

[46] Förstermann U. Nitric oxide and oxidative stress in vascular disease. Pflugers Arch 2010; 459(6):923-39.

[47] Förstermann U. Oxidative stress in vascular disease: causes, defense mechanisms and potential therapies. Nat Clin Pract Cardiovasc Med 2008; 5(6):338-49. http://www.ncbi.nlm.nih.gov/pubmed/18461048

[48] Förstermann U, Li H. Therapeutic effect of enhancing endothelial nitric oxide synthase (eNOS) expression and preventing eNOS uncoupling. Br J Pharmacol 2011;164(2):213-23. http://www.ncbi.nlm.nih.gov/pubmed/21198553

[49] Kawasaki K, Smith RS Jr, Hsieh CM, Sun J, Chao J, Liao JK. Activation of the phosphatidylinositol 3-kinase/protein kinase Akt pathway mediates nitric oxide-induced endothelial cell migration and angiogenesis. Mol Cell Biol 2003; 23(16):5726-37. http://www.ncbi.nlm.nih.gov/pubmed/12897144

[50] Jones MK, Tsugawa K, Tarnawski AS, Baatar D. Dual actions of nitric oxide on angiogenesis: possible roles of PKC, ERK, and AP-1. Biochem Biophys Res Commun 2004;318(2):520-8. http://www.ncbi.nlm.nih.gov/pubmed/15120632

[51] Fukumura D, Kashiwagi S, Jain RK. The role of nitric oxide in tumour progression. Nat Rev Cancer. 2006 Jul;6(7):521-34. http://www.ncbi.nlm.nih.gov/pubmed/16794635

[52] Jadeski LC, Lala PK. Nitric oxide synthase inhibition by N(G)-nitro-L-arginine methyl ester inhibits tumor-induced angiogenesis in mammary tumors. Am J Pathol 1999;155(4):1381-90. http://www.ncbi.nlm.nih.gov/pubmed/10514420

[53] Zorov DB, Juhaszova M, Sollott SJ. Mitochondrial ROS-induced ROS release: an update and review. Biochim Biophys Acta 2006;1757(5-6):509-17.

[54] Murphy MP. How mitochondria produce reactive oxygen species. Biochem J 2009;417(1):1-13. http://www.ncbi.nlm.nih.gov/pubmed/19061483

[55] Zhang DX, Gutterman DD. Mitochondrial reactive oxygen species-mediated signaling in endothelial cells. Am J Physiol Heart Circ Physiol 2007; 292(5):H2023-31.

[56] Rohlena J, Dong LF, Ralph SJ, Neuzil J. Anticancer drugs targeting the mitochondrial electron transport chain. Antioxid Redox Signal 2011;15(12):2951-74. http://www.ncbi.nlm.nih.gov/pubmed/21777145

[57] Fukai T, Ushio-Fukai M.Superoxide dismutases: role in redox signaling, vascular function, and diseases. Antioxid Redox Signal 2011;15(6):1583-606. http://www.ncbi.nlm.nih.gov/pubmed/21473702

[58] Oshikawa J, Urao N, Kim HW, Kaplan N, Razvi M, McKinney R, Poole LB, Fukai T, Ushio-Fukai M. Extracellular SOD-derived H2O2 promotes VEGF signaling in caveolae/lipid rafts and post-ischemic angiogenesis in mice. PLoS One 2010;5(4):e10189. http://www.ncbi.nlm.nih.gov/pubmed/20422004

[59] Morikawa K, Shimokawa H, Matoba T, Kubota H, Akaike T, Talukder MA, Hatanaka M, Fujiki T, Maeda H, Takahashi S, Takeshita A. Pivotal role of Cu,Zn-superoxide dismutase in endothelium-dependent hyperpolarization. J Clin Invest 2003;112(12): 1871-9. http://www.ncbi.nlm.nih.gov/pubmed/14679182

[60] Marikovsky M, Nevo N, Vadai E, Harris-Cerruti C. Cu/Zn superoxide dismutase plays a role in angiogenesis. Int J Cancer 2002;97(1):34-41. http://www.ncbi.nlm.nih.gov/pubmed/11774241

[61] Groleau J, Dussault S, Haddad P, Turgeon J, Ménard C, Chan JS, Rivard A. Essential role of copper-zinc superoxide dismutase for ischemia-induced neovascularization

via modulation of bone marrow-derived endothelial progenitor cells. Arterioscler Thromb Vasc Biol 2010;30(11):2173-81. http://www.ncbi.nlm.nih.gov/pubmed/20724700

[62] Boon EM, Downs A, Marcey D. "Proposed Mechanism of Catalase". Catalase: H2O2: H2O2 Oxidoreductase: Catalase Structural Tutorial. Retrieved 2007-02-11.

[63] Ho YS, Xiong Y, Ma W, Spector A, Ho D. "Mice Lacking Catalase Develop Normally but Show Differential Sensitivity to Oxidant Tissue Injury". J Biol Chem 2004;279(31): 32804–12. http://dx.doi.org/10.1074%2Fjbc.M404800200

[64] Grover AK, Hui J, Samson SE. Catalase activity in coronary artery endothelium protects smooth muscle against peroxide damage. Eur J Pharmacol 2000;387(1):87-91. http://www.ncbi.nlm.nih.gov/pubmed/10633165

[65] Ellis A, Pannirselvam M, Anderson TJ, Triggle CR. Catalase has negligible inhibitory effects on endothelium-dependent relaxations in mouse isolated aorta and small mesenteric Br J Pharmacol 2003;140(7):1193-200. http://www.ncbi.nlm.nih.gov/pubmed/14597598

[66] Glorieux C, Dejeans N, Sid B, Beck R, Calderon PB, Verrax J. Catalase overexpression in mammary cancer cells leads to a less aggressive phenotype and an altered response to chemotherapy. Biochem Pharmacol 2011;82(10):1384-90. http://www.ncbi.nlm.nih.gov/pubmed/21689642

[67] Wood ZA, Schröder E, Robin Harris J, Poole LB. Structure, mechanism and regulation of peroxiredoxins Trends Biochem Sci 2003;28(1):32-40. http://linkinghub.elsevier.com/retrieve/pii/S0968-0004(02)00003-8

[68] Rhee SG, Kang SW, Chang TS, Jeong W, Kim K. Peroxiredoxin, a novel family of peroxidases. IUBMB Life 2001;52(1-2):35-41. http://www.ncbi.nlm.nih.gov/pubmed/11795591

[69] Miki H, Funato Y. Regulation of intracellular signalling through cysteine oxidation by reactive oxygen species. J Biochem 2012;151(3):255-61. http://www.ncbi.nlm.nih.gov/pubmed/22287686

[70] Neumann CA, Krause DS, Carman CV, Das S, Dubey DP, Abraham JL, Bronson RT, Fujiwara Y, Orkin SH, Van Etten RA. Essential role for the peroxiredoxin Prdx1 in erythrocyte antioxidant defence and tumour suppression. Nature 2003;424 (6948): 561–5. http://dx.doi.org/10.1038%2Fnature01819

[71] Han YH, Kim SU, Kwon TH, Lee DS, Ha HL, Park DS, Woo EJ, Lee SH, Kim JM, Chae HB, Lee SY, Kim BY, Yoon do Y, Rhee SG, Fibach E, Yu DY. Peroxiredoxin II is essential for preventing hemolytic anemia from oxidative stress through maintaining hemoglobin stability. Biochem Biophys Res Commun 2012;426(3):427-32.

[72] Lee S, Kim SM, Lee RT. Thioredoxin and Thioredoxin Target Proteins: From Molecular Mechanisms to Functional Significance. Antioxid Redox Signal. 2012.

[73] Matsui M, Oshima M, Oshima H, Takaku K, Maruyama T, Yodoi J, Taketo MM. Early embryonic lethality caused by targeted disruption of the mouse thioredoxin gene. Dev Biol. 1996; 178(1):179-85.

[74] Nonn L, Williams RR, Erickson RP, Powis G. The absence of mitochondrial thioredoxin 2 causes massive apoptosis, exencephaly, and early embryonic lethality in homozygous mice. Mol Cell Biol. 2003 Feb;23(3):916-22.

[75] Dunn LL, Buckle AM, Cooke JP, Ng MK. The emerging role of the thioredoxin system in angiogenesis. Arterioscler Thromb Vasc Biol. 2010;30(11):2089-98.

[76] Biaglow JE, Miller RA. The thioredoxin reductase/thioredoxin system: novel redox targets for cancer therapy. Cancer Biol Ther. 2005; 4(1):6-13.

[77] Lubos E, Loscalzo J, Handy DE. Glutathione peroxidase-1 in health and disease: from molecular mechanisms to therapeutic opportunities. Antioxid Redox Signal. 2011;15(7):1957-97. http://www.ncbi.nlm.nih.gov/pubmed/21087145

[78] Thomas JP, Geiger PG, Maiorino M, Ursini F, Girotti AW. Enzymatic reduction of phospholipid and cholesterol hydroperoxides in artificial bilayers and lipoproteins.Biochim Biophys Acta1990;1045(3):252-60. http://www.ncbi.nlm.nih.gov/pubmed/2386798

[79] Ursini F, Maiorino M, Valente M, Ferri L, Gregolin C. Purification from pig liver of a protein which protects liposomes and biomembranes from peroxidative degradation and exhibits glutathione peroxidase activity on phosphatidylcholine hydroperoxides. Biochim Biophys Acta. 1982 Feb 15;710(2):197-211.

[80] Godeas C, Tramer F, Micali F, Soranzo M, Sandri G, Panfili E. Distribution and possible novel role of phospholipid hydroperoxide glutathione peroxidase in rat epididymal spermatozoa. Biol Reprod 1997;57(6):1502-8. http://www.ncbi.nlm.nih.gov/pubmed/9408261

[81] Olson GE, Whitin JC, Hill KE, Winfrey VP, Motley AK, Austin LM, Deal J, Cohen HJ, Burk RF. Extracellular glutathione peroxidase (Gpx3) binds specifically to basement membranes of mouse renal cortex tubule cells. Am J Physiol Renal Physiol 2010;298(5):F1244-53.

[82] Yu YP, Yu G, Tseng G, Cieply K, Nelson J, Defrances M, Zarnegar R, Michalopoulos G, Luo JH. Glutathione peroxidase 3, deleted or methylated in prostate cancer, suppresses prostate cancer growth and metastasis. Cancer Res 2007;67(17):8043-50.

[83] Esworthy RS, Mann JR, Sam M, Chu FF. Low glutathione peroxidase activity in Gpx1 knockout mice protects jejunum crypts from gamma-irradiation damage. Am J Physiol Gastrointest Liver Physiol 2000;279(2):G426-36. http://www.ncbi.nlm.nih.gov/pubmed/10915653

[84] Lei XG, Cheng WH, McClung JP. Metabolic regulation and function of glutathione peroxidase-1. Annu Rev Nutr 2007;27:41-61. http://www.ncbi.nlm.nih.gov/pubmed/17465855

[85] De Haan JB, Crack PJ, Flentjar N, Iannello RC, Hertzog PJ, Kola I. An imbalance in antioxidant defense affects cellular function: the pathophysiological consequences of a reduction in antioxidant defense in the glutathione peroxidase-1 (Gpx1) knockout mouse. Redox Rep 2003;8(2):69-79. http://www.ncbi.nlm.nih.gov/pubmed/12804009

[86] Wong CH, Abeynaike LD, Crack PJ, Hickey MJ. Divergent roles of glutathione peroxidase-1 (Gpx1) in regulation of leukocyte-endothelial cell interactions in the inflamed cerebral microvasculature. Microcirculation 2011;18(1):12-23. http://www.ncbi.nlm.nih.gov/pubmed/21166922

[87] Lubos E, Loscalzo J, Handy DE. Glutathione peroxidase-1 in health and disease: from molecular mechanisms to therapeutic opportunities. Antioxid Redox Signal 2011;15(7):1957-97.

[88] Bors W, Heller W, Michel C and Saran M. Flavonoids as antioxidants: determination of radical Scavenging efficiencies. Methods in Enzymology 1990; 186: 343-55.

[89] Duffy SJ, Keaney JF Jr, Holbrook M, Gokce N, Swerdloff PL, Frei B, Vita JA. Short- and long-term black tea consumption reverses endothelial dysfunction in patients with coronary artery disease. Circulation 2001;104(2):151-6.

[90] Scoditti E, Calabriso N, Massaro M, Pellegrino M, Storelli C, Martines G, De Caterina R, Carluccio MA. Mediterranean diet polyphenols reduce inflammatory angiogenesis through MMP-9 and COX-2 inhibition in human vascular endothelial cells: A potentially protective mechanism in atherosclerotic vascular disease and cancer. Arch Biochem Biophys 2012; 527(2):819.

[91] Bagchi D, Sen CK, Bagchi M. Anti-angiogenic, antioxidant, and anti-carcinogenic properties of a novel anthocyanin-rich berry extract formula. Atalay M. Biochemistry 2004;69(1):75-80.

[92] Yant LJ, Ran Q, Rao L, Van Remmen H, Shibatani T, Belter JG, Motta L, Richardson A, Prolla TA. The selenoprotein GPX4 is essential for mouse development and protects from radiation and oxidative damage insults. Free Radic Biol Med 2003;34(4): 496-502.

[93] Riccioni G, D'Orazio N, Salvatore C, Franceschelli S, Pesce M, Speranza L. Carotenoids and vitamins C and E in the prevention of cardiovascular disease. Int J Vitam Nutr Res 2012;82(1):15-26.

[94] Emmanuele V, López LC, Berardo A, Naini A, Tadesse S, Wen B, D'Agostino E, Solomon M, DiMauro S, Quinzii C, Hirano M. Heterogeneity of coenzyme Q10 deficiency: patient study and literature review. Arch Neurol 2012;69(8):978-83.

[95] Dulak J, Loboda A, Jozkowicz A. Effect of heme oxygenase-1 on vascular function and disease. Curr Opin Lipidol 2008;19(5):505-12.

[96] Zhou S, Ye W, Zhang M, Liang J. The effects of nrf2 on tumor angiogenesis: a review of the possible mechanisms of action. Crit Rev Eukaryot Gene Expr 2012;22(2):149-60.

[97] Shibuya M. Tyrosine Kinase Receptor Flt/VEGFR Family: Its Characterization Related to Angiogenesis and Cancer. Genes Cancer 2010;1(11):1119-23.

[98] Carmeliet P. VEGF as a key mediator of angiogenesis in cancer. Oncology 2005;69 Suppl 3:4-10.

[99] Manalo DJ, Rowan A, Lavoie T, Natarajan L, Kelly BD, Ye SQ, Garcia JG, Semenza GL. Transcriptional regulation of vascular endothelial cell responses to hypoxia by HIF-1. Blood 2005;105(2):659-69.

[100] Tuder RM, Flook BE, Voelkel NF. Increased gene expression for VEGF and the VEGF receptors KDR/Flk and Flt in lungs exposed to acute or to chronic hypoxia. Modulation of gene expression by nitric oxide. J Clin Invest 1995;95(4):1798-807.

[101] Loges S, Mazzone M, Hohensinner P, Carmeliet P. Silencing or fueling metastasis with VEGF inhibitors: antiangiogenesis revisited. Cancer Cell 2009;15(3):167-70.

[102] Reiss Y. Angiopoietins. Recent Results Cancer Res 2010;180:3-13.

[103] Kim YM, Kim KE, Koh GY, Ho YS, Lee KJ. Hydrogen peroxide produced by angiopoietin-1 mediates angiogenesis. Cancer Res 2006;66(12):6167-74.

[104] Zhu P, Tan MJ, Huang RL, Tan CK, Chong HC, Pal M, Lam CR, Boukamp P, Pan JY, Tan SH, Kersten S, Li HY, Ding JL, Tan NS. Angiopoietin-like 4 protein elevates the prosurvival intracellular O2(-):H2O2 ratio and confers anoikis resistance to tumors. Cancer Cell 2011;19(3):401-15.

[105] Dejana E, Giampietro C. Vascular endothelial-cadherin and vascular stability. Curr Opin Hematol 2012;19(3):218-23.

[106] Walsh TG, Murphy RP, Fitzpatrick P, Rochfort KD, Guinan AF, Murphy A, Cummins PM. Stabilization of brain microvascular endothelial barrier function by shear stress involves VE-cadherin signaling leading to modulation of pTyr-occludin levels. J Cell Physiol 2011;226(11):3053-63.

[107] Carmeliet P, Collen D. Molecular basis of angiogenesis. Role of VEGF and VE-cadherin.Ann N Y Acad Sci 2000;902:249-62.

[108] Lin MT, Yen ML, Lin CY, Kuo ML. Inhibition of vascular endothelial growth factor-induced angiogenesis by resveratrol through interruption of Src-dependent vascular endothelial cadherin tyrosine phosphorylation. Mol Pharmacol 2003;64(5):1029-36.

[109] Simão F, Pagnussat AS, Seo JH, Navaratna D, Leung W, Lok J, Guo S, Waeber C, Salbego CG, Lo EH. Pro-angiogenic effects of resveratrol in brain endothelial cells: nitric

oxide-mediated regulation of vascular endothelial growth factor and metalloproteinases. J Cereb Blood Flow Metab. 2012;32(5):884-95.

[110] Distler JH, Hirth A, Kurowska-Stolarska M, Gay RE, Gay S, Distler O. Angiogenic and angiostatic factors in the molecular control of angiogenesis. Q J Nucl Med 2003;47(3):149-61.

[111] Karin M. Nuclear factor-kappaB in cancer development and progression. Nature 2006;441(7092):431-6.

[112] Santoro MM, Samuel T, Mitchell T, Reed JC, Stainier DY. Birc2 (cIap1) regulates endothelial cell integrity and blood vessel homeostasis. Nat Genet 2007;39(11):1397-402.

[113] Schreck R, Rieber P, Baeuerle PA. Reactive oxygen intermediates as apparently widely used messengers in the activation of the NF-kappa B transcription factor and HIV-1. EMBO J 1991;10(8):2247-58.

[114] Meyer M, Schreck R, Baeuerle PA. H2O2 and antioxidants have opposite effects on activation of NF-kappa B and AP-1 in intact cells: AP-1 as secondary antioxidant-responsive factor. EMBO J 1993;12(5):2005-15.

[115] Ebadi M, Sharma SK, Wanpen S, Amornpan A. Coenzyme Q10 inhibits mitochondrial complex-1 down-regulation and nuclear factor-kappa B activation. J Cell Mol Med 2004;8(2):213-22.

[116] Suzuki YJ, Mizuno M, Packer L. Signal transduction for nuclear factor-kappa B activation. Proposed location of antioxidant-inhibitable step. J Immunol 1994;153(11): 5008-15.

[117] Gloire G, Legrand-Poels S, Piette J. NF-kappaB activation by reactive oxygen species: fifteen years later. Biochem Pharmacol 2006;72(11):1493-505.

[118] Trachootham D, Alexandre J, Huang P. Targeting cancer cells by ROS-mediated mechanisms: a radical therapeutic approach? Nat Rev Drug Discov 2009;8(7):579-91.

[119] Weyemi U, Redon CE, Parekh PR, Dupuy C, Bonner WM. NADPH Oxidases NOXs and DUPXs As Putative Targets for Cancer Therapy. Anticancer Agents Med Chem 2012 Aug 27.

[120] Tertil M, Jozkowicz A, Dulak J. Oxidative stress in tumor angiogenesis- therapeutic targets.Curr Pharm Des 2010;16(35):3877-94.

[121] Pani G, Galeotti T, Chiarugi P. Metastasis: cancer cell's escape from oxidative stress.Cancer Metastasis Rev 2010;29(2):351-78.

Chapter 4

Accessory Cells in Tumor Angiogenesis — Tumor-Associated Pericytes

Yoshinori Minami, Takaaki Sasaki,
Jun-ichi Kawabe and Yoshinobu Ohsaki

Additional information is available at the end of the chapter

http://dx.doi.org/10.5772/54523

1. Introduction

In contrast to the normal tissue vasculature, tumor vessels are structurally and functionally abnormal [1-3]. These abnormal tumor vessels are characterized by an irregular, disorganized, and tortuous architecture with a highly dysfunctional and leaky endothelial cell (EC) layer [1, 3]. ECs are often loosely connected with each other and are covered by fewer and abnormal mural pericytes (PCs) [2-4].

Research into the molecular mechanisms and physiology of PCs associated with tumor angiogenesis is a critical field in cancer research. In this chapter, we will focus on the pathophysiology of PCs in tumor angiogenesis, the role of PCs in resistance to anti-angiogenesis therapy, and PCs as a therapeutic target.

2. Pathophysiology of pericytes in tumor angiogenesis

Despite the increasing evidence that PCs plays important roles in the angiogenic process, the origin of PCs is still not fully understood. They are commonly described as originating from various types of progenitors depending on their anatomical location in the body. For example, epicardial, mesenchymal, and neural crest cells are believed to be a source for pericytes in the cardiac coronary vasculature, dorsal aorta, and cardiac outflow tract, respectively [5].

Pericytes play an important role in stabilizing blood vessels in the microvasculature [6, 7]. A feature of pericyte function is their ability to provide vascular stability through crosstalk be-

INTECH
open science | open minds

© 2013 The Author(s). Licensee InTech. This chapter is distributed under the terms of the Creative Commons Attribution License http://creativecommons.org/licenses/by/3.0), which permits unrestricted use, distribution, and reproduction in any medium, provided the original work is properly cited.

tween PCs and endothelial cells (ECs). PCs deposit matrix or releasing factors that can promote EC differentiation or quiescence [8].

2.1. Crosstalk between ECs and PCs

In blood vessels, the crosstalk between ECs and PCs plays a critical role in the regulation of vascular formation, maturation, remodeling, stabilization and function [9]. PCs communicate with ECs by direct physical contact and paracrine signaling pathways.

Gap junctions provide direct contact between PCs and ECs that enable the exchange of ions and small molecules. Adhesion plaques anchor PCs to ECs, while peg-and-socket junctions enable the cells to penetrate the vascular basement membrane [10].

A variety of signaling factors mediate PC–EC interactions, including platelet-derived growth factor subunit B (PDGFB) and angiopoietin/Tie 2 [11].

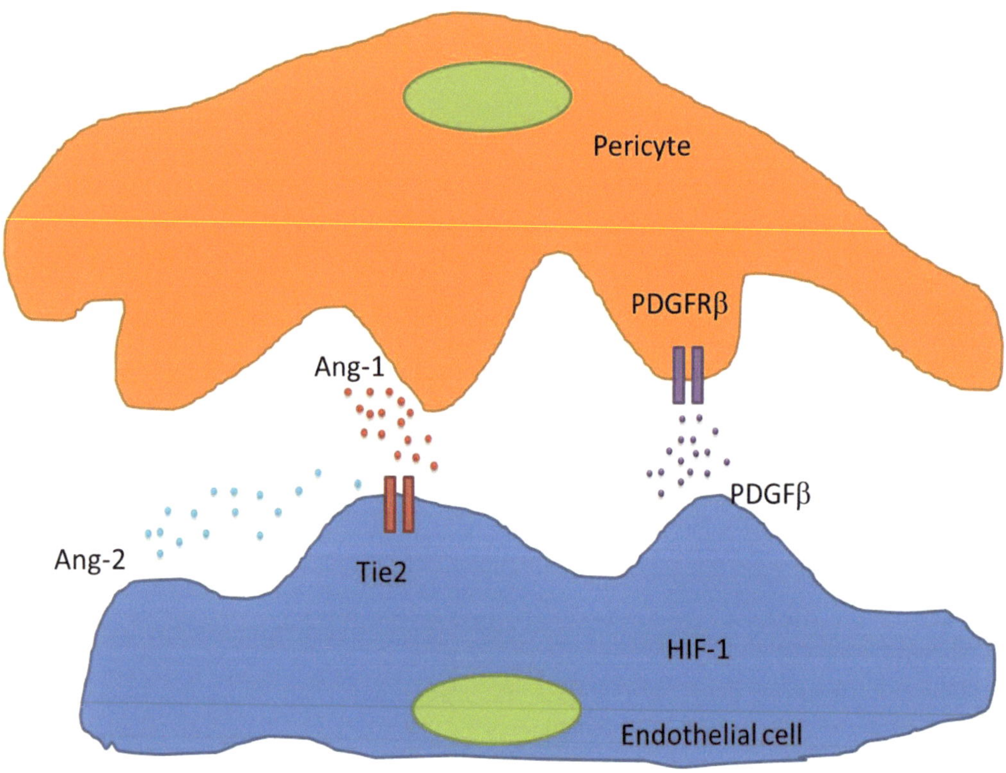

Figure 1. Crosstalk between endothelial cells and pericytes

2.1.1. PDGF/PDGFR family

Pericyte homeostasis in normal biology is regulated in significant part by signaling through the PDGF ligand and receptor system (Fig. 1) [12, 13]. PDGF is a potent mitogen for pericytes and fibroblasts. PDGF consists of A, B, C, and D polypeptide chains, and it forms the homodimers PDGF-AA, BB, CC, and DD, and the heterodimer PDGF-AB [14]. The specific tyrosine kinase receptors of the PDGFR family consist of PDGFR-α and PDGFR-β [15, 16]. PDGFR-α binds to PDGF-AA, BB, AB, and CC, whereas PDGFR-β binds with BB and DD [17].

Previous studies have shown that a <90% reduction in pericyte coverage in mice is compatible with postnatal survival [18], whereas loss of >95% of pericytes is lethal [18, 19], suggesting that a rather low threshold of pericyte density is required for basal function of microvasculature.

Activated ECs secrete PDGF-BB to attract PCs and PC progenitors, which are either tissue-resident cells and/or cells derived from bone marrow, and express PDGFRs [20], suggesting a paracrine signaling circuit [12, 18]. Pericyte deficiency, seen in knockout mice lacking PDGF-BB and its receptor, PDGFR-β, resulted in various changes in microvasculature, including endothelial hyperplasia, vessel dilation, tortuosity, leakage, and rupture, leading to wide-spread and lethal microhemorrhages and edema in late gestation [19, 21].

Studies of implanted tumors have shown that pericytes initially accumulate at the interface of tumor and host tissue and later around new blood vessels, exhibiting close contacts with ECs. Maturation of the tumor-associated vasculature is accompanied quantitatively by a reduced PC volume and qualitatively by morphological changes in whichPCs become flattened and elongated [22].

There is evidence that overexpression of PDGF-BB in tumor cells dramatically increases the PC coverage [23]. Moreover, Song et al. have also shown that tumor-derived PDGF-BB increases tumor PC coverage by activation of stromal-derived factor 1 alpha (SDF-1α) [24]. Thus, PDGF-BB appears to be a critical player in the recruitment of PCs to newly formed vessels [25].

2.1.2. Angiopoietin/Tie family

The angiopoietin (Ang) family consists of several members including Ang-1, Ang-2, Ang-3 (murine specific), and Ang-4 (human specific), which have two tyrosine kinase receptors, Tie-1 and Tie-2.

Ang-1 was initially identified as an activating ligand for Tie-2, which is expressed by perivascular cells [26]. Genetic deletion of Ang-1 resulted in prenatal lethality, due to severe heart and vascular defects, very similar in phenotype to Tie-2-deficient mice [27]. Ang-1 is predominantly secreted by PCs and can bind with Tie-2 on ECs in a paracrine pattern. Ang-1 enhances PC-EC interactions, represses the proliferation and migration of ECs, and promotes the maturation of newly formed blood vessels [27, 28]. Constitutive Ang-1/Tie-2 signaling is required to maintain the quiescent vasculature [29-31] (Fig. 1).

Ang-2 was initially identified as a homologue of Ang-1 [32]. Ang-2 was found to bind to Tie-2 with an affinity similar to that of Ang-1. However, unlike Ang-1, exogenous Ang-2 produces only a very weak activation of Tie-2 on ECs. When ECs are activated by tumor-derived pro-angiogenic factors, Ang-2 acts as an autocrine antagonist of Ang-1/Tie-2 signaling [33]. Moreover, Ang-2 activates the downstream pathways including PI3K/Akt, and thus functions as a promoter of angiogenesis [32]. Nasarre et al. have shown that tumors implanted into genetically Ang-2-ablated mice grew more slowly than those implanted into wild-type mice [34], which suggests that Ang-2 is a potent target for anti-tumor therapies (Fig. 1).

Tie-2 receptor expression recently has been identified in mesenchymal cells that are present in the stroma, implicating a repository for tumor vessel pericytes [35].

2.2. PCs in tumor angiogenesis

Many tumors express the pro-angiogenic vascular endothelial growth factor (VEGF) at high levels [36]. In contrast to ECs in normal tissues, ECs in the tumor vasculature are dependent on VEGF for survival [37]. Excessive VEGF signaling through VEGF receptor 2 (VEGFR2) loosens tight junctions of ECs, increasing permeability in the interstitial tumor microenvironment. Interestingly, in tumors with reduced levels of VEGF and other angiogenic regulatory factors, tumor vessels are less torturous, with normalized blood flow due to improved PC coverage, the so-called "vascular normalization" [3, 38, 39].

PCs stabilize ECs and mediate EC survival and maturation in normal vasculature, through both direct cell contact with ECs and paracrine signaling. It was reported that PCs in tumor vasculature are abnormal [40]. Low PC coverage correlates with poor clinical outcome in several different tumor types [41-43], but so far, the active involvement of PCs in tumor progression remains unclear. PCs are usually absent in tumor vasculature or have loose associations with ECs, leaving most of the tumor microvessels immature, the significance of which has been revealed in studies in which genetic or pharmacologic ablation of PC coverage facilitates metastatic dissemination of tumor cells [43, 44].

Activated PCs loosely attach to microvessels and develop cytoplasmic extensions into the tumor parenchyma [45]. Compared to quiescent PCs, activated PCs can change their genomic expression profiles [9], leading to phenotypes that are highly proliferative with the pluripotency to differentiate into other PCs, matrix-forming cells, smooth muscle cells, or adipocytes.

2.3. Molecular marker of PCs

The challenges of defining a PC have not been made easier by the fact that a general pan-PC molecular marker has not been found. Because of the diverse characteristics, functions, and locations of PCs in various organs, it probably never will be discovered. There are, however, a few dynamic molecular markers that are present in PCs, albeit not exclusively, and that are commonly used for their detection. The expression patterns of these markers can vary in a tissue-specific manner or be dependent on the developmental or angiogenic stage of a blood vessel. Desmin and alpha-smooth-muscle actin (α-SMA) are contractile filaments, and regulator of G protein signaling 5 (RGS-5) is a GTPase-activating protein; all three are intracellular proteins. Neuron-glial 2 (NG2), a chondroitin sulfate proteoglycan, and platelet-derived growth factor receptor beta (PDGFRβ), a tyrosine-kinase receptor, are cell-surface proteins. Antibodies against these proteins (except RGS-5) are commonly used to identify PCs in tissue

http://dx.doi.org/10.5772/54523

sections (Table 1). Desmin is a muscle-specific class III intermediate filament found in mature skeletal, cardiac, and smooth-muscle cells.

Molecular Marker	Alternative name		Mouse	Human
a-SMA	α-Smooth muscle actin	Expressed only locally by pericytes in tumor vasculature contractile filaments	+	+
PDGFR-β	Platelet-derived growth factor β	Tyrosine kinase receptor	+	+
Desmin		Reactive to developing and developed pericyte contractile filaments	+	+
Nestin	-		+	+
Smooth muscle myosin	-		+	+
Tropomyosin	-		+	+
NG2	Neuron-glial 2 (chondroitin sulfate proteoglycan) High-molecular-weight melanoma-associated antigen (HMWMAA)	Tyrosine kinase receptor Expressed in pericytes in early stages of angiogenesis	+	+
Aminopeptidase A	CD249, BP1		+	+
Aminopeptidase N	CD13		+	+
MMP9	Matrix metalloproteinase-9, gelatinase B		+	+
Sulphatide	3'-sulphogalactosylceramide		-	+
VEGFR1	vascular endothelial growth factor receptor-1		+	+
RGS5	Regulator of G-protein signaling-5	Novel marker for pericytes and vascular smooth muscle cells GTPase-activating protein	+	+
3G5 Ganglioside antigen	-	Specific for a pericyte surface ganglioside	-	+

Table 1. Markers of pericytes for microscopic imaging (antibody availability)

2.4. Role of bone marrow-derived PC progenitors

Bone marrow–derived hematopoietic cells expressing the PC marker NG2 were identified in close contact with tumor blood vessels in animal models of melanoma [46], pancreatic islet carcinomas [47], and brain tumors [48, 49]. Thus, PC progenitor cells appear to be recruited to sites of angiogenesis from the bone marrow niche; however, intravenously injected PC progenitor cells may fail to migrate and integrate into the tumor vasculature [50].

Tumor hypoxia due to the vascular regression following anti-angiogenic therapy appears to induce recruitment of various bone marrow-derived cells to the tumor microenvironment [51]. Rajantie et al. demonstrated the significant contribution of bone marrow–derived cells using an inducible hypoxia-inducible factor 1 alpha subunit (HIF1-α) animal model. In response to hypoxia in glioblastomas [52, 53], not only Tie-2-, VEGFR1-, CD11b-, and F4/80-positive cells but ECs and PC progenitor cells are released into the circulation from the bone marrow through the HIF1-α signal pathway. Then, they contribute to the neovascularization of glioblastoma [51]. In an HIF1-α knock-down mouse model, fewer bone marrow-derived cells are recruited to the tumors, which severely impairs tumor growth. These data suggest paradoxical induction of tumor angiogenesis via bone marrow-derived vessel progenitor cells after anti-angiogenic therapy.

3. Role of PCs in resistance to anti-angiogenic therapies

Although an anti-VEGF therapy, bevacizumab, has shown clinical efficacy in the treatment of several tumor types, its efficacy will ultimately be limited by acquired drug resistance. [54]. Putative mechanisms of resistance to anti-VEGF therapy include (1) activation and/or up-regulation of alternative pro-angiogenic pathways including PDGF/PDGFR signaling in the tumor [55], (2) recruitment of bone marrow-derived pro-angiogenic cells that differentiate into PCs, and (3) increased PC coverage of tumor microvasculature partially mediated by PDGFR signaling [56, 57].

Studies have shown that vessels without PC coverage are more dependent on VEGF signaling for survival [9] and that inhibition of VEGF leads to increased PC coverage of the tumor vasculature [58]. PCs may protect ECs from VEGF withdrawal, leading to PC-mediated resistance to anti-angiogenic therapies.

4. Targeting PCs as an anti-angiogenic therapy

Although a series of anti-angiogenic strategies targeting VEGF or its receptor VEGFR2 have been shown to efficiently prevent the growth of many types of tumors [59, 60], reports have shown that targeting VEGF signaling alone is often ineffective at inducing vascular regression or preventing the rapid regrowth of tumor vessels [58, 61-63]. One possible explanation for this failure is that the anti-angiogenic inhibitors mainly target immature ECs lacking PCs coverage, while showing a limited effect on the PC-associated mature vessels [63-65].

Although tumor PCs are less abundant and more loosely attached to vessels than those in healthy tissues, they have emerged as a critical therapeutic target for anti-angiogenic therapy.

http://dx.doi.org/10.5772/54523

Preclinical and clinical studies have largely focused on the role of tumor PCs in promoting EC survival and stabilizing the tumor vasculature through a variety of signaling networks. As noted earlier, PC recruitment to tumor neovessels is dependent on signaling through the PDGF-BB/PDGFRβ and Ang-1/Tie-2 networks.

4.1. Targeting PDGF-BB/ PDGFRβ signaling

PDGF-BB/PDGFRβ signaling appears to be critical for maintaining the PC–EC contacts needed for vessel stabilization. Vascular regression could also lead to the normalization of tumor microvessels and the opening of previously collapsed vessels [66] via decreased interstitial fluid pressure [67]. These data suggest that PDGF/PDGFR pathway inhibition is a potent target for anti-tumor therapies by leading to improved drug delivery [68-70].

Drug Name	Target	Type	Clinical stage
Sunitinib (Sutent)	PDGFRs, VEGFRs, FLT-3, CSF1R	Small molecule inhibitor	Approved for metastatic RCC, imatinib-resistant GIST, PNET
Sorafenib (Nexavar)	PDGFRs, VEGFRs, Raf, cKit	Small molecule inhibitor	Approved for metastatic RCC, HPCC
Pazopanib (Votrient)	PDGFRs, VEGFRs, cKit	Small molecule inhibitor	Approved for metastatic RCC
Vandetanib (Caprelsa)	PDGFRs, VEGFRs, EGFR	Small molecule inhibitor	Approved for metastatic medullary thyroid cancer
Axitinib (Inlyta)	PDGFRs, VEGFRs, cKit	Small molecule inhibitor	Approved for metastatic RCC
Motesanib	PDGFRs, VEGFRs, cKit	Small molecule inhibitor	Phase III
Cediranib (Recentin)	PDGFRs, VEGFRs, cKit	Small molecule inhibitor	Phase III
Cabozantinib	PDGFRs, VEGFRs, cMet, RET, cKit	Small molecule inhibitor	Phase III
Tivozanib	PDGFRs, VEGFRs, cKit	Small molecule inhibitor	Phase III
Regorafenib	PDGFRs, VEGFRs, Raf, cKit	Small molecule inhibitor	Phase III

Table 2. PDGF/PDGFR inhibitors that are approved and/or in clinical development

Combining PDGFRβ tyrosine kinase inhibition with VEGF inhibition more efficiently blocked tumor angiogenesis than VEGF inhibition alone in several experimental models [63, 71-74]. Bergers et al. have shown that combined treatment by anti-PDGFR agents together with anti-VEGF significantly reduces PC coverage and increases the success of anti-tumor treatment in the RIP1-TAG2 mouse model [63]. Similarly, PDGF inhibition disrupts PC support and sensitizes ECs to anti-angiogenic chemotherapy, resulting in regression of pre-existing tumor vasculature in a mouse model [13]. Long-term blockade of PDGF signaling by anti-PDGFRβ antibody reduces the concentration of PCs within the tumor tissue and also increases the apoptosis of ECs [73].

Several studies have tested the effects of combining anti-tumor agents with anti-PC agents that target PDGF or other PC markers, such as NG2 proteoglycan [75]. Involvement of the SDF-1α/CXCR4 axis in PC recruitment within PDGF-BB–overexpressing tumors suggests that a blockade of this axis may provide an additional target in anti-angiogenic tumor therapy [24].

Most recently, treatment of primary tumors in an animal model of breast cancer with combination VEGF and PDGF receptor therapy led to decreased PC coverage and an increased number of metastases. The observed promotion of metastasis by imatinib is consistent with previous reports demonstrating the key role of PDGFRβ signaling in PC recruitment and the importance of PCs in limiting tumor cell metastasis [43]. These findings provide the mechanistic basis for the differential effects these agents have on metastasis promotion.

However, a human clinical trial for renal carcinoma showed that inhibition of both the VEGF and PDGF pathways resulted in no therapeutic benefit when compared to inhibition of the VEGF pathway alone; in fact, the combined regimen exhibited toxicity [76]. Given these results, further preclinical studies are needed to clarify the mechanism(s) by which PDGF-targeted agents affect PC–EC interactions, and additional clinical studies are needed to clarify the potential benefits and risks associated with anti-PC tumor therapy.

4.2. Targeting Ang/Tie signaling

PCs have been shown to stabilize blood vessels and provide EC survival signals through the Ang-1/Tie-2 pathway [73, 77]. Therefore, by targeting tumor PCs it may be possible to overcome PC-mediated resistance to VEGF pathway inhibition and achieve more effective tumor vessel destabilization through disruption of the PC–EC association or directly through PC loss.

Trebananib (AMG 386) is a peptide-Fc fusion protein that inhibits angiogenesis by neutralizing the interaction between the Tie-2 receptor and Ang-1 and Ang-2 [78]. In phase I testing, it was found to be well tolerated in combination with chemotherapy [79] and to reduce tumor blood flow or permeability [80]. In a phase II trial of trebananib in combination with paclitaxel in patients with recurrent ovarian cancer, although a statistically significant improvement in progression-free survival for the treatment arm was not observed, the objective response rates and progression-free survival at the higher dose are suggestive of an antitumor effect [81]. The toxicity profile, including peripheral edema but not bowel perforations, is consistent with a mechanism distinct from that of VEGF inhibitors. Trebananib plus paclitaxel is now being investigated in an ongoing phase III study (TRINOVA-1 [Trial in Ovarian Cancer-1]) for the treatment of recurrent ovarian cancer. Phase II trials in breast, colorectal, kidney, stomach, and liver cancers are underway.

CVX060 (PF-04856884) is a recombinant humanized monoclonal antibody fused to two Ang-2 binding peptides [82, 83]. In preclinical studies, CVX-060 was anti-angiogenic and decreased tumor proliferation. In phase I testing, this agent significantly decreased tumor blood flow and affected circulating serum Ang-2 levels. This agent is being evaluated in combination with sunitinib in renal cell carcinoma. Currently, a phase II trial for kidney and a phase I trial for other solid tumors are underway.

Other agents in development include monoclonal antibodies directed against Ang-2 (MEDI-3617, AMG 780, REGN910) and multi-targeted tyrosine kinase inhibitors inhibiting Tie-2 (CEP11981, ARRY614) [84].

4.3. Other approaches

At least two alternative therapeutic approaches appear plausible given the role of PCs in promoting tumor angiogenesis. The first approach is to promote excessive PC recruitment, thereby causing vessel stabilization and restricting vessel sprouting. This approach may limit tumor angiogenesis in blood vessels with normal PC investment of the EC and may prevent the dissemination of tumor cells into the circulation by reducing the leakiness of intratumoral blood vessels and, perhaps, by also blocking extravasation of circulating tumor cells.

The second approach involves the use of PC progenitor cells as a cellular vehicle for gene delivery. This idea is supported by previous work using progenitor ECs [85-87], and more recently, PCs [50] to deliver anti-angiogenic gene therapy.

Neither of these approaches promoting PC recruitment to the tumor vasculature has been tested in preclinical models or clinical trials; both are highly speculative and no proof-of-principle studies have been conducted in animal models.

5. Conclusions

Based on the crucial role of PCs in microvessel maturity and the concomitant histological evaluation of EC-PC interactions and tumor microvessel morphology, combining different chemotherapeutic agents and anti-angiogenic treatments that normalize tumor vasculature seems to be inevitable. Many new angiogenic inhibitors target pathways that are involved in the recruitment of PCs to tumor microvessels. Therefore, it is essential to assess PCs in parallel with ECs when studying tumor vasculature. This evaluation, which can be performed in a diagnostic pathology laboratory, can be used as a decision-making tool to select patients who might benefit from anti-angiogenic therapies.

Acknowledgements

Y. Ohsaki was supported by a Grant-in-aid for scientific research (C) #20590910 for the study of cancer treatment by regulating bone marrow-derived endothelial progenitor cells.

Author details

Yoshinori Minami[1], Takaaki Sasaki[1*], Jun-ichi Kawabe[2] and Yoshinobu Ohsaki[1]

*Address all correspondence to: takaaki6@asahikawa-med.ac.jp

1 Respiratory Center, Asahikawa Medical University, Asahikawa, Japan

2 Department of Cardiovascular Regeneration and Innovation, Asahikawa Medical University, Asahikawa, Japan

References

[1] De Bock, K., et al., Endothelial oxygen sensors regulate tumor vessel abnormalization by instructing phalanx endothelial cells. J Mol Med (Berl), 2009. 87(6): p. 561-9.

[2] Jain, R.K., Determinants of tumor blood flow: a review. Cancer Res, 1988. 48(10): p. 2641-58.

[3] Jain, R.K., Normalization of tumor vasculature: an emerging concept in antiangiogenic therapy. Science, 2005. 307(5706): p. 58-62.

[4] Mazzone, M., et al., Heterozygous deficiency of PHD2 restores tumor oxygenation and inhibits metastasis via endothelial normalization. Cell, 2009. 136(5): p. 839-51.

[5] Bergwerff, M., et al., Neural crest cell contribution to the developing circulatory system: implications for vascular morphology? Circ Res, 1998. 82(2): p. 221-31.

[6] Nehls, V. and D. Drenckhahn, The versatility of microvascular pericytes: from mesenchyme to smooth muscle? Histochemistry, 1993. 99(1): p. 1-12.

[7] Sims, D.E., The pericyte--a review. Tissue Cell, 1986. 18(2): p. 153-74.

[8] Armulik, A., A. Abramsson, and C. Betsholtz, Endothelial/pericyte interactions. Circ Res, 2005. 97(6): p. 512-23.

[9] Benjamin, L.E., I. Hemo, and E. Keshet, A plasticity window for blood vessel remodelling is defined by pericyte coverage of the preformed endothelial network and is regulated by PDGF-B and VEGF. Development, 1998. 125(9): p. 1591-8.

[10] Rucker, H.K., H.J. Wynder, and W.E. Thomas, Cellular mechanisms of CNS pericytes. Brain Res Bull, 2000. 51(5): p. 363-9.

[11] Jain, R.K. and M.F. Booth, What brings pericytes to tumor vessels? J Clin Invest, 2003. 112(8): p. 1134-6.

[12] Hellstrom, M., et al., Role of PDGF-B and PDGFR-beta in recruitment of vascular smooth muscle cells and pericytes during embryonic blood vessel formation in the mouse. Development, 1999. 126(14): p. 3047-55.

[13] Pietras, K. and D. Hanahan, A multitargeted, metronomic, and maximum-tolerated dose "chemo-switch" regimen is antiangiogenic, producing objective responses and survival benefit in a mouse model of cancer. J Clin Oncol, 2005. 23(5): p. 939-52.

[14] Andrae, J., R. Gallini, and C. Betsholtz, Role of platelet-derived growth factors in physiology and medicine. Genes Dev, 2008. 22(10): p. 1276-312.

[15] Heldin, C.H., A. Ostman, and L. Ronnstrand, Signal transduction via platelet-derived growth factor receptors. Biochim Biophys Acta, 1998. 1378(1): p. F79-113.

[16] Kelly, J.D., et al., Platelet-derived growth factor (PDGF) stimulates PDGF receptor subunit dimerization and intersubunit trans-phosphorylation. J Biol Chem, 1991. 266(14): p. 8987-92.

[17] Betsholtz, C., L. Karlsson, and P. Lindahl, Developmental roles of platelet-derived growth factors. Bioessays, 2001. 23(6): p. 494-507.

[18] Enge, M., et al., Endothelium-specific platelet-derived growth factor-B ablation mimics diabetic retinopathy. EMBOJ, 2002. 21(16): p. 4307-16.

[19] Lindahl, P., et al., Pericyte loss and microaneurysm formation in PDGF-B-deficient mice. Science, 1997. 277(5323): p. 242-5.

[20] Lamagna, C. and G. Bergers, The bone marrow constitutes a reservoir of pericyte progenitors. J Leukoc Biol, 2006. 80(4): p. 677-81.

[21] Hellstrom, M., et al., Lack of pericytes leads to endothelial hyperplasia and abnormal vascular morphogenesis. J Cell Biol, 2001. 153(3): p. 543-53.

[22] Verhoeven, D. and N. Buyssens, Desmin-positive stellate cells associated with angiogenesis in a tumour and non-tumour system. Virchows Arch B Cell Pathol Incl Mol Pathol, 1988. 54(5): p. 263-72.

[23] McCarty, M.F., et al., Overexpression of PDGF-BB decreases colorectal and pancreatic cancer growth by increasing tumor pericyte content. J Clin Invest, 2007. 117(8): p. 2114-22.

[24] Song, N., et al., Overexpression of platelet-derived growth factor-BB increases tumor pericyte content via stromal-derived factor-1alpha/CXCR4 axis. Cancer Res, 2009. 69(15): p. 6057-64.

[25] Betsholtz, C., Insight into the physiological functions of PDGF through genetic studies in mice. Cytokine Growth Factor Rev, 2004. 15(4): p. 215-28.

[26] Davis, S., et al., Isolation of angiopoietin-1, a ligand for the TIE2 receptor, by secretion-trap expression cloning. Cell, 1996. 87(7): p. 1161-9.

[27] Suri, C., et al., Requisite role of angiopoietin-1, a ligand for the TIE2 receptor, during embryonic angiogenesis. Cell, 1996. 87(7): p. 1171-80.

[28] Iivanainen, E., et al., Angiopoietin-regulated recruitment of vascular smooth muscle cells by endothelial-derived heparin binding EGF-like growth factor. FASEB J, 2003. 17(12): p. 1609-21.

[29] Jones, N., et al., Tie receptors: new modulators of angiogenic and lymphangiogenic responses. Nat Rev Mol Cell Biol, 2001. 2(4): p. 257-67.

[30] Dumont, D.J., et al., Dominant-negative and targeted null mutations in the endothelial receptor tyrosine kinase, tek, reveal a critical role in vasculogenesis of the embryo. Genes Dev, 1994. 8(16): p. 1897-909.

[31] Thurston, G., Role of Angiopoietins and Tie receptor tyrosine kinases in angiogenesis and lymphangiogenesis. Cell Tissue Res, 2003. 314(1): p. 61-8.

[32] Maisonpierre, P.C., et al., Angiopoietin-2, a natural antagonist for Tie2 that disrupts in vivo angiogenesis. Science, 1997. 277(5322): p. 55-60.

[33] Feng, Y., et al., Impaired pericyte recruitment and abnormal retinal angiogenesis as a result of angiopoietin-2 overexpression. Thromb Haemost, 2007. 97(1): p. 99-108.

[34] Nasarre, P., et al., Host-derived angiopoietin-2 affects early stages of tumor development and vessel maturation but is dispensable for later stages of tumor growth. Cancer Res, 2009. 69(4): p. 1324-33.

[35] De Palma, M., et al., Tie2 identifies a hematopoietic lineage of proangiogenic monocytes required for tumor vessel formation and a mesenchymal population of pericyte progenitors. Cancer Cell, 2005. 8(3): p. 211-26.

[36] Senger, D.R., et al., Tumor cells secrete a vascular permeability factor that promotes accumulation of ascites fluid. Science, 1983. 219(4587): p. 983-5.

[37] Zhang, Z., et al., VEGF-dependent tumor angiogenesis requires inverse and reciprocal regulation of VEGFR1 and VEGFR2. Cell Death Differ, 2010. 17(3): p. 499-512.

[38] Goel, S., et al., Normalization of the vasculature for treatment of cancer and other diseases. Physiol Rev, 2011. 91(3): p. 1071-121.

[39] De Bock, K., S. Cauwenberghs, and P. Carmeliet, Vessel abnormalization: another hallmark of cancer? Molecular mechanisms and therapeutic implications. Curr Opin Genet Dev, 2011. 21(1): p. 73-9.

[40] Raza, A., M.J. Franklin, and A.Z. Dudek, Pericytes and vessel maturation during tumor angiogenesis and metastasis. Am J Hematol, 2010. 85(8): p. 593-8.

[41] Yonenaga, Y., et al., Absence of smooth muscle actin-positive pericyte coverage of tumor vessels correlates with hematogenous metastasis and prognosis of colorectal cancer patients. Oncology, 2005. 69(2): p. 159-66.

[42] O'Keeffe, M.B., et al., Investigation of pericytes, hypoxia, and vascularity in bladder tumors: association with clinical outcomes. Oncol Res, 2008. 17(3): p. 93-101.

[43] Cooke, V.G., et al., Pericyte depletion results in hypoxia-associated epithelial-to-mesenchymal transition and metastasis mediated by met signaling pathway. Cancer Cell, 2012. 21(1): p. 66-81.

[44] Xian, X., et al., Pericytes limit tumor cell metastasis. J Clin Invest, 2006. 116(3): p. 642-51.

[45] Morikawa, S., et al., Abnormalities in pericytes on blood vessels and endothelial sprouts in tumors. Am J Pathol, 2002. 160(3): p. 985-1000.

[46] Rajantie, I., et al., Adult bone marrow-derived cells recruited during angiogenesis comprise precursors for periendothelial vascular mural cells. Blood, 2004. 104(7): p. 2084-6.

[47] Song, S., et al., PDGFRbeta+ perivascular progenitor cells in tumours regulate pericyte differentiation and vascular survival. Nat Cell Biol, 2005. 7(9): p. 870-9.

[48] Bababeygy, S.R., et al., Hematopoietic stem cell-derived pericytic cells in brain tumor angio-architecture. Stem Cells Dev, 2008. 17(1): p. 11-8.

[49] Jodele, S., et al., The contribution of bone marrow-derived cells to the tumor vasculature in neuroblastoma is matrix metalloproteinase-9 dependent. Cancer Res, 2005. 65(8): p. 3200-8.

[50] Bexell, D., et al., Bone marrow multipotent mesenchymal stroma cells act as pericyte-like migratory vehicles in experimental gliomas. Mol Ther, 2009. 17(1): p. 183-90.

[51] Du, R., et al., HIF1alpha induces the recruitment of bone marrow-derived vascular modulatory cells to regulate tumor angiogenesis and invasion. Cancer Cell, 2008. 13(3): p. 206-20.

[52] Li, Z., et al., Cardiovascular lesions and skeletal myopathy in mice lacking desmin. Dev Biol, 1996. 175(2): p. 362-6.

[53] Milner, D.J., et al., Disruption of muscle architecture and myocardial degeneration in mice lacking desmin. J Cell Biol, 1996. 134(5): p. 1255-70.

[54] Jubb, A.M. and A.L. Harris, Biomarkers to predict the clinical efficacy of bevacizumab in cancer. Lancet Oncol, 2010. 11(12): p. 1172-83.

[55] Sasaki, T., et al., Administration of VEGF receptor tyrosine kinase inhibitor increases VEGF production causing angiogenesis in human small-cell lung cancer xenografts. Int J Oncol, 2008. 33(3): p. 525-32.

[56] Bergers, G. and D. Hanahan, Modes of resistance to anti-angiogenic therapy. Nat Rev Cancer, 2008. 8(8): p. 592-603.

[57] Crawford, Y., et al., PDGF-C mediates the angiogenic and tumorigenic properties of fibroblasts associated with tumors refractory to anti-VEGF treatment. Cancer Cell, 2009. 15(1): p. 21-34.

[58] Benjamin, L.E., et al., Selective ablation of immature blood vessels in established human tumors follows vascular endothelial growth factor withdrawal. J Clin Invest, 1999. 103(2): p. 159-65.

[59] Hanahan, D. and J. Folkman, Patterns and emerging mechanisms of the angiogenic switch during tumorigenesis. Cell, 1996. 86(3): p. 353-64.

[60] O'Reilly, M.S., et al., Endostatin: an endogenous inhibitor of angiogenesis and tumor growth. Cell, 1997. 88(2): p. 277-85.

[61] Baluk, P., H. Hashizume, and D.M. McDonald, Cellular abnormalities of blood vessels as targets in cancer. Curr Opin Genet Dev, 2005. 15(1): p. 102-11.

[62] Bergers, G. and S. Song, The role of pericytes in blood-vessel formation and maintenance. Neuro Oncol, 2005. 7(4): p. 452-64.

[63] Bergers, G., et al., Benefits of targeting both pericytes and endothelial cells in the tumor vasculature with kinase inhibitors. J Clin Invest, 2003. 111(9): p. 1287-95.

[64] Bono, A.V., et al., Sorafenib's inhibition of prostate cancer growth in transgenic adenocarcinoma mouse prostate mice and its differential effects on endothelial and pericyte growth during tumor angiogenesis. Anal Quant Cytol Histol, 2010. 32(3): p. 136-45.

[65] Huang, J., et al., Vascular remodeling marks tumors that recur during chronic suppression of angiogenesis. Mol Cancer Res, 2004. 2(1): p. 36-42.

[66] Padera, T.P., et al., Pathology: cancer cells compress intratumour vessels. Nature, 2004. 427(6976): p. 695.

[67] Rodt, S.A., et al., A novel physiological function for platelet-derived growth factor-BB in rat dermis. J Physiol, 1996. 495 (Pt 1): p. 193-200.

[68] Baranowska-Kortylewicz, J., et al., Effect of platelet-derived growth factor receptor-beta inhibition with STI571 on radioimmunotherapy. Cancer Res, 2005. 65(17): p. 7824-31.

[69] Jayson, G.C., et al., Blockade of platelet-derived growth factor receptor-beta by CDP860, a humanized, PEGylated di-Fab', leads to fluid accumulation and is associated with increased tumor vascularized volume. J Clin Oncol, 2005. 23(5): p. 973-81.

[70] Pietras, K., et al., Inhibition of PDGF receptor signaling in tumor stroma enhances antitumor effect of chemotherapy. Cancer Res, 2002. 62(19): p. 5476-84.

[71] Shaheen, R.M., et al., Tyrosine kinase inhibition of multiple angiogenic growth factor receptors improves survival in mice bearing colon cancer liver metastases by inhibition of endothelial cell survival mechanisms. Cancer Res, 2001. 61(4): p. 1464-8.

[72] Reinmuth, N., et al., Induction of VEGF in perivascular cells defines a potential paracrine mechanism for endothelial cell survival. FASEB J, 2001. 15(7): p. 1239-41.

[73] Erber, R., et al., Combined inhibition of VEGF and PDGF signaling enforces tumor vessel regression by interfering with pericyte-mediated endothelial cell survival mechanisms. FASEB J, 2004. 18(2): p. 338-40.

[74] Farhadi, M.R., et al., Combined inhibition of vascular endothelial growth factor and platelet-derived growth factor signaling: effects on the angiogenesis, microcirculation, and growth of orthotopic malignant gliomas. J Neurosurg, 2005. 102(2): p. 363-70.

[75] Maciag, P.C., et al., Cancer immunotherapy targeting the high molecular weight melanoma-associated antigen protein results in a broad antitumor response and reduction of pericytes in the tumor vasculature. Cancer Res, 2008. 68(19): p. 8066-75.

[76] Hainsworth, J.D., et al., Treatment of advanced renal cell carcinoma with the combination bevacizumab/erlotinib/imatinib: a phase I/II trial. Clin Genitourin Cancer, 2007. 5(7): p. 427-32.

[77] Abramsson, A., P. Lindblom, and C. Betsholtz, Endothelial and nonendothelial sources of PDGF-B regulate pericyte recruitment and influence vascular pattern formation in tumors. J Clin Invest, 2003. 112(8): p. 1142-51.

[78] Coxon, A., et al., Context-dependent role of angiopoietin-1 inhibition in the suppression of angiogenesis and tumor growth: implications for AMG 386, an angiopoietin-1/2-neutralizing peptibody. Mol Cancer Ther, 2010. 9(10): p. 2641-51.

[79] Mita, A.C., et al., Phase 1 Study of AMG 386, a Selective Angiopoietin 1/2–Neutralizing Peptibody, in Combination with Chemotherapy in Adults with Advanced Solid Tumors. Clin Cancer Res, 2010. 16(11): p. 3044-3056.

[80] Herbst, R.S., et al., Safety, Pharmacokinetics, and Antitumor Activity of AMG 386, a Selective Angiopoietin Inhibitor, in Adult Patients With Advanced Solid Tumors. J of Clin Oncol, 2009. 27(21): p. 3557-3565.

[81] Karlan, B.Y., et al., Randomized, Double-Blind, Placebo-Controlled Phase II Study of AMG 386 Combined With Weekly Paclitaxel in Patients With Recurrent Ovarian Cancer. J of Clin Oncol, 2012. 30(4): p. 362-371.

[82] Huang, H., et al., Specifically Targeting Angiopoietin-2 Inhibits Angiogenesis, Tie2-Expressing Monocyte Infiltration, and Tumor Growth. Clin Cancer Res, 2011. 17(5): p. 1001-1011.

[83] Doppalapudi, V.R., et al., Chemical generation of bispecific antibodies. Proc Nat AcadSci, 2010. 107(52): p. 22611-22616.

[84] Cascone, T. and J.V. Heymach, Targeting the Angiopoietin/Tie2 Pathway: Cutting Tumor Vessels With a Double-Edged Sword? J Clin Oncol, 2012. 30(4): p. 441-444.

[85] Dudek, A.Z., et al., Systemic inhibition of tumour angiogenesis by endothelial cell-based gene therapy. Br J Cancer, 2007. 97(4): p. 513-22.

[86] Somani, A., et al., The establishment of murine blood outgrowth endothelial cells and observations relevant to gene therapy. Transl Res, 2007. 150(1): p. 30-9.

[87] Milbauer, L.C., et al., Blood outgrowth endothelial cell migration and trapping in vivo: a window into gene therapy. Transl Res, 2009. 153(4): p. 179-89.

Chapter 5

Endothelial and Accessory Cell Interactions in Neuroblastoma Tumor Microenvironment

Jill Gershan, Andrew Chan,
Magdalena Chrzanowska-Wodnicka,
Bryon Johnson, Qing Robert Miao and
Ramani Ramchandran

Additional information is available at the end of the chapter

http://dx.doi.org/10.5772/55486

1. Introduction

Early childhood tumors that originate from the adrenal medulla and sympathetic nervous system are classified as neuroendocrine tumors [2]. Based on immunohistological criteria, neuroendocrine tumors can be broadly categorized as either neural or epithelial. As the name implies, tumors of the neural subtype display various degrees of neuronal differentiation and they stain positive for the neuroendocrine markers, synaptophysin and chromogranin A [3, 4]. Less well-differentiated or more primitive neural tumors are referred to as neuroblastoma (NB) while tumors with more differentiated features, such as ganglion and nerve bundles, are referred to as ganglioneuroblastoma and ganglioneuroma. This chapter focuses on NB, a form of cancer that occurs in infants and young children. NB is by far the most common cancer in infants, and the fourth most common type of cancer in children [5]. There are approximately 650 new cases each year in the United States, and NB accounts for 15% of all cancer deaths in children. At present, NB patients have limited options for therapy and there is a pressing need to find better treatment options. To develop better treatment options, it is critical to understand the origins of this disease, and mechanisms involved in disease progression. The first section of this chapter is dedicated to a review of neuroendocrine embryology in order to shed some light on the cell that may be responsible for NB. The exact NB progenitor cell has not been identified, however there is evidence that these cells are derived from the neural crest (NC). Understanding the differentiation of NC to cell types that constitute the peripheral nervous system, and the mechanisms utilized during this process is critical to our knowledge of NB

INTECH
open science | open minds

© 2013 The Author(s). Licensee InTech. This chapter is distributed under the terms of the Creative Commons Attribution License http://creativecommons.org/licenses/by/3.0), which permits unrestricted use, distribution, and reproduction in any medium, provided the original work is properly cited.

progression. In particular, migration of NC cells along the dorsal-ventral axis of the developing embryo, and the role of matrix in this process is likely to benefit our understanding of mechanisms of cancer metastasis in general. Subsequent sections of this chapter will address NB progression and the many factors (including genetic alterations such as *N-Myc* (*MYCN*) amplification) and cues from the surrounding microenvironment that determine tumor cell proliferation, survival, migration and angiogenesis. The tumor microenvironment is composed of endothelial cells, immune cells, and stromal cells, and, based on their phenotype, either contribute or prevent the progression or metastasis of tumor. We will focus on the contributions of Schwann cells, extracellular matrix, endothelial and immune cells to NB progression and pathogenesis to highlight the intricacies of how the microenvironment affects tumor development.

2. Neuroblastoma developmental mechanisms

Two branching networks that often develop side-by-side during embryonic development include nerves and blood vessels [6]. During embryogenesis, the neural network comprised of both the central nervous system (CNS) and peripheral nervous system (PNS) develops first, and is composed of specialized cells called neurons that relay and transmit signals across different parts of the body [7]. The CNS includes the brain, spinal cord and retina while the PNS consists of sensory neurons, ganglia and the interconnecting nerves that connect to the CNS. Neurons project long cable like cellular extensions called axons that, via electrochemical waves, transmit signals by the release of neurotransmitters at axonal junctions or synapses.

2.1. NB: A peripheral nervous system tumor

NB is a PNS tumor derived from embryonic neural precursor cells. To understand the ontogeny of NB, the development and differentiation of neural precursor cells that are involved in PNS development will be discussed to obtain a better appreciation of the cells, signaling pathways and mechanisms involved in NB. Within the PNS there are somatic and visceral neurons. The somatic neurons innervate skin, bone joints and muscles, and their cell bodies often lie in the dorsal root ganglia of the spinal cord. The visceral neurons innervate internal organs, blood vessels and glands. The visceral component of the PNS is called the autonomic nervous system (ANS), and consists of two parts: the sympathetic nervous system (SNS) and the parasympathetic nervous system (PSNS). Both the SNS and PSNS often work in complementary but opposite fashions to maintain homeostasis in most organs. Two types of neurons, namely the pre-and post-ganglion, represent the majority of ANS, and are responsible for regulating the function of target organs. The pre-ganglionic neurons of the SNS are short while those of the PSNS are long. As a general principle, neurotransmitters are secreted at a synapse that usually occurs at the junction of two axons emerging from two neurons. One exception to this rule is observed in the chromaffin cells of the adrenal medulla. These neuroendocrine cells do not possess axons and directly release neurotransmitters (catecholamines, noradrenalin, adrenaline) into systemic circulation thereby affecting multiple organs. The chromaffin cells play an important role in the fight-or-flight response and are found in small numbers in structures

http://dx.doi.org/10.5772/55486

such as the carotid aorta, vagus nerve, bladder and prostate in addition to the adrenal medulla. The origin of these chromaffin cells has been attributed to a common precursor population called sympathoadrenal (SA) cells that give rise to both sympathetic neurons and chromaffin cells. Because NB is often associated with the SA cell or its progenitors [8], the development of these cells in embryogenesis provides clues to the disease inception and progression. During early PNS development there are three overlapping stages in which NBs could arise [9]. These are (1) the formation and fate specification of NC into sympathoadrenal (SA) progenitors, (2) bilateral migration and differentiation of SA cells and their coalescence near the aorta, and (3) differentiation of PNS neurons into fully developed ganglia and the establishment of synaptic connections.

2.2. Signaling mechanisms guiding neural crest development

Since chromaffin cells and neurons of the SA system arise from neural crest (NC) cells, it has been proposed that NC cells may be the origin for NB. The NC is a transient embryonic population of cells that arise from the dorsal region of the newly formed neural tube [10]. NC cells undergo epithelial-to-mesenchymal (EMT) transition, and begin to migrate through the developing mesenchyme to differentiate into the craniofacial skeleton, melanocytes as well as the SA system.

a. Formation and fate specification of NC into SA progenitors: The NC cells form at the border between neural and non-neural tissue in the vertebrate embryo. As the neural fold elevates, cells induced to become NC are located in the dorsal neural tube. The specification of NC cells is intricately linked to neural induction since these two processes also dictate the neural-non-neural boundary. It is well accepted from evidence in multiple model systems that loss of bone morphogenetic protein (BMP) signaling coincides with neural induction and thereby NC induction. BMP signaling alone is not sufficient for NC induction, as members of the Wnt and fibroblast growth factor (FGF) families have also been associated with NC induction [11]. Studies in mice, chicken, frog and zebrafish have implicated a cascade of transcription factors that confer NC cell identity. These include NC specifier genes such as Slug, Zic5, Sox9, Sox10, FoxD3, c-Myc and AP2 [12]. These factors are expressed in premigratory, and, or early migratory NC cells and are likely involved in the induction and survival of these cells. The differentiation of NC cells into the SA progenitor pathway is poorly understood. Single cell labeling studies in zebrafish [13] support the premise that Neurogenin-2 in pre- and early migrating NC cells promotes the sensory neuron differentiation at the expense of sympathetic neurons [13]. These data imply that the SA lineage is specified at an early migratory stage; however, it is unclear which molecular mechanisms trigger expression of Neurogenin-2 in a subset of NC cells. Cells during this early less differentiated stage could contribute to NB since alteration in the transcriptional signaling cascade may lead to precocious precursor cell proliferation or lack of further differentiation of these cells into the next phase of NC development.

b. Bilateral migration and differentiation of SA cells: Once specified, NC cells must delaminate from the neural tube in order to migrate to their final destination (Figure 1). Delamination is a process of tissue splitting into separate populations regardless of cellular mechanisms [14, 15]. With reference to NC, delamination is often used interchangeably with epithelial-to-mesenchymal transition. EMT is a series of molecular events that orchestrate changes from an epithelial cell phenotype into a mesenchymal (migratory) phenotype [16]. Several EMT-inducing transcription factors such as Snail, SoxE and Foxd3 function during multiple steps of NC development. In addition, EMT induces changes in junctional proteins such as N-cadherin and cadherin6B. These processes are reminiscent of events during general tumorigenesis whereby cancer cells undergo EMT and lose the ability to adhere to substratum leading to loss of contact-mediated inhibition. Therefore, NC cells provide a relevant model to investigate different aspects of tumorigenesis and metastasis especially with respect to NB.

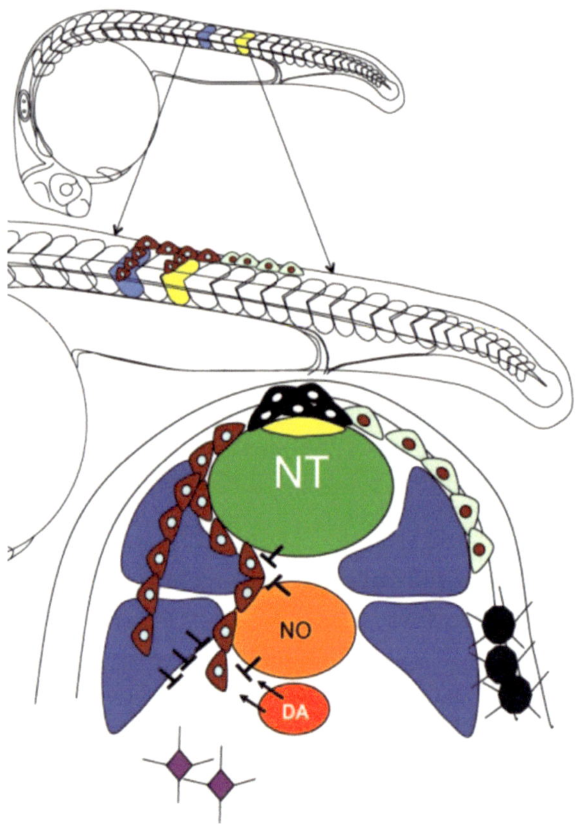

Figure 1. Neural crest cell development in zebrafish. A high power image of the trunk neural crest cell migration is depicted. A cartoon of the cross-section of the trunk region is indicated. Black cells overlying the ectoderm are neural crest cells that specify from the dorsal roof plate (yellow region) of the neural tube (NT). NC cells that migrate dorso-ventrally (teal color) will differentiate into melanocytes (black shaped cells). NC cells that migrate ventromedially differentiate into sympathetic ganglia (purple cells). NC cells (red) that migrate through the somite form Schwann cells and sensory neurons and glia of DRG. NC cells that migrate between the somite and the neural tube as indicated differentiate into sympathetic ganglia.and chromaffin cells. Inhibitory signals (inverted T) and activation signals (arrows) guide the migration of the NC cells from the dorsal to ventral region. DA: dorsal aorta, NO: notochord, and blue structures are somites.

http://dx.doi.org/10.5772/55486

As NC cells delaminate from the neural tube, tissues surrounding the neural tube produce both positive and negative cues that guide NC along defined pathways [17]. Trunk NC migration is guided by signals emerging from adjacent somites [18], which falls under three distinct phases, (1) Directed migration resulting from contact with the ectoderm and cues from the microenvironment, (2) Contact-mediated guidance facilitating homing to the target site, and (3) Contact-inhibition of movement upon entry and colonization of the target site (i.e. the trunk for SA) [15]. These migratory behaviors occur as streams of cells, and once in the trunk, NC cells migrate either ventromedially or dorsolaterally (Figure 1) [8]. NC cells migrating via the ventromedial route (without invading the somite) become neurons and glia of the sympathetic ganglia and adrenal chromaffin cells. NC cells that take the ventromedial route and invade and remain in the sclerotome coalesce to form Schwann cells, and the sensory neurons and glia of the dorsal root ganglia (DRG). We will discuss the role of Schwann cells in NB Pathogenesis later in this chapter. NC cells that take a dorsolateral route, in between the dorsal Ectoderm and the dermamyotome, differentiate into melanocytes (Figure 1) [17]. Because NBs often emerge in the sympathetic ganglia, it is conceivable that during the migratory process, NC cells that carry mutations in critical genes implicated in NBs, such as MYCN, may lose contact inhibition and prematurely proliferate in response to molecular signals that emanate from surrounding tissue. In terms of molecular cues, trunk NC cells that migrate via the ventromedial route enter the somite via attraction cues from CXCR4/CXCL12 signaling, which has also been implicated in breast cancer metastasis [19, 20]. These NC cells are confined to the rostral sclerotome by Neuropilin2/Semaphorin3F repulsion molecules working in concert with Eph/ephrin signalling, F-spondin and proteoglycans, which, reinforce this migration route. Similarly, signaling through CXCR4/CXCl12, ErbB2 and 3/Neuregulin, and GFRá3/artemin mediate NC cell attraction past the somite and work in concert with Neuropilin1/Semaphorin4A repulsion cues from surrounding tissues that restricts NC cell migration to the dorsal aorta [17].

c. Differentiation of PNS neurons into fully developed ganglia: Once the migrated partially differentiated NC cells (SA progenitors) reach the vicinity of dorsal aorta, bone morphogenetic proteins secreted by SA cells trigger a molecular signaling cascade that is essential and sufficient to initiate the differentiation into both the noradrenergic sympathetic neurons and the cholinergic parasympathetic neurons of the ANS. Interestingly, BMP signaling is used at the first (NC induction) and third (NC differentiation into PNS neurons) stage of NC development implying its critical role in this pathway, and perhaps in NB. BMP-2 treatment of human NB cell lines (RTBM1 and SH-SY5Y) leads to growth arrest and differentiation [21]. BMP receptor IA expressed on SA progenitors responds to BMP inducing the expression of the proneural gene mammalian achaete-scute homolog (*Mash-1*) and the paired-like homebox2B (*PHOX2B*) transcription factors. PHOX2B is essential for maintaining Mash-1 expression and proliferation of SA progenitors. Human NB cell lines show high Hash-1 expression, and retinoic acid treatment decreases Hash-1 expression and promotes neurite extension [22, 23]. Germline mutations of *PHOX2B* in both a familial case of NB and in a patient with a genetically determined congenital malformation of NC-derived cells-namely, Hirschsprung disease (HSCR) exemplifies the underlying contribution of late stage genes in NC development to NB pathogenesis [24].

2.3. Model system contribution to neuroblastoma pathogenesis

Much information contributing to the pathogenesis of NB has been generated from in vitro studies performed on cell lines derived from patients [8]. Similar to other tumors, oncogene amplification or allelic loss has been linked to NB progression. Proto-oncogenes v-myc myelocytomatosis viral related oncogene (*MYCN)*, anaplastic lymphoma kinase (*ALK*) and, more recently, transforming tyrosine kinase receptor type A *(TrkA)* [25] have been widely suspected as likely contributors in NB pathogenesis. In fact, *MYCN* amplification is one of the few predictors of a poor clinical outcome for patients with NB. Tumors without *MYCN* amplification that correlate with poor survival frequently show an aberrant up regulation of genes in the *MYC* pathway, and down regulation of genes in the SA lineage differentiation pathway emphasizing the importance of MYC signaling in NB pathogenesis. BMP signal transducers in SA cells, namely transcription factors *PHOX2A* and *PHOX2B*, bind and activate noradrenergic marker genes, tyrosine hydroxylase (TH) and dopamine-β-hydroxylase that are essential enzymes for noradrenaline production. Evidence shows that *MYCN* overexpression under the tyrosine hydroxylase promoter in mice drives tumor formation that resembles human NB [26]. Recently, a dopamine-β-hydroxylase promoter driving *MYCN* and *ALK* genes in zebrafish [27] also resulted in NB formation. In this fish model, the authors demonstrated that upregulated *MYCN* mediated sympathetic neuroblast proliferation, which is eventually mitigated by a developmentally timed apoptosis of neuroblast cells. The concomitant activation of ALK blocks the neuroblast apoptosis at a critical window in development thereby establishing a novel synergistic mechanism for these two oncogenes in NB pathogenesis. These tumor models clearly imply that turning on oncogenes in cells that are undergoing transitions during NC development is at the heart of NB ontogeny and progression.

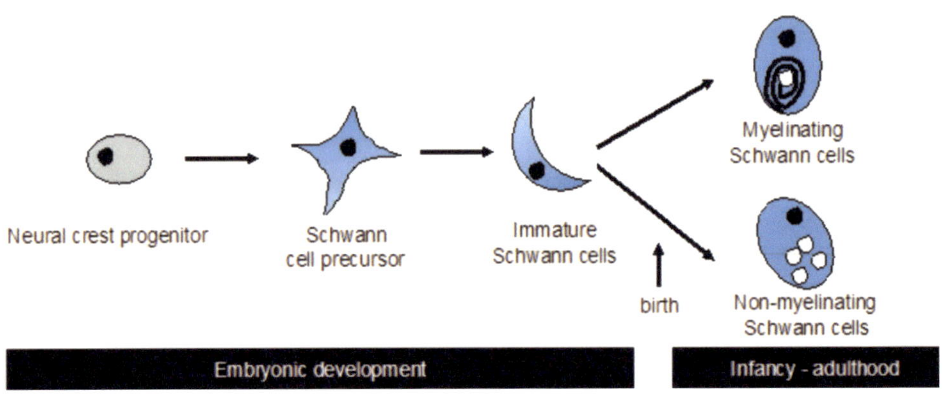

Figure 2. Schwann cell development. Schematic representation of different developmental stages of Schwann cells showing the transitory cell types being involved during embryogenesis and after birth.

http://dx.doi.org/10.5772/55486

3. Role of Schwann cells in NB tumor microenvironment

NB is characterized by the co-existence of both stromal Schwann cells and neuroblastic tumor cells. The NC origin of Schwann cells suggests that they may co-evolve with tumor cells from common neural progenitors. However, the origin and functional relevance of tumor-associated Schwann cells remain controversial. Although widely assumed to be infiltrating normal Schwann cells, the finding of common genetic alterations shared with neuroblastic tumor cells argues for the same origin as tumor cells. It is well established that stroma-rich NB is associated with differentiated tumors of favorable prognosis. On the contrary, stroma-poor NB is associated with metastatic diseases and poor outcomes. Among the various organs, a high fraction of NB disseminates to the bone and bone marrow. How Schwannian stroma affect tumor dissemination has not been extensively studied. To this end, several soluble factors have been isolated from Schwann cells that have proliferative, survival and angiogenic activities in the tumor microenvironment. These include Chemokine C-X-C motif ligand 13 (CXCL13), Secreted Protein Acidic and Rich in Cysteine (SPARC), and Pigment Epithelium-Derived Factor (PEDF). Determining their roles in NB progression will aid in future development of novel treatments for this childhood malignancy, and will be discussed in detail here.

3.1. Schwann cells in normal development and NB

In the PNS, Schwann cells serve as the major glial cell type for individual neurons. During development, NC progenitors differentiate into multiple lineages including neurons, glial cells, pigment cells, endocrine cells and mesenchymal cells [28]. Based on the hierarchical organization of lineage segregation, NC-derived stem cells (NCSC) first undergo gliogenesis to generate a pool of Schwann cell precursors (SCP)(Figure 2). The helix-loop-helix transcription factor, Sox10, is required for this event by promoting the survival of NCSC and glial cell specification [29-31]. Sox10 also plays an instructive role in determining how NCSC response to neuregulin-1 (NRG-1)[32, 33]. In the PNS, NRG-1 stimulates Schwann cell proliferation, migration, and myelination [34]. NRG-1 also regulates the migratory behavior of NC cells [35, 36].

The maturation of SCP gives rise to immature Schwann cells, which in E15 mouse embryos, encapsulate bundles of axons through a process of radial sorting [37-39]. At this stage the ratio of Schwann cells to axons is 1:1 and this fine balance is partly achieved by axon-driven proliferation of immature Schwann cells. A host of factors are implicated that includes NRG-1 [40], transforming growth factor-β (TGF-β) [41-44], and laminins. Further differentiation of immature Schwann cells generates myelinating Schwann cells which surround large diameter axons, while smaller diameter axons are covered with nonmyelinating Schwann cells [45]. The functional importance of Schwann cells in neuronal survival is well established. For example, mice lacking the NRG-1 receptor, ErbB3, are devoid of SCP and have extensive neuronal cell death in the dorsal root ganglia [46]. Apart from NRG-1, additional trophic factors implicated in neuronal survival include brain-derived neurotrophic factor (BDNF), ciliary neurotrophic factor (CNTF), leukemia inhibitory factor (LIF), and hepatocyte growth factor (HGF) [47].

In early childhood, tumors originating from the adrenal medulla and sympathetic nervous system are classified as neuroendocrine tumors. Based on immunohistological criteria, neuroendocrine tumors can be broadly categorized into two types – neural and epithelial. As its name implies, tumors of the neural subtype display various degrees of neuronal differentiation and they stained positive for neuroendocrine markers, synaptophysin and chromogranin A [3, 4]. Less well-differentiated or more primitive neural tumors are referred to as NB while tumors with more differentiated features, such as ganglion and nerve bundles, are referred to as ganglioneuroblastoma (GNB) and ganglioneuroma (GN) (Figure 3A). Overall, GNB and GN show greater immunoreactivities towards the three neurofilament (NF) phosphoisoforms, NF-L (light), NF-M (medium), and NF-H (heavy)[48]. Also, well-differentiated tumors have higher expression of neuronal markers such as microtubule associated proteins (MAPS) and tau. Furthermore, in GNB and GN, both glial cell markers, glial fibrillary acidic protein (GFAP) and myelin basic protein (MBP) are detected, providing evidence of differentiation into non-myelinating and myelinating Schwann cells, respectively [48].

A

Histologic group	Stroma-poor		Stroma-rich		
Tumor type	Neuroblastoma		Ganglioneuroblastoma		Ganglioneuroma
MYCN amplification	24%		10%		
Histologic subtype	Undifferentiated	Differentiating	Well-differentiated	Intermixed	Focal nodular
Survival	36%	72%	100%	92%	18%

B

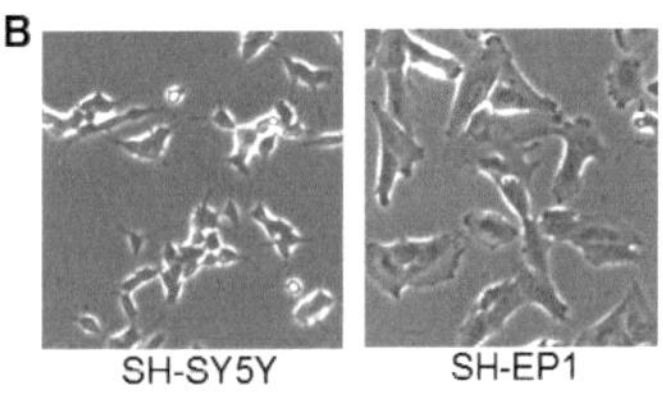

Figure 3. Neural crest tumor typesA. The different histologic groups and subtypes of neural crest tumors with their characteristics depicted [1]. **B.** Brightfield photomicrographs of neuroblastic SH-SY5Y and Schwannian SH-EP1 cell lines (gifts from Dr. Robert A. Ross).

3.2. Histology and origin of Schwannian stroma in NB

The relevance of Schwannian stroma in the diagnosis and prognosis of NB has been addressed by the seminal study by Shimada *et. al.* [1]. In general, NB can be subdivided into stroma-poor and stroma-rich groups. Stroma-poor tumors have diffuse growth patterns of neuroblastic tumor cells divided by thin septa of fibrovascular tissues. This subgroup represents the classical NB and has either an undifferentiated or differentiating histology with various degrees of mitoses and karyorrhexis or nuclear fragmentation (MKI). In general, stroma-poor tumors are considered as favorable if diagnosed <1.5 yr old, with a low MKI and a differentiating histology. This group has a survival rate of 84%. On the contrary, stroma-poor tumors that are unfavorable have a high MKI (for <1.5 yr old), undifferentiated histology (1.5-5 yr old) and occur in patients greater than 5 years of age. This group has a survival rate of only 4.5%.

Tumors of the stroma-rich group have extensive Schwannian stroma and are representative of the GNB and GN histological types. This group can be further classified into three histological subtypes – well-differentiated, intermixed and focal nodular (Figure 3A). The overall survival for stroma-rich tumors is 67% as compared to 47% for stroma-poor counterparts. Expectedly, patients with stroma-rich tumors that are well-differentiated or intermixed have

90-100% survival survival. Interestingly, patients with the focal nodular subtype has the poorest survival of only 18%. Thus, tumors with good prognosis are the favorable stroma-poor and well-differentiated or intermixed stroma-rich. These tumors have non-advanced staging. In contrast, unfavorable stroma-poor and focal nodular stroma-rich lead topoor prognosis, and they are frequently stage III and IV diseases.

At the molecular level, stroma-poor tumors have a higher frequency (24%) of *MYCN* gene amplification as opposed to 10% for stroma-rich tumors [49, 50]. In this case, the overexpression of *MYCN* most likely leads to the expansion of the NC progenitor population. Indeed, silencing *MYCN* in NB cell lines promotes differentiation [51-53]. *MYCN* expression appears to be differentially regulated in neuroblastic and Schwannian S-type cells. For instance, LA1-55n, a neuroblastic tumor subline, has readily detectable *MYCN* expression while this oncoprotein was not present in the S-type counterpart, LA1-5s [54]. Similarly, ALK mutant protein can be detected in the neuroblastic subline of SK-N-SH while absent in several S-type sublines [55]. Thus, while *MYCN* amplification drives the expansion neuronal progenitors [56], this oncogenic event does not appear to impede differentiation into either neuronal or Schwann cell lineages [57, 58].

The common NC origin of Schwann cells and neurons would argue that Schwannian stroma in NB is derived from a common cancer initiating cell [59]. However, this assertion is not without controversy. An earlier study using cytogenetic analysis of 19 NBs demonstrated that 18 of these tumors displayed near-triploidy while no chromosomal aberrations were detected in Schwann cells [60]. This leads to the conclusion that Schwann cells in tumor stroma are reactive in nature and most likely from infiltrating normal Schwann cells. With the advent of laser-capture microdissection and allelotyping techniques, Mora *et. al.* have demonstrated in 27 of 28 NBs, S100-positive Schwann cells have identical allelic compositions as the neuroblastic tumor cells [59, 61]. Also, Schwannian stromal cells isolated from bone metastases have identical marker chromosomes as neuroblastic tumor cells [62]. Finally, the Schwannian S-type cell line, SH-EP1, harbors a F1174L mutation in the *ALK* gene that is also present in the neuroblastic N-type tumor cell line, SH-SY5Y (author's unpublished results)(Figure 3B). Both cell lines are derived from the widely used SK-N-SH NB cells [63]. All these data provide evidence that Schwann cells are tumor-derived.

3.3. The role of trophic factors in Schwannian stromal and NB pathogenesis

Since Schwannian stroma-rich tumors are associated with favorable prognosis, it is logical to assume that Schwann cells harbor tumor-suppressing properties. To this end, experiments aiming to address the biological relevance of Schwann cells in NB are limited and confined mostly to *in vitro* studies. By co-cultivation experiments, neuroblastic tumor cells have been shown to stimulate the proliferation of Schwann cells [64]. This observation may explain the rapid expansion of Schwannian stromal during NB maturation. In the same study, Schwann cells also promote neurite outgrowth in neuroblastic tumor cells. Similar survival and differentiation promoting activities were also reported when Schwann cell conditioned medium was tested on four NB cell lines [55, 65]. These results are consistent with the differentiated histology associated with stroma-rich tumors. One caveat is that Schwann cells used in these studies were isolated from normal human peripheral nerves. It will be of interest to compare tumor-derived versus normal Schwann cells in their abilities to promote differentiation and survival of neuroblastic tumor cells. Several trophic factors have been implicated in neuronal homeostasis. These include NGF, BDNF, LIF, and CNTF [66]. The biological effects of conditioned medium mentioned above are most likely the results of a combination of these soluble factors. Clearly defining their specific biological activities, for example, differentiation versus survival may have therapeutic implications. For instance, factors that only promote differentiation but not growth can have therapeutic effects in stroma-poor tumors. Alternatively, targeting the receptors for survival promoting factors such as the TrkB receptor for BDNF may be a plausible treatment strategy [25].

The paracrine effects of trophic factors produced by Schwann cells are not restricted to neuroblastic tumor cells. For instance, three factors secreted by Schwann cells are known to inhibit angiogenesis. These include tissue inhibitor of metalloproteinase-2 (TIMP-2)[67], PEDF [68] and SPARC [69]. TIMP-2 was identified as a potential anti-angiogenic mediator in the conditioned medium of Schwann cells derived from both adult nerves and stroma-rich GN [67]. The negative effects of TIMP-2 on angiogenesis are independent of its ability to inhibit metalloproteinase (MMP) activities [70]. Instead TIMP-2 binds directly to endothelial cells through $\alpha3\beta1$ integrin and dampens $\beta1$-mediated signaling and cell proliferation. PEDF, on the other hand, is a 50 kDa glycoprotein that belongs to the SERPIN family of serine protease inhibitors [71], and it binds to a PLA2/nutrin/patatin-like phospholipase domain-containing 2 (PNPLA2) receptor [72]. PEDF suppresses angiogenesis by inducing apoptosis in endothelial cells, blocking motility and tube formation [73]. In NB, PEDF enhances Schwann cell growth and inhibits basic fibroblast growth factor (bFGF) and vascular endothelial growth factor (VEGF) induced endothelial cell migration [68]. Consistent with these activities, the least differentiated NB show weak staining for PEDF while high levels are observed in well-differentiated GNB and GN. Finally, SPARC is a matricellular protein implicated in adipogenesis [74]. Surface receptors such as Stabilin-1 and $\alpha5\beta3$ integrin have been implicated in mediating SPARC biological activities [75, 76]. Its anti-angiogenic activities are mediated by the direct binding to a host of angiogenic mediators such as VEGF, and platelet-derived growth factor (PDGF)[77, 78]. High levels of SPARC are associated with favorable outcomes in NB [69]. *In vivo* experimental proof further supports the anti-tumorigenic role of Schwannian stroma. Using an NB xenotransplant model, NB cells implanted in sciatic nerve have greater number of infiltrating Schwann cells, more differentiated neuroblasts and reduced vascularity when compared to tumor cells injected outside of the sciatic nerves [79]. All these findings reinforce the notion that the favorable prognosis in stroma-rich NB is the consequence of a host of anti-angiogenic factors produced by the Schwannian stromal compartment.

3.4. Plasticity of Schwannian stroma

During NB progression, there is evidence of dynamic remodeling of the Schwannian tumor microenvironment that involves additional stromal cell types. One such cell type is cancer-associated fibroblasts (CAFs). CAFs are frequently detected in epithelial tumors such as breast carcinomas [80]. CAFs are "reactive" in nature and differ from normal fibroblasts by having a more motile or myogenic phenotype [81, 82]. In addition, CAFs also confer a pro-tumorigenic microenvironment by remodeling the extracellular matrices and producing pro-angiogenic and pro-mitogenic trophic factors. In one study, an evaluation of 60 NBs revealed an inverse correlation between the existence of CAFs and Schwannian stroma [83]. In stroma-rich GNs, alpha-smooth muscle actin (α-sma)-positive and h-Caldesmon-negative CAFs are rarely detected. On the contrary, ~90% of stromal cells in Schwannian stroma-poor NB stained positive for CAFs. Indeed, the presence of CAFs in NB is associated with microvascular proliferation. All these findings reiterate the role of Schwann cells in conferring homeostasis in NB tumor microenvironment and this may be achieved by blocking the expansion of CAFs. However, it is unclear how the relative fractions of Schwann cells versus CAFs are being regulated and whether neuroblastic tumor cells can play an instructive role in these events.

One plausible link between Schwann cells and CAFs is the well-established role of bone marrow-derived human mesenchymal stem cells (hMSCs) in the formation of tumor stroma. hMSCs are pluripotent and can differentiate into multiple cell types such as bone, cartilages, and adipose tissues [84]. hMSCs when co-mixed with weakly metastatic breast cancer cells greatly enhance their metastatic potential [85]. Interestingly, hMSCs co-mixed with NB undergo a conversion to a cell type expressing the Schwann cell markers, S100 and Egr-2 [86]. Similarly, prolonged exposure of hMSCs to tumor-derived conditioned media also results in their transition to myofibroblasts [87]. Thus, it is plausible that neuroblastic tumor cells may dictate the composition of tumor stroma by instructing hMSCs to differentiate into either Schwann cells or CAFs. Another interesting aspect of hMSCs in NB is that bone marrow is a common site of metastatic spread [88]. The ability of the chemokine, stromal-derived factor (SDF-1/CXCL12), in bone marrow homing by binding to its receptor, CXCR4, on neuroblastic tumor cells has been reported [89]. Following seeding in the bone marrow, neuroblastic tumor cells may instruct hMSCs to differentiate into Schwann cells, thereby creating a favorable metastatic niche in an otherwise non-permissive environment.

An additional intriguing finding is that Schwann cells isolated from quail sciatic nerves can undergo transdifferentiation into myofibroblasts [90]. In vitro, TGF-β drastically enhanced the conversion of cultured Schwann cells to α-sma$^+$ and sox10$^+$ myofibroblasts. When transplanted into the first branchial arch of E2 chick embryos, these Schwann cells incorporate into the perivascular space of developing vessel walls as α-sma$^+$ cells [90]. Based on these observations, it is tempting to speculate that neuroblastic tumor cells secrete TGF-β to remodel tumor stromal by converting Schwannian-rich to a CAF-rich tumor microenvironment. In summary, this level of plasticity in stromal remodeling may allow tumor cells to adapt to local hypoxic environment or in seeding of metastatic cells.

3.5. The role of Schwannian stromal in NB therapy

From a treatment standpoint, NB in infants has a more favorable prognosis with low-grade tumors that resolved spontaneously. However, the overall survival for patients greater than 4 year old remains around 40%. Also, there are few options once tumors are refractory to conventional chemo- and radiation-therapies. How can studying the role of Schwann cells in

NB can translate into better treatment? As mentioned above, the ability of NB to differentiate into neurons and Schwann cells even in the presence of *MYCN* gene amplification can be explored in the clinical settings. Resident cancer initiating (stem) cells or "intermediate I-type" cell lines such as NUB-7 and BE(2)-C can be differentiated into neurons by retinoic acid (RA) exposure or into Schwann cells by 5-bromo-2′-deoxyuridine (BrdU) exposure [58, 91, 92]. The current standard therapy for high risk NB includes initial induction chemotherapy, followed by autologous hematopoietic stem cell transplantation, and residual disease is treated with a maintenance dose of 13-cis-RA [93, 94]. Under this aggressive treatment regimen, only one-third of patients survived [95]. It will be of interest to test if a combination of RA and BrdU is more effective in differentiating residual NB. In fact, the role of BrdU as a radiosensitizing agent is well established [96, 97].

Another treatment modality is inhibition of angiogenesis. Bevacizumab (Avastin), a humanized monoclonal antibody against VEGF has been shown to enhance the efficacy of topotecan in a NB xenograft model [98]. It has moderate toxicity with overall severe adverse events of 17% [99]. Extensive clinical trial data of Bevacizumab for NB is lacking and its therapeutic efficacy in treating this pediatric tumor is yet to be determined. Nevertheless, the fact that Schwann cells secrete a host of soluble anti-angiogenic factors can be harnessed for therapeutic use. For example, PEDF is effective in blocking growth in a wide variety of tumors [73, 100, 101]. In fact, the delivery of PEDF by adenoviral-mediated gene transfer in NB suppresses angiogenesis and blocks tumor growth [102].

One of the overarching concerns in treatment-resistant high risk NB is the involvement of developmental plasticity inSchwann cells. Indeed, Schwann cells have the capacity to dedifferentiate into less mature progenitors *in vivo* under regenerative conditions. This level of plasticity in Schwann cells has been observed in injured axons wherethis activity requires an active Raf kinase [103]. One scenario is that following intense chemotherapies, while most hyperproliferative neuroblastic tumor cells are expected to be eradicated, residual stromal cells survive and undergo dedifferentiation into neural progenitors to repopulate the primary tumor site. Alternatively, as reported by our group, treatment of the ALK-positive tumor cell line SK-N-SH with an ALK inhibitor leads to the outgrowth of S-type cell populations while N-type cells are mostly eliminated [55]. Conditioned media from these Schwann-like cells confer striking survival toward N-type cells. Thus, tumor-associated Schwann cells or CAFs may provide a chemoresistant niche to support tumor recurrence from the few neuroblastic tumor cells that survive.

In summary, while Schwannian stroma have been considered as a benign byproduct of maturing NB, their presence is intimately linked to the survival and differentiation of neuroblastic tumor cells. The development of transgenic animal models that can recapitulate features of stroma-rich and stroma-poor tumors will be necessary to better understand this interaction. These *in vivo* models will be useful for deciphering the biological effects of Schwannian stroma on tumor cells, the paracrine factors involved and their intracellular signaling. Although Schwannian stroma is an attractive target for NB therapy, the NB tumor stroma/microenvironment, which is composed of the extracellular matrix plays an equally important role in NB pathogenesis, which is discussed next.

http://dx.doi.org/10.5772/55486

4. Cell-matrix and cell-cell molecular interactions in the neuroblastoma tumor microenvironment

In 1986 Harold F. Dvorak coined the phrase: "Tumors are wounds that never heal". His comment was based on similarities in the content of new blood vessels, lymphocytes, macrophages, and connective tissue components (including cellular and extracellular matrix elements) present in healing wounds and tissue surrounding tumor cells [104]. During tumor (parenchyma) development, the wound repair resolution stage fails, resulting in a microenvironment (stroma) that never "heals". Multiple factors in the "wounded" tumor microenvironment promote NB progression. In this section, we highlight the role of the extracellular matrix (ECM) in this process.

4.1. Biochemical and biophysical cues from the extracellular matrix

4.1.1. ECM stiffness conveys differentiation signals

The NB tumor microenvironment provides biochemical and mechanical signals similar to the microenvironments of other tumor types, but there is specificity in how NB tumor cells respond to these signals. It is well recognized that the interaction of tumor with stroma occurs via biochemical signaling and that the ECM provides a source of signals that instruct cellular behavior. Our understanding of how biomechanical signaling generated by shear stress, compression, and tension affect survival, proliferation, migration, and gene expression is increasing [105]. Changes in tension homeostasis occur in cancer, with breast cancer as one of the best studied examples [106]. Mechanical cues from the ECM may influence retinoic acid-mediated differentiation, which in turn may regulate clinically relevant aspects of NB biology. Recent studies show that ECM stiffness provides a physical cue that reduces NB proliferation and promotes differentiation [107]. Increasing ECM stiffness enhances neurite extension (neuritogenesis) and suppresses cell proliferation. Increased ECM stiffness also reduces expression of the oncogenic *MYCN* transcription factor. Furthermore, the addition of RA enhances ECM stiffness. Together, the data suggest that the mechanical signals from the cellular microenvironment influence NB differentiation in synergy with the RA biochemical differentiation factor [107].

4.1.2. SPARC and cell survival

One of the matrix proteins with a documented role in tumor progression is SPARC (osteonectin or BM-40). SPARC is a 34 kDa calcium-binding glycoprotein shown to associate with the cell membrane and membrane receptors [108, 109]. SPARC appears to have a cancer-type specific effect on tumor metastasis. In prostate cancer, SPARC is linked with increased migration and prostate cancer metastasis to bone. This occurs via activation of integrins $\alpha v\beta 3$ and $\alpha v\beta 5$ expressed on tumor cells [110]. In contrast, SPARC appears to act as a tumor suppressor in NB. This tumor suppressor effect has been studied in the context of radiation therapy. Irradiation of NB tumor cells was shown to inhibit SPARC expression. Interestingly, SPARC expression was significantly decreased in radiation-therapy resistant cancer cells [111]. Exogenous overexpression of SPARC significantly suppressed the activity of AKT. This suppression was accompanied by an increase in the PTEN tumor suppressor protein both in vitro and in vivo, [112] and sensitized NB cells to radiation by inhibiting irradiation-induced cell cycle arrest. Therefore, SPARC expression restored NB radiosensitivity. In addition to this function, SPARC expressed by NB cells appears to affect endothelial cells in the immediate vicinity. Interestingly, SPARC overexpression and secretion by NB cells induced endothelial cell apoptosis, inhibited angiogenesis and suppressed expression of the pro-angiogenic molecules, VEGF, FGF, PDGF and MMP-9 in endothelial cells. This suppressed expression of growth factors was mediated by inhibition of the Notch signaling pathway [113]. Therefore, promoting SPARC expression may be a plausible anti-NB therapy.

4.2. Role of cell adhesion molecules in NB progression

4.2.1. NCAM and NB progression

Intercellular communication is a fundamental biological property that is regulated during cellular growth and differentiation. In general terms, abnormalities in gap junction intracellular communication (GJIC) and cell-cell adhesion correlate with poor prognosis for cancer treatment [114-117]. Loss of either cell-cell adhesion or GJIC occurs in cancers, and gain of communication or adhesion suppresses tumor growth [118, 119]. Cell adhesion molecules (CAMs) have been reported to regulate tumor progression and metastasis, acting as oncogenes or tumor suppressors [120-122], and one such molecule namely Neural cell adhesion molecule (NCAM) is of particular importance for both, normal brain development [123] and NB regulation. NCAM is the main protein carrier of polysialic acid (polySia), a major regulator of cell-cell interactions in the developing nervous system that is required for neuronal plasticity. Studies in NCAM knockout mice showed that the effects of polySia occur via the expression of NCAM [123]. During normal neuronal differentiation or upon RA induced differentiation of a NB cell line, NCAM appears in non-polysialated form. This allows for its hemophilic interactions, and in turn triggers enhanced ERK signaling and MAPK-dependent neuritogenesis [124]. Therefore, it can be expected that inhibition of polysialation will promote neuronal differentiation and may inhibit NB progression.

4.2.2. N-cadherin and NB progression

Clinical studies suggest that tumor invasiveness, not the ability to detach from the primary tumor are determinants of the progression to metastasis [125]. In epithelial-derived tumors, metastasis is often preceded by the loss of E-cadherin cell-cell adhesion [126, 127]. The loss of E-cadherin is often accompanied by de novo expression of N-cadherin, which promotes cell motility and migration; a phenomenon called "the cadherin switch" [128-130]. Further, N-cadherin homophilic interactions between tumor cells and surrounding tissue such as tumor vessel endothelium and stroma facilitate the transit and survival of tumor cells in distant organs [131-133]. N-cadherin thus may play a role in preventing metastasis in NB through such homotypic and heterotypic cell-cell interactions. In line with this hypothesis, N-cadherins are expressed on various NB tumors and NB cell lines, with lowest levels in patients undergoing metastasis. Therefore, its expression negatively correlates with metastasis [134].

http://dx.doi.org/10.5772/55486

4.2.3. *Reelin signaling in NB*

Reelin is an extracellular secreted protein of the Cajal-Retzius cells located in the marginal zone of the developing cerebral cortex, and is required for the organization of the cortex into layers of neurons [135]. In the absence of reelin, neurons exhibit a broader and irregular pattern of positioning [136]. Although reelin interacts with integrins and cadherins, signals from reelin are transduced by cell membrane receptors: ApoER2 and Very Low Density Lipoprotein Receptor (VLDLR) and by the intracellular regulatory protein disabled-1 (Dab1) [137, 138]. Downstream signaling involves adapter protein crk and the small GTPase Rap1 [139]. Reelin triggers the activation of Rap1 in migrating cerebral cortical neurons when they are midway through their migration path (from the ventricular zone toward the cortical plate). This activation of Rap1 by reelin is critical for neuronal multipolar polarization and migration along glia, and therefore, normal cerebral cortex organization [140-143]. However, reelin expression is not limited to the normal tissues such as brain, but is also detected in several different tumor pathologies where it has been linked with tumor aggressiveness [144]. A recent study suggests that reelin signaling regulates a migratory switch promoting metastasis in NB [145]. Reelin expression is negatively regulated by miR-128, a brain-enriched microRNA. miR-128 is downregulated in untreated NB patients, and ectopic miR-128 overexpression reduced NB cell motility and invasiveness and impaired cell growth. Furthermore, a small series of primary human NBs showed an association between high levels of miR-128 expression and favorable features, such as a favorable stage score based on the International Neuroblastoma Staging System Classification (Shimada category, [146]). In addition to the autocrine function in differentiating tumors, reelin acts as a chemoattractant for several NB cell lines. It is also expressed in blood vessels in several NB cell lines, but not in normal tissue. Therefore, it is postulated that in addition to the autocrine function, paracrine reelin presented by NB blood vessels may act as a chemoattractant and promote hematogenic and lymphogenic dissemination in NB progression [145].

4.2.4. *Gap junctions – Cellular connectivity and suppression of growth*

Cell-cell interactions are mediated by specialized connections between membranes of adjacent cells called gap junctions. Gap junctions form by connecting two hemichannels (connexons) on neighboring cells, with each hemichannel comprised of a hexamer of connexin. Of the 20 known connexins, connexin 43 is the most ubiquitously expressed [147]. Gap junctional coupling in NB is negatively regulated by protein kinase C (PKC) [148]. PKC isozymes regulate various aspects of proliferation and PKC inhibitors are under study in clinical trials as potential anti-cancer therapy. Tamoxifen, an estrogen receptor antagonist, exerts some of its anti-tumor effects via PKC signaling [149, 150]. However, the exact cellular mechanisms targeted by PKC inhibitors are not known. Recently, it was shown that inhibition of PKC in NB cell lines increases GJIC via a mechanism that does not depend on the redistribution of connexin 43 or its phosphorylation [148]. Furthermore, PKC inhibition promoted cell-cell adhesion, a finding that suggests that suppression of tumor growth by PKC inhibition may be due to effects on increased GJIC and cell-cell adhesion [148].

Overall, these studies suggest that the extracellular matrix and CAMs play an important role in the biochemical and biophysical regulation of NB. The careful examination of NB environment-specific cues to fully define their effects on NB tumor progression offers an opportunity for NB targeted therapy.

5. Role of endothelial cells in NB microenvironment pathogenesis

5.1. Role of angiogenesis in NB pathogenesis

In 1962, Dr. Judah Folkman described the seminal observation that tumor angiogenesis is dependent on de novo blood vessel formation [151]. The sprouting of new blood vessels from pre-existing ones is a multi-step process consisting of endothelial cell proliferation, migration and tube formation [152]. Tumor angiogenesis is not only induced by growth factors and cytokines secreted from tumor cells [153], but also modulated by cell-cell interaction [152]. Aberrant angiogenesis is associated with excessive growth-promoting signals and a lack of sufficient "pruning," cues that spatially and temporally modulate vessel growth, remodeling and stabilization [152]. As compared to normal blood vessels, tumor vessels are more dilated and tortuous, form arteriovenous shunts, and lack the normal artery-capillary-vein hierarchy [154]. Tumor vasculature not only provides oxygen and nutrients to promote tumor proliferation and progression, but also facilitates tumor metastatic spreading. Thus, tumor angiogenesis represents an attractive new target for tumor therapy because it is well accepted that new blood vessel formation promotes tumor growth and metastatic spread [152, 155, 156].

In terms of NB, current evidence suggests that advanced and aggressive stages of NB are dependent on angiogenesis [157-159]. Meitar et al [160] demonstrated the association of the tumor angiogenesis and poor outcome in human NB. Like most solid tumors, several well-known pro-angiogenic growth factors such as VEGF-A, VEGF-B, bFGF, angiopoietin-2 (Ang-2), transforming growth factor alpha (TGF-α) and PDGF were found in advanced-stage NB tumors [161]. Human NBs produce extracellular matrix-degrading enzymes, that induce endothelial cell proliferation and are angiogenic in vivo [162]. Integrins $\alpha v\beta 3$ and $\alpha v\beta 5$ are more highly expressed in blood vessels of high-risk versus low-risk NB tumors [163]. In addition, lymphatic vessels are observed in NB [164] with higher expression of the VEGF-C lymphangiogenesis growth factor observed in advanced stage of NB [161]. These evidences suggest that tumor angiogenesis likely contributes to NB pathogenesis.

5.2. Contributions of *MYCN* amplification and trks-mediated signaling pathways to NB tumor angiogenesis

NB is an embryonic tumor that is derived from cells of the primitive NC [165]. In general, genetic abnormalities play a key role in determining tumor phenotype, [165, 166]. *MYCN* amplification is one of the first identified genetic defects in NB, and high levels of *MYCN* are associated with aggressive tumor behavior and poor survival [167]. *MYCN* is member of the MYC family of basic helix-loop-helix transcription factors that control a broad regulatory network implicated in cell cycle, DNA damage response, differentiation and apoptosis [168]. There is evidence that *MYCN* amplification is also associated with tumor angiogenesis. Several studies demonstrated that *MYCN* amplification in NB suppressed the expression of angiogenesis inhibitors, such as activin A, interleukin-6 and leukemia inhibitory factor [169, 170]. Activin A represses NB growth, endothelial cell proliferation and angiogenesis [171, 172]. In addition, highly expressed activin A in differentiated NB strongly correlates with a favorable NB outcome [173]. Interestingly, inhibition of PI3K/rapamycin results in the degradation of *MYCN* in NB tumor cells and results in blockage of angiogenesis indirectly [174].

A second gene family implicated in NB is the TRK family of neurotrophin receptors (NTRK) that play critical roles in the development of the CNS and PNS [25, 175]. The 3 characterized members are TrkA (NTRK1), TrkB (NTRK2) and TrkC (NTRK3) with nerve growth factor (NGF), BDNF and neurotrophin-3 (NT-3) as their primary ligands, respectively [175]. The sequential Trk expression is important for complete differentiation of normal sympathetic neurons, and the *Trk* genes expressed reflect the stage of neuronal differentiation [176]. High expression of TrkA and TrkC are associated with the ability for NB to differentiate and spontaneous regress, and are predominately found in clinically favorable NB. One mechanism that could explain this is that high expression of TrkA reduces the expression of angiogenic factors in NB cells and suppresses NB tumor xenograft growth associated with reduced angiogenic factor expression and vascularization of tumors [177]. In contrast, TrkB and its ligand, BDNF, are highly expressed in aggressive NB associated with increased cell survival, angiogenesis and drug resistance [25, 175].

5.3. Anti-angiogenesis treatments in NB - conventional anti-VEGF/VEGFR2 signaling pathways

Although targeting of the tumor vasculature represents a promising tool for cancer therapy, there are no current clinical trials of anti-angiogenesis therapy for NB [157-159]. There are several pre-clinical studies in NB animal models [157-159], and depending on the unique aspects of NB, several different approaches for anti-angiogenesis therapy is feasible. VEGF and its cognate receptor 2 (VEGFR2) are major regulators of angiogenesis. Anti-VEGF/VEGFR2 signaling pathways and inhibition of endothelial cell proliferation and migration are the most common anti-angiogenesis therapeutic approaches. The recently approved anti-angiogenesis drug, bevacizumab (Avastin), is a recombinant monoclonal antibody that binds VEGF-A and subsequently blocks the activation of its receptors. Bevacizumab reduces NB tumor growth by reducing angiogenesis [178]. In addition, treatment with bevacizumab can transiently induce tumor vasculature remodeling allowing for improved delivery and efficacy of chemotherapy in NB tumor xenografts [98]. A VEGFR-2 tyrosine kinase inhibitor Sugen 5416 (SU5416, Semoxinal) is a specific VEGFR-1 (Flt-1) and VEGFR-2 (Flk-1) tyrosine kinase inhibitor that has shown efficacy in inhibiting angiogenesis in vivo models of NB [179]. Efficacy of inhibiting tumor growth was increased when SU5416 was given in combination with irradiation or chemotherapy [180, 181]. In addition to VEGF inhibitors, other angiogenesis inhibitors have shown efficacy on NB tumor angiogenesis and growth, which is discussed in detail elsewhere [157, 159, 182]. TNP-470 is a synthetic analog of fumagillin, an antibiotic isolated from the fungus Aspergillus fumigatus fresenius with antineoplastic activity. TNP-470 is a potent selective inhibitor of Methionine aminopeptidase-2 (MetAP-2) resulting in endothelial cell cycle arrest late in G1 phase and leading to inhibition of tumor angiogenesis [183]. TNP-470 treatment in a NB tumor xenograft model reduced the tumor growth rate and decreased capillary density [184-188], and increased the efficacy of chemotherapy [181]. Taken together, these results suggest that anti-angiogenesis is an effective approach for reducing NB growth and burden. In addition to direct approaches targeting the vasculature in NB, indirect anti-angiogenesis approaches have also shown efficacy in NB. For the most part, these approaches rely on the induction of differentiation of NB. For example, retinoids have been shown to exert their effects by inducing differentiation of NB cells. Retinoids and fenretinide, a synthetic retinoid, have demonstrated anti-angiogenic effects in NB tumor xenografts [189, 190]. The inhibitory effects were mediated by retinoic acid induced expression of thrombospondin-1 (TSP-1) in NB cells. TSP-1 is an important endogenous angiogenesis inhibitor that inhibits endothelial cell proliferation and migration. Interestingly, TSP-1 is silenced in a subset of undifferentiated advanced-stage NB tumors and NB cell lines due to promoter methylation [191]. Remarkably, ABT-510, a peptide derived from TSP-1, suppressed the growth of NB tumor xenografts [192]. In combination with valproic acid, ABT-510 showed potent inhibitory effects on the growth of NB tumor xenografts. Taken together, these results suggest that both direct and indirect approaches of targeting angiogenesis are feasible therapeutic approaches for NB.

6. Molecular and cellular mechanistic interface between endothelial and immune cells in NB

The statement that "tumors are wounds that never heal" [21] has relevance for which phenotype of immune cells are present in the tumor microenvironment, and whether these cells interact to promote or prevent tumor. During the initial stage of wound healing there is an inflammatory response that is produced by an influx of immune cells that release inflammatory mediators. The next stage of tissue remodeling is characterized by a down-regulation of the immune response, cell proliferation, and revascularization of the wound via angiogenesis [193-195]. In the resolution stage of tissue remodeling, cell proliferation is halted and vessels are stabilized. In the tumor microenvironment, there is a perpetual state of inflammation, cell proliferation and angiogenesis similar to an unhealed wound. Chronic hypoxia in the tumor microenvironment is a contributing factor as to why tumors are wounds that never heal. The cellular response to hypoxia is controlled by the expression of hypoxia inducible factors (HIF) [196]. Low oxygen tension prevents the ubiquitination and subsequent proteosomal degradation of HIF-α proteins allowing them to translocate to the nucleus and dimerize with HIF-β forming functional transcription factors (HIF-1α/HIF-β or HIF-2α/HIF-β) that promote up-regulation of angiogenic target genes. There is also evidence that HIF-1α regulates energy homeostasis and plays a role in the differentiation of immune cells that can have pro or anti-tumor effects [197]. Notably, HIF-2α expression is required to maintain an undifferentiated state of NB tumor-initiating cells, and expression of HIF-2α is associated with poor outcome in NB [197, 198]. Hypoxia and chronic inflammation are key characteristics of the tumor microenvironment that promote immune suppression and vascularization. In NB as well as other solid tumors, cytokine and chemokine mediators as well as angiogenic factors influence the differentiation state of immune cells which ultimately determines whether or not these cells can be activated to contribute to anti-tumor immunity. This section highlights how immune cells are affected by factors in the tumor microenvironment to become both tolerogenic and pro-angiogenic with an emphasis on the interconnection between angiogenesis and tumor immunity. In addition, future prospects for treating NB with combinations of anti-angiogenic agents and immune-based therapies as a strategy to reverse the immune suppression in the tumor microenvironment is discussed.

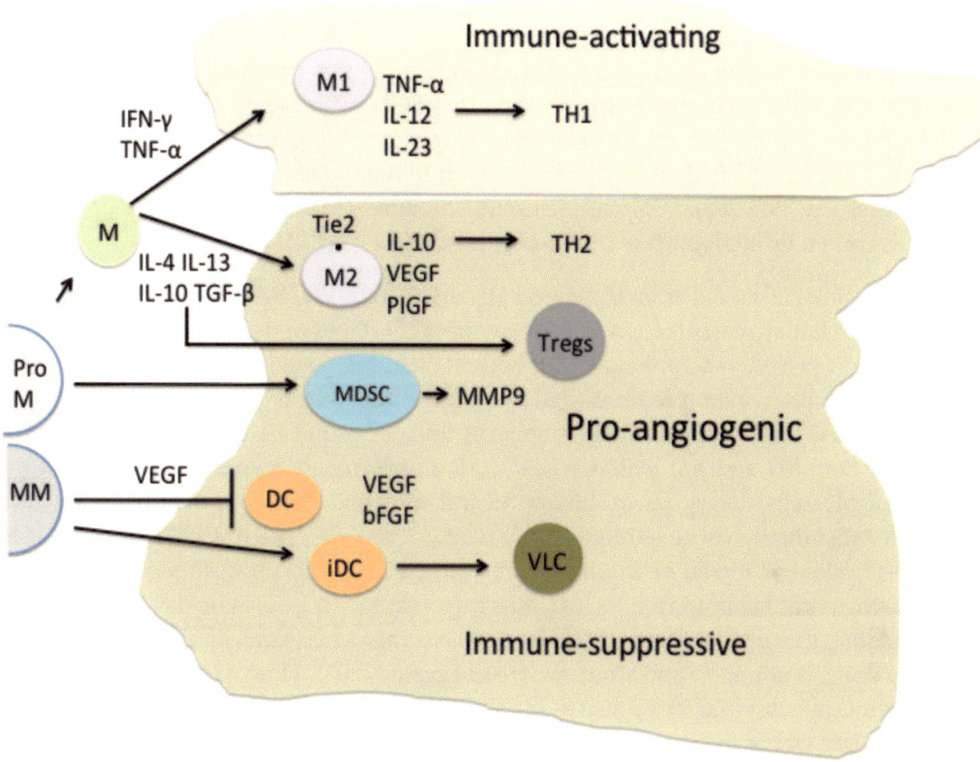

Figure 4. The contribution of immune cells in the tumor microenvironment. Pro M: pro-monocyte; MM: myelomonocytic stem cell; M: monocyte; M1 and M2: type 1 and 2 macrophages; MDSC: myeloid-derived suppressor cell; DC: dendritic cell; iDC: immature dendritic cell; VLC: vascular leukocyte cell; Tregs: T regulatory cells; IFN-γ: interferon gamma; TNF-α: tumor necrosis factor alpha; TGF-β: transforming growth factor beta; VEGF: vascular endothelial growth factor; bFGF: basic fibroblast growth factor; PIGF: placental growth factor; and MMP9: matrix metalloproteinase 9.

6.1. Myeloid cells

Innate immune cells of the myeloid lineage, including monocytes, macrophages and dendritic cells have been implicated as drivers of angiogenesis (Figure 4). Of these cells, the contribution to angiogenesis has been best characterized for macrophages. Studies in both human tumors and murine tumor models have shown that the presence of tumor associated macrophages (TAMs) correlates with enhanced vessel density, tumor progression and metastasis [199]. During inflammation, monocytes are attracted by chemo-attractants to damaged tissues, where they differentiate into macrophages. These macrophages are phenotypically plastic, and depending on the environmental signals within wounds or tumors, they differentiate into functional subsets with different activation states [200]. At sites of inflammation, interferon gamma (IFN-γ) and TNF-α facilitate macrophage differentiation into cytotoxic "M1" cells that secrete pro-inflammatory cytokines (TNF-α, IL-1, IL-6, IL-12 and IL-23). M1 macrophages are phagocytic, sustain tissue inflammation, and promote a T helper-1 (TH1) anti-tumor immune response [201, 202]. Alternatively, when induced in the presence of IL-4, IL-13, IL-10 and TGF-β, macrophages differentiate into "M2" cells that secrete IL-10 and participate in tissue remodeling and immune suppression. M2 macrophages also produce angiogenic factors. These factors include VEGF, placental growth factor (PIGF), arginase and the Tie2 angiopoietin cell surface receptor [203, 204]. Monocytes/macrophages that express Tie2 (referred to as TEMS) are a source of VEGF and have been found in human and murine spontaneous and orthotopic tumors [205, 206]. TEMS reside in close proximity to the tumor vasculature and are possibly recruited by angiopoietin-2-expressing endothelial cells [199].

Using a physiologic model of skin wound repair, CCR2^{hi}/VEGF-expressing macrophages were shown to initiate vascular sprouts during the early stages of tissue repair [195]. During the early repair period, macrophages with both M1 and M2 gene profiles were present, but cells with a M2 phenotype predominated during the later stages of repair. Results of this study imply that VEGF-expressing macrophages initiate wound-tissue vascularization. The presence of both M1 and M2 macrophages during early repair may be a reflection of the presence of M1 cells during the resolution of inflammation and the presence of M2 cells associated with initiation of an immune-suppressive tissue repair program. The data obtained from this physiologic model of wound healing parallels the process that occurs within the tumor microenvironment. In tumors, M1 cells are often found in sites of chronic inflammation, simulating the inflammatory stage of wound healing, while M2 cells are associated with vascularization, immune suppression and tissue repair [207]. However, this paradigm of tissue repair is not absolute for tumors as demonstrated by an aggressive inflammatory form of breast cancer where there is up-regulation of both VEGF and the IL-6 pro-inflammatory (M1) cytokine [208].

Dendritic cells (DCs) are professional antigen-presenting cells by nature, and they are intimately involved in the activation of tumor-specific T cells. DCs originate from CD34^{+} bone marrow precursors, and they differentiate into heterogeneous subsets due to differentiation plasticity. Within this heterogeneity there are functionally 2 major distinct subtypes of dendritic cells classified as myeloid DC (mDCs) and plasmacytoid DC (pDCs). Plasmacytoid DCs produce anti-angiogenic type I interferons [209], and mDC have the capacity to function as potent antigen-presenting cells. The maturation state of DCs adds another layer of complexity as immature DCs have high endocytic activity, but they lack expression of the co-stimulatory molecules that are necessary for T cell activation. Based on these properties, immature DCs are considered as immune-tolerogenic rather than immune-activating. VEGF affects the development and maturation of DCs. Binding of VEGF to the VEGFR-1 receptor on

CD34⁺ bone marrow progenitor cells limits differentiation along the DC lineage [210], and engagement of VEGFR-2 inhibits the maturation of DCs [210-212]. Furthermore, high levels of tumor-derived VEGF are associated with the presence of DCs with decreased co-stimulatory molecule expression [213]. There is evidence that tumor-infiltrating immature DCs also promote angiogenesis by secreting VEGF and bFGF [214, 215], and that immature DCs participate in de novo formation of blood vessels or neovascularization in the tumor micro-environment. Under the influence of VEGF or angiogenic factors, immature mDCs trans-differentiate into endothelial-like DCs (called vascular leukocytes, VLC) expressing both DC and endothelial markers such as von Willebrand factor, VEGFR-2, and VE-cadherin (CD31) [216]. Remarkably, human VLC were able to form perfusable blood vessels when transplanted into immune-deficient mice, indicating a potential to support neovascularization.

In addition to macrophages and DCs, neutrophils, eosinophils and mast cells can contribute to tumor angiogenesis. Tumor-infiltrating neutrophils and mast cells secrete VEGF and MMP-9 [217]. Secretion of MMP-9 facilitates the availability of pro-angiogenic factors through a remodeling of the extracellular matrix. Interestingly, an increase in the number of neutrophils in the tumor microenvironment correlates with increased micro-vessel density [218]. The presence of mast cells in murine models of melanoma [219], squamous cell carcinoma [220] and pancreatic islet tumors [221] has been associated with increased angiogenesis. Mast cells are present in the tumor microenvironment prior to vessel formation [222], and they congre-gate near tumor-derived vessels [220, 223]. Since mast cells contain pro-angiogenic factors in their secretory granules, it has been hypothesized that secretion of these factors by mast cells promotes tumor angiogenesis [199]. There is indirect evidence that eosinophils promote tumor angiogenesis, as they have been detected in human tumors [199], and they are also a source of pro-angiogenic factors [224].

Myeloid-derived suppressor cells (MDSC) are immature myeloid progenitors of monocytes, neutrophils and DCs. As tumor-resident cells, MDSC facilitate tumor progression by their immunosuppressive properties. However, these cells may also have a role in promoting angiogenesis. Studies have shown that tumor angiogenesis is decreased when the MDSC chemo-attractant, BV8 (PROK2), was neutralized [225], and tumor blood vessel density increased when MDSC were co-injected with colorectal cancer cells into mice [226]. MDSC also secrete matrix metalloproteases.

6.2. T cells

Cancer patients have a decrease in immune function that can be attributed in part to the tolerogenic differentiation of innate immune cells. However, there is evidence that VEGF also interferes with T cell development. Effective T cells have the ability to specifically recognize and kill tumors. In fact, the most significant predictor of survival from solid tumors is the presence of CD8 T cells in the tumor core and invasive margins [227]. In vivo administration of a supraphysiologic concentration of recombinant VEGF blocks bone marrow-derived progenitor cells from seeding in the thymus reducing T cell production [228]. These data imply that VEGF secreted from tumors or cells in the tumor microenvironment may contribute to a systemic decrease in T cells.

As previously described, cells of the innate immune system have an important pro-angiogenic role in the tumor microenvironment. However, cells that mediate adaptive immunity also contribute to angiogenesis. The tumor microenvironment is immune suppressive due to the presence of multiple tolerogenic mechanisms. One of the most potent immune suppressive mediators arises through the differentiation of $CD4^{+}CD25^{-}$ T cells into $CD4^{+}CD25^{+}FoxP3^{+}$ regulatory T cells (Tregs) [229]. In addition to promoting tumorigenesis through immunosuppression, there is evidence that Tregs contribute to tumor angiogenesis. Accumulation of Tregs in the tumor microenvironment is associated with increased angiogenesis and increased microvessel density [230]. $CD4^{+}CD25^{+}$ Tregs secrete higher amounts of VEGF than $CD4^{+}CD25^{-}$ CD4 T cells, and when Tregs are depleted from the tumor microenvironment there is less VEGF and angiogenesis present [231]. Therefore, elimination of Tregs as a form of tumor immunotherapy may provide two benefits: a release from immune suppression and decreased angiogenesis.

To summarize the pro-tumorigenic role of immune cells in the tumor microenvironment, there is now convincing evidence that suppressive immune cells can contribute to tumor angiogenesis. This angiogenic activity may be a reflection of the natural wound healing process, as wounds naturally switch from an immune-activating acute inflammatory environment to one that is immune suppressive and pro-angiogenic. As an unhealed wound, the tumor microenvironment may continually cycle between one of inflammation and immune suppression. An understanding of how immune cells, tumor cells, endothelial cells and other cells in the microenvironment contribute to immune suppression and angiogenesis is key in order to devise therapies that can reprogram cells in this environment to be both immune activating and anti-angiogenic. Given the parallels between suppressed anti-tumor immunity and angiogenesis, therapies designed to relieve anti-tumor immune suppression may halt the angiogenic program, or vice versa. Studies to test synergy between immune-based and anti-angiogenic therapies have recently emerged; however, for NB, this field is in its infancy.

6.3. Anti-angiogenic and immune therapies to treat NB

The current standard of care for high-risk NB patients includes myeloablative chemotherapy followed by autologous hematopoietic stem cell transplant (AHSCT) and isotretinoin (13-*cis*-retinoic acid). While these treatments have improved the survival of patients with high-risk disease, approximately 60% of these patients will relapse and die of their disease. Recently, immune therapy has been added to standard treatment protocols as a strategy to improve survival. Post-transplant treatment with an antibody that targets the highly expressed GD2 disialoganglioside on NB tumor cells, in combination with interleukin-2 (IL-2) and granulocyte macrophage colony-stimulating factor (GM-CSF), has resulted in a 2-year 20% increase in event-free survival compared to patients treated with standard therapy alone [232]. Despite this multimodal therapy, the mortality rate remains high for patients with metastatic NB. Indicators of disease associated with a poor prognosis include a paucity of stromal Schwann cells, *MYCN* amplification, expression of the TrkB receptor tyrosine kinase and a high vascular index [233]. Infiltration of immune cell subsets has also been associated with high-risk disease.

TAMs expressing CD68 and IL-6, as well as IL-6-expressing $CD33^{+}CD14^{+}$ myelomonocytic cells in the bone marrow, are indicators of poor survival [234]. Expression of inflammation-associated genes (IL-6, IL-6R, IL-10 and TGFβ1) also correlates with a poor 5-year event-free survival [235]. In search of new therapies aimed at targeting these high-risk factors, both preclinical and clinical studies designed to test either immune or anti-angiogenic therapies are in progress.

The goal of immune therapy is to summon immune effector cells to the tumor microenvironment and promote activation against the tumor. Much of the effort in cancer immunotherapy has focused on the activation of effector T cells, but in order to achieve an effective anti-tumor T cell response, tumor antigen, mature antigen-presenting DCs and tumor antigen-reactive T cells must be present [236]. Autologous or allogeneic whole tumor cell vaccines, tumor lysate vaccines, antigen–primed DC vaccines, and induction of endogenous tumor cell lysis are all strategies to provide a source of tumor antigens. Agents such as GM-CSF, toll-like receptor (TLR) ligands, or agonistic anti-CD40 antibody are administered to promote DC migration and maturation. Blockade of T cell inhibitory receptors with anti-CTLA-4 or anti-PD-1 antibodies, administration of T cell survival chemokines (IL-2, IL-12 or IL-15), Treg blockade, or adoptive transfer of immune cells are therapies that can promote T cell activation. Recent attention has been directed to targeting immune suppressive factors in the tumor microenvironment using molecular inhibitors or antibodies. As previously noted, the functional complexity of immune cells, and their modulation by the tumor microenvironment to become immune suppressive, is recognized as key factor in the failure of effective anti-tumor immunity.

For NB, the efficacy of several different immune therapies has been examined in both preclinical murine tumor models (Table 1) and clinical trials (Table 2). Preclinical therapies include whole-cell tumor vaccines secreting immune activating cytokines (GM-CSF, IFN-γ, IL-21) or expressing immune co-stimulatory molecules (CD54 (ICAM), CD80, CD86, CD137L). In the N2a murine tumor model, our laboratory and others have shown that depletion of Tregs using anti-CD4 or anti-CD25 mAbs increases vaccine-induced anti-tumor immunity [242, 246]. Another immune therapy designed to augment the number of anti-tumor T cells involves the adoptive cell transfer (ACT) of lymphocytes or T cells. For this therapy, autologous T cells are expanded ex vivo and returned to the patient after they have been activated against tumor antigens. Tumor-specific T cell receptors genetically attached to T cell activating domains (chimeric antigen receptors or CARS) have been transduced into T cells as a method to increase the anti-tumor cytolytic activity provided by ACT. In a preclinical model, adoptive transfer of T cells expressing an anti-GD2 CAR and the CCR2b chemokine receptor promoted trafficking of T cells to the tumor and resulted in tumor regression [245]. Of 11 patients enrolled in a clinical trial testing ACT of Epstein-Barr virus (EBV)-specific T cells expressing the anti-GD2 CAR, 2 patients had tumor regression and 2 patients experience stable disease (Table 2). One of the earliest pre-clinical strategies used a combination of anti-human GD2 antibody and IL-2 treatment in a human-mouse NB xenograft model [237]. After over a decade of study, a combination of anti-GD2, IL-2, GM-CSF and cis-retinoic acid, given in the context of autologous hematopoietic stem cell transplantation, has now been shown to improve the event-free survival of treated patients [232].

Model	Therapy	Response	References
SCID (immune deficient) mouse	Human/mouse chimeric anti-GD2 and IL-2 (ch14.8-IL-2) plus IL-2-activated human PBMCs	Suppressed dissemination of human SK-N-AS NB injected under the splenic capsule	[237]
N2a syngeneic mouse	IL-2-secreting N2a tumor vaccine	Induced protective immunity against N2a and prolonged survival of N2a-bearing mice	[238]
N2a syngeneic mouse	GM-CSF or GM-CSF and IFN-γ secreting N2a tumor vaccine	Regression of tumor in retroperitoneal inoculated N2a-bearing mice	[239]
AGN2a (N2a subclone) syngeneic mouse	AGN2a tumor vaccine transiently transfected to express CD54, CD80, CD86 and CD137L	Protection from AGN2a tumor challenge	[240]
AGN2a (N2a subclone) syngeneic mouse	Anti-CD25 mAb followed by AGN2a CD80, CD86-expressing tumor vaccine	Enhanced protection to AGN2a tumor challenge	[241]
N2a syngeneic mouse	IL-21-secreting AGN2a tumor vaccine	Protective anti-tumor immunity and detection of survivin-specific CTLs	[242]
NXS2 syngeneic mouse	Survivin DNA minigene vaccine	Increase in CD8 T cells at the tumor site and reduced tumor growth	[243]
NXS2	Tyrosine hydroxylase DNA minigene vaccine	Induced tyrosine hydroxylase-specific CTLs and eradicated primary tumor	[244]
SCID	ACT of T cells expressing anti-GD2 CAR and CCR2b	Reduction in growth of huNB xenograft and increased trafficking of CD2 CAR CCR2b T cells to the tumor	[245]
N2a	IL-21-secreting N2a tumor vaccine and anti-CD4 mAb	Reduced dissemination of intravenous inoculated N2a tumor.	[242]
AGN2a (N2a subclone)	ACT of CD25-depleted T cells following TBI and HSCT and AGN2a tumor vaccine expressing CD54, CD80, CD86, and CD137L	Increase in survival of AGN2a-bearing mice	[246]

Table 1. Immunotherapies for neuroblastoma (pre-clinical)

Therapy	Response	Reference
IL-2	No objective tumor response.	[247]
Autologous NB transfected to produce IL-2	Of 10 patients, 1CR, 1PR and 3SD; 4 patients with anti-tumor CTLs	[248]
Allogeneic NB secreting IL-2	No cytotoxicity against the vaccinating cell line; 1PR, 7SD and 4PD	[248]
Allogeneic NB secreting IL-2 and lymphotactin	Of 21 patients with relapsed or refractory disease: 2CR 1PR; increased NK cytolytic activity	[249]
Anti-GD2 (hu14.18)/IL-2 fusion protein	Of 27 patients there were no CR or PR, 3 patients had anti-tumor activity	[250]
Anti-LI-CAM CAR	Of 6 patients, 1 with limited disease had a PR	[251]
Autologous IL-2-secreting tumor vaccine	In patients with minimal disease there was a rise in circulating CD4 and CD8 T cells specific for autologous tumor	[252]
ACT of EBV-specific T cells transduced with anti-GD2 CAR	Of 11 patients 2CR and 2SD	[253]
Anti-GD2 (hu14.18)/IL-2 fusion protein	Of 23 patients with non-bulky tumor there were 5CR	[254]
Anti-GD2 (ch14.18) GM-CSF, IL-2 and cis-retinoic acid following myeloablative conditioning and AHSCT	Improved event-free survival Incorporated into standard of care	[232]

Table 2. Immunotherapies for neuroblastoma (clinical)

In addition to infiltration of specific immune cellular subsets, a high NB vascular index also correlates with aggressive disease [255]. High expression of pro-angiogenic factors (HIF-2α, VEGF-A, bFGF, TGF-α, PDGF-A, angiopoietin-2, MMP-2, MMP-9, and integrins $\alpha v\beta 3$ and $\alpha v\beta 5$) as well as down-regulation the endothelial cell growth inhibitor, activin A, have been reported in advance stage or high risk NB [256-260]. Given these findings, studies have been designed to target angiogenesis with (1) Agents that directly target endothelial cells (endostatin, thrombospondin-1, thalidomide), (2) Agents that indirectly block the production or activity of pro-angiogenic molecules (antibodies to VEGF or VEGF receptors), or (3) Or agents that target both endothelial and tumor cells (receptor tyrosine kinase inhibitors (RTK) and interferon alpha (IFN-α)). For a complete review, refer to [233]. TPN-470 is an agent that inhibits the proliferation of endothelial cells by inactivating methionine aminopeptidase; however, biochemical instability may limit its application [261]. Fenretinide (N-(4-hydroxyphenyl or 4HPR) is a synthetic analog of retinoic acid that represses endothelial cell proliferation and is associated with a reduction in VEGFR-2 and FGF-2R-2 receptor expression on endothelial cells [262]. Retinoids are promising anti-tumor agents because they also induce the differentiation of NB cells and promote the survival of tumor-reactive CD8 T cells [233, 263]. As mentioned previously, the isotretinoin retinoid has recently been added to standard care protocols for the treatment of refractory NB. Bevacizumab is an anti-VEGF monoclonal antibody that binds to VEGF receptors, blocking signaling through these receptors. A VEGF Trap decoy is another agent used to block VEGFR. This agent is composed of VEGFR-1 and VEGFR-2 segments fused to an IgG1 molecule [264]. The receptor tyrosine kinase inhibitors, SUGEN, axitinib, imatinib mesylate, sunitinib, sorafenib and ZD6474 differentially target various receptors including PDGFR, VEGFR, the stem cell factor receptor (c-KIT), the FMS-related tyrosine kinase 3, epidermal growth factor receptor (EGFR) and RET on endothelial and tumor cells [265, 266]. Preclinical studies testing the effects of these agents on human-mouse NB xenografts have been performed. For these studies, human NB cell lines were grafted (orthotopically or subcutaneously) into immune compromised mice. Tumor growth, apoptosis of tumor and endothelial cells, and tumor vascularization were examined after treatment with the anti-angiogenic agent(s). It is important to note that these mouse models cannot accurately assess impact of the immune system on tumor growth because they lack an intact human immune system. A summary of NB anti-angiogenic preclinical studies is shown in Table 3.

Model	Therapy	Response	Reference
NB xenografts into immune-compromised (Nude, SCID, NOD-SCID)	TNP-470 (AMG-1470)	Inhibited endothelial cell proliferation and migration	[267]
	Fenretinide	Prevented the induction of endothelial cell proliferation and angiogenesis	[268]
	High dose VEGF Trap decoy	Disrupted early vessel formation and vessel remodeling	[264]
	Imatinib mesylate (Gleevec)	Inhibited NB growth and suppressed PDGFR and c-Kit phosphorylation	[269]
	SUGEN (SU11657)	Reduced angiogenesis, tumor growth and increased apoptosis of NB	[265]
	Bevacizumab	Decrease in tumor micro-vessel density, tumor growth and angiogenesis	[270, 271]

Model	Therapy	Response	Reference
	Combined treatment with a thrombospondin-1 peptide and valproic acid histone deacetylase inhibitor	Inhibited growth of NB xenografts and stabilized the growth of large tumors	[272]
	ZD6474 RTK	Inhibited tumor growth and induced endothelial cell apoptosis	[266]
	Sunitinib and sorafenib	Inhibited angiogenesis and tumor growth	[273]
	Bevacizumab and cyclophosphamide	Synergistic anti-tumor effect	[274]
	Axitinib	Tumor growth delay, but no regression	[275]

Table 3. Neuroblastoma pre-clinical anti-angiogenic therapies

Since the infiltration of immune-suppressive cells and a high vascular index both correlate with aggressive NB, interventions designed to reverse both immune suppression and angiogenesis represent promising treatment approaches. However, studies testing such combination therapies for the treatment of NB or other cancers are relatively scarce (Table 4). One ongoing phase I NB trial combines immune therapy with anti-angiogenic therapy. For this study, an iodine ^{131}I-conjugated anti-GD2 monoclonal antibody is administered in combination with bevacizumab [276]. Combination therapies for other cancers (renal cell carcinoma) have included treatment with bevacizumab and IFN-α [277] or IL-2 [278]. Surprisingly, combinations of anti-tumor immune and anti-angiogenic therapies have not been tested preclinically in NB, and there are relatively few preclinical studies in other tumor models (Table 4). However, there is evidence that these therapies can act synergistically to elicit anti-tumor responses: (1) Combinations of cytokine-secreting tumor cell-based vaccines and agents that block VEGFR signaling were tested in melanoma and breast cancer models; (2) Immune-activating cytokines, endostatin, and pigment epithelium-derived factor were tested in a hepatocellular carcinoma model; (3) Adoptive transfer of tumor-antigen specific T cells with anti-VEGF and IL-2 was tested in a melanoma tumor model; and (4) Vaccination with a viral vector encoding immune stimulatory molecules and treatment with sunitinib was tested in a colon cancer transgenic mouse model.

While it is almost certain that a combination of therapies (chemotherapy, radiation, targeted therapies, immune and/or anti-angiogenic) will be required to mount an effective anti-tumor response, the appropriate combination will likely vary among the different cancer types. For

System	Therapy	Response	Reference
Neuroblastoma clinical trial	^{131}I-labeled anti-GD2 mAb and bevacizumab	In progress	Clinicaltrials.gov
Clinical trials in other tumor models			
Renal cell carcinoma	Bevacizumab and IFN-α	Significant increase in progression-free survival compared to IFN-α alone	[277]
Renal cell carcinoma	Bevacizumab and IL-2	No clinical benefit	[278]
Preclinical Studies in other tumor models			
B16F10 melanoma	GM-CSF secreting tumor vaccine with a recombinant adeno-associated virus vector expressing a soluble VEGF receptor	A significant increase in tumor-free survival associated with a reduction in tumor-infiltrating immature DC and Tregs and an increase in effector T cells	[279]
Her2/neu breast cancer	Her2/neu expressing GM-CSF secreting tumor vaccine in combination with anti-VEGFR-1, DC101 mAb	In non-tolerant WT syngeneic mice there was accelerated tumor regression associated with expansion of CD4 and CD8 T cells. In tolerant neu transgeneic mice there was delayed tumor growth, but no regression	[280]
Woodchuck hepatocellular carcinoma	Adenovirus vectors encoding IL-12, GM-CSF, endostatin and pigment epithelium-derived factor	Regression of large tumor (>8,000 mm^2) required infusion of all vectors	[281]
B-16 melanoma	Adoptive transfer of Pmel-1 transgenic T cells with anti-VEGF, a tumor vaccine expressing melanoma tumor antigen, gp100, and IL-2 after non-myeloablative total body irradiation	There was a significant increase in survival in tumor-bearing mice when anti-VEGF was administered prior to irradiation and immune therapy	[282]
MC38-CEA colon carcinoma in CEA-transgenic mice	Sunitinib plus primary vaccination with CD80, ICAM1, LFA-3 and CEA expressing vaccinia virus and a boost with fowlpox virus	Treatment with sunitinib prior to vaccination resulted in a significant reduction in tumor growth	[283]

Table 4. Combined immune and anti-angiogenic therapy

http://dx.doi.org/10.5772/55486

NB, the ideal combination is yet to be determined. Bevacizumab (Avastin®) is FDA-approved for other solid tumors and represents a promising addition to augment immune and chemotherapeutic anti-tumor efficacy for NB. Receptor tyrosine kinase inhibitors, including imatinib mesylate (Gleevec®), sorafenib (Nexavar®), and sunitinib (Sutent®) have shown some anti-tumor efficacy in NB preclinical studies, and these agents are also FDA-approved for the treatment of some solid tumors. The results from studies using combined anti-angiogenic and anti-tumor immune therapy are encouraging and offer a new avenue to explore more effective eradication of NB and other cancers. Given the multiple types of immunotherapy and anti-angiogenic agents, as well as different platforms of delivery, more studies using combinations of these therapies are warranted.

7. Conclusion

NB is an enigmatic childhood cancer that has developmental origins in NC cell lineage. MYCN, ALK and TRKA are the key target genes for NB prognosis. Extracellular matrix and cell adhesion molecules that participate in interactions and signaling across endothelial cells, immune and Schwann cells in the NB microenvironment have potential for targeting. The future for NB biology and therapy looks bright and multiple modalities affecting various cell types and signals in NB microenvironment are anticipated.

Nomenclature

ALK: anaplastic lymphoma kinase; ANS: autonomic nervous system; Ang-2: angiopoietin-2; ACT: adoptive cell transfer; BMP: bone morphogenic protein; BDNF: brain-derived neurotrophic factor; bFGF: basic fibroblast growth factor; BrdU: 5-bromo-2′-deoxyuridine; CNS: central nervous system; CNTF: ciliary neurotrophic factor; CAFs: cancer-associated fibroblasts; CAM: cell adhesion molecules; CAR: chimeric antigen receptor; CR: complete response; DRG: dorsal root ganglia; DC: dendritic cell; EMT: epithelial to mesenchymal transition; ECM: extracellular matrix; EBV: Epstein-Barr virus; EGFR: epidermal growth factor receptor; FDA: Federal Drug Administration; FGF: fibroblast growth factor; GNB: ganglioneuroblastoma; GN: ganglioneuroma; GFAP: glial fibrillary acidic protein; GJIC: gap junction intracellular communication; GM-CSF: granulocyte macrophage colony-stimulating factor; HGF: hepatocyte growth factor; hMSC: human mesenchymal stem cells; HIF: hypoxia inducible factor; IFN-γ: interferon gamma; IFN-α: interferon alpha; LIF: leukemia inhibitory factor; MYCN: v-myc myelocytomatosis viral-related protein; MAPs: microtubule associated proteins; MBP: myelin basic protein; MKI: mitosis-karyorrhexis index; MMP: metalloproteinase; mDC: myeloid dendritic cell; MDSC: myeloid-derived suppressor cell; NB: neuroblastoma; NC: neural crest; NCSC: neural crest-derived stem cell; NRG-1 neuregulin-1; NF: neurofilament; NCAM: neural cell adhesion molecule; NGF: nerve growth factor; NT-3: neurotropin-3; PBMC: peripheral blood mononuclear cell; PNS: peripheral nervous system; PSNS: parasympathetic nervous system; PEDF: pigment epithelium-derived factor; PDGF: platelet-derived growth factor; PolySia: polysialic acid; PIGF: placental growth factor; pDC: plasmacytoid dendritic cell; PD: progressive disease; PR: partial response; RA: retinoic acid; RTK: receptor tyrosine kinase; SA: sympathoadrenal; SPARC: Secreted Protein Acidic and Rich in Cysteine; SC: Schwann cell; SCP: Schwann cell precursor; SAE: severe adverse effect; SD: stable disease; Trk: tyrosine kinase receptor; TH: tyrosine hydroxylase; TGF-β : transforming growth factor-beta; TIMP-2: tissue inhibitor of metalloproteinase-2; TGF-α: transforming growth factor-alpha; TSP-1: thrombospondin-1; TAMs: tumor-associated macrophages; TNF-α: tumor necrosis factor-alpha; TH1: T helper-1; TEMS: Tie2 monocytes/ macrophages; Tregs: T regulatory cells; TLR: toll-like receptor; VLC: vascular leukocytes; VEGF: vascular endothelial growth factor

Acknowledgements

We thank members of our respective labs for supporting our programs in developmental, vascular, tumor and immune biology. We also thank Marjorie Siebert Aylen Foundation for supporting RR's research on NB. MC-W is supported by NHLBI grant HL111582. BJ is supported by NIH grant CA100030. RR is supported by NHLBI grant HL090712, and seed funds from Children's Research Institute. QRM is supported by NHLBI grant HL108938 and start-up funds from MCW. We thank MACC fund and the BloodCenter of Wisconsin for their generous contribution to the research programs of the authors (BJ, AC and JG; MC-W).

Author details

Jill Gershan[1], Andrew Chan[2], Magdalena Chrzanowska-Wodnicka[3], Bryon Johnson[4], Qing Robert Miao[5] and Ramani Ramchandran[6*]

*Address all correspondence to: rramchan@mcw.edu

1 Department of Pediatrics, Medical College of Wisconsin, Milwaukee, WI, USA

2 School of Biomedical Sciences, The Chinese University of Hong Kong, Shatin, NT, Hong Kong

3 Blood Research Institute, Milwaukee, WI, USA

4 Department of Pediatrics, Medical College of Wisconsin, Milwaukee, WI, USA

5 Divisions of Pediatric Surgery and Pediatric Pathology, Departments of Surgery and Pathology, Medical College of Wisconsin, Milwaukee, WI, USA

6 Department of Pediatrics, Medical College of Wisconsin, Milwaukee, WI, USA

References

[1] Shimada H, Chatten J, Newton WA, Jr., Sachs N, Hamoudi AB, Chiba T, Marsden HB, Misugi K: Histopathologic prognostic factors in neuroblastic tumors: definition of subtypes of ganglioneuroblastoma and an age-linked classification of neuroblastomas. J Natl Cancer Inst 1984; 73(2) 405-416.

[2] Maris JM, Hogarty MD, Bagatell R, Cohn SL: Neuroblastoma. Lancet 2007; 369(9579) 2106-2120.

[3] Wiedenmann B, Franke WW, Kuhn C, Moll R, Gould VE: Synaptophysin: a marker protein for neuroendocrine cells and neoplasms. Proc Natl Acad Sci U S A 1986; 83(10) 3500-3504.

[4] Lloyd RV, Wilson BS: Specific endocrine tissue marker defined by a monoclonal antibody. Science 1983; 222(4624) 628-630.

[5] Grimmer MR, Weiss WA: Childhood tumors of the nervous system as disorders of normal development. Curr Opin Pediatr 2006; 18(6) 634-638.

[6] Carmeliet P, Tessier-Lavigne M: Common mechanisms of nerve and blood vessel wiring. Nature 2005; 436(7048) 193-200.

[7] Brodal P: The Central Nervous System, vol. Fourth Edition, 4th edn: Oxford University Press; 2010.

[8] Brodeur GM: Neuroblastoma: biological insights into a clinical enigma. Nat Rev Cancer 2003; 3(3) 203-216.

[9] Stewart RA, Lee JS, Lachnit M, Look AT, Kanki JP, Henion PD: Studying peripheral sympathetic nervous system development and neuroblastoma in zebrafish. Methods Cell Biol 2010; 100 127-152.

[10] Bronner-Fraser M, Stern CD, Fraser S: Analysis of neural crest cell lineage and migration. J Craniofac Genet Dev Biol 1991; 11(4) 214-222.

[11] Nieto MA: The early steps of neural crest development. Mech Dev 2001; 105(1-2) 27-35.

[12] Adams MS, Gammill LS, Bronner-Fraser M: Discovery of transcription factors and other candidate regulators of neural crest development. Dev Dyn 2008; 237(4) 1021-1033.

[13] Zirlinger M, Lo L, McMahon J, McMahon AP, Anderson DJ: Transient expression of the bHLH factor neurogenin-2 marks a subpopulation of neural crest cells biased for a sensory but not a neuronal fate. Proc Natl Acad Sci U S A 2002; 99(12) 8084-8089.

[14] Gammill LS, Roffers-Agarwal J: Division of labor during trunk neural crest development. Dev Biol 2010; 344(2) 555-565.

[15] Theveneau E, Mayor R: Neural crest delamination and migration: from epithelium-to-mesenchyme transition to collective cell migration. Dev Biol 2012; 366(1) 34-54.

[16] Kerosuo L, Bronner-Fraser M: What is bad in cancer is good in the embryo: importance of EMT in neural crest development. Semin Cell Dev Biol 2012; 23(3) 320-332.

[17] Kulesa PM, Gammill LS: Neural crest migration: patterns, phases and signals. Dev Biol 2010; 344(2) 566-568.

[18] Krull CE, Collazo A, Fraser SE, Bronner-Fraser M: Segmental migration of trunk neural crest: time-lapse analysis reveals a role for PNA-binding molecules. Development 1995; 121(11) 3733-3743.

[19] Fernandis AZ, Prasad A, Band H, Klosel R, Ganju RK: Regulation of CXCR4-mediated chemotaxis and chemoinvasion of breast cancer cells. Oncogene 2004; 23(1) 157-167.

[20] Schmid BC, Rudas M, Rezniczek GA, Leodolter S, Zeillinger R: CXCR4 is expressed in ductal carcinoma in situ of the breast and in atypical ductal hyperplasia. Breast Cancer Res Treat 2004; 84(3) 247-250.

[21] Nakamura Y, Ozaki T, Koseki H, Nakagawara A, Sakiyama S: Accumulation of p27 KIP1 is associated with BMP2-induced growth arrest and neuronal differentiation of human neuroblastoma-derived cell lines. Biochem Biophys Res Commun 2003; 307(1) 206-213.

[22] Ichimiya S, Nimura Y, Seki N, Ozaki T, Nagase T, Nakagawara A: Downregulation of hASH1 is associated with the retinoic acid-induced differentiation of human neuroblastoma cell lines. Med Pediatr Oncol 2001; 36(1) 132-134.

[23] Soderholm H, Ortoft E, Johansson I, Ljungberg J, Larsson C, Axelson H, Pahlman S: Human achaete-scute homologue 1 (HASH-1) is downregulated in differentiating neuroblastoma cells. Biochem Biophys Res Commun 1999; 256(3) 557-563.

[24] Trochet D, Bourdeaut F, Janoueix-Lerosey I, Deville A, de Pontual L, Schleiermacher G, Coze C, Philip N, Frebourg T, Munnich A *et al*: Germline mutations of the paired-like homeobox 2B (PHOX2B) gene in neuroblastoma. Am J Hum Genet 2004; 74(4) 761-764.

[25] Brodeur GM, Minturn JE, Ho R, Simpson AM, Iyer R, Varela CR, Light JE, Kolla V, Evans AE: Trk receptor expression and inhibition in neuroblastomas. Clinical cancer research : an official journal of the American Association for Cancer Research 2009; 15(10) 3244-3250.

[26] Weiss WA, Aldape K, Mohapatra G, Feuerstein BG, Bishop JM: Targeted expression of MYCN causes neuroblastoma in transgenic mice. EMBO J 1997; 16(11) 2985-2995.

[27] Zhu S, Lee JS, Guo F, Shin J, Perez-Atayde AR, Kutok JL, Rodig SJ, Neuberg DS, Helman D, Feng H *et al*: Activated ALK collaborates with MYCN in neuroblastoma pathogenesis. Cancer cell 2012; 21(3) 362-373.

[28] Woodhoo A, Sommer L: Development of the Schwann cell lineage: from the neural crest to the myelinated nerve. Glia 2008; 56(14) 1481-1490.

[29] Paratore C, Goerich DE, Suter U, Wegner M, Sommer L: Survival and glial fate acquisition of neural crest cells are regulated by an interplay between the transcription factor Sox10 and extrinsic combinatorial signaling. Development 2001; 128(20) 3949-3961.

[30] Bremer M, Frob F, Kichko T, Reeh P, Tamm ER, Suter U, Wegner M: Sox10 is required for Schwann-cell homeostasis and myelin maintenance in the adult peripheral nerve. Glia 2011; 59(7) 1022-1032.

[31] Finzsch M, Schreiner S, Kichko T, Reeh P, Tamm ER, Bosl MR, Meijer D, Wegner M: Sox10 is required for Schwann cell identity and progression beyond the immature Schwann cell stage. J Cell Biol 2010; 189(4) 701-712.

[32] Britsch S, Goerich DE, Riethmacher D, Peirano RI, Rossner M, Nave KA, Birchmeier C, Wegner M: The transcription factor Sox10 is a key regulator of peripheral glial development. Genes Dev 2001; 15(1) 66-78.

[33] Garratt AN, Voiculescu O, Topilko P, Charnay P, Birchmeier C: A dual role of erbB2 in myelination and in expansion of the schwann cell precursor pool. J Cell Biol 2000; 148(5) 1035-1046.

[34] Birchmeier C: ErbB receptors and the development of the nervous system. Exp Cell Res 2009; 315(4) 611-618.

[35] Britsch S, Li L, Kirchhoff S, Theuring F, Brinkmann V, Birchmeier C, Riethmacher D: The ErbB2 and ErbB3 receptors and their ligand, neuregulin-1, are essential for development of the sympathetic nervous system. Genes Dev 1998; 12(12) 1825-1836.

[36] Meyer D, Yamaai T, Garratt A, Riethmacher-Sonnenberg E, Kane D, Theill LE, Birchmeier C: Isoform-specific expression and function of neuregulin. Development 1997; 124(18) 3575-3586.

[37] Davies AM: Paracrine and autocrine actions of neurotrophic factors. Neurochem Res 1996; 21(7) 749-753.

[38] Benninger Y, Thurnherr T, Pereira JA, Krause S, Wu X, Chrostek-Grashoff A, Herzog D, Nave KA, Franklin RJ, Meijer D *et al*: Essential and distinct roles for cdc42 and rac1 in the regulation of Schwann cell biology during peripheral nervous system development. J Cell Biol 2007; 177(6) 1051-1061.

[39] Nodari A, Zambroni D, Quattrini A, Court FA, D'Urso A, Recchia A, Tybulewicz VL, Wrabetz L, Feltri ML: Beta1 integrin activates Rac1 in Schwann cells to generate radial lamellae during axonal sorting and myelination. J Cell Biol 2007; 177(6) 1063-1075.

[40] Morrissey TK, Levi AD, Nuijens A, Sliwkowski MX, Bunge RP: Axon-induced mitogenesis of human Schwann cells involves heregulin and p185erbB2. Proc Natl Acad Sci U S A 1995; 92(5) 1431-1435.

[41] Guenard V, Rosenbaum T, Gwynn LA, Doetschman T, Ratner N, Wood PM: Effect of transforming growth factor-beta 1 and -beta 2 on Schwann cell proliferation on neurites. Glia 1995; 13(4) 309-318.

[42] Ridley AJ, Davis JB, Stroobant P, Land H: Transforming growth factors-beta 1 and beta 2 are mitogens for rat Schwann cells. J Cell Biol 1989; 109(6 Pt 2) 3419-3424.

[43] Yang D, Bierman J, Tarumi YS, Zhong YP, Rangwala R, Proctor TM, Miyagoe-Suzuki Y, Takeda S, Miner JH, Sherman LS *et al*: Coordinate control of axon defasciculation and myelination by laminin-2 and -8. J Cell Biol 2005; 168(4) 655-666.

[44] Yu WM, Feltri ML, Wrabetz L, Strickland S, Chen ZL: Schwann cell-specific ablation of laminin gamma1 causes apoptosis and prevents proliferation. J Neurosci 2005; 25(18) 4463-4472.

[45] Jessen KR, Mirsky R, Salzer J: Introduction. Schwann cell biology. Glia 2008; 56(14) 1479-1480.

[46] Riethmacher D, Sonnenberg-Riethmacher E, Brinkmann V, Yamaai T, Lewin GR, Birchmeier C: Severe neuropathies in mice with targeted mutations in the ErbB3 receptor. Nature 1997; 389(6652) 725-730.

[47] Davies AM: Neuronal survival: early dependence on Schwann cells. Curr Biol 1998; 8(1) R15-18.

[48] Molenaar WM, Baker DL, Pleasure D, Lee VM, Trojanowski JQ: The neuroendocrine and neural profiles of neuroblastomas, ganglioneuroblastomas, and ganglioneuromas. Am J Pathol 1990; 136(2) 375-382.

[49] Shimada H, Stram DO, Chatten J, Joshi VV, Hachitanda Y, Brodeur GM, Lukens JN, Matthay KK, Seeger RC: Identification of subsets of neuroblastomas by combined histopathologic and N-myc analysis. J Natl Cancer Inst 1995; 87(19) 1470-1476.

[50] Goto S, Umehara S, Gerbing RB, Stram DO, Brodeur GM, Seeger RC, Lukens JN, Matthay KK, Shimada H: Histopathology (International Neuroblastoma Pathology Classification) and MYCN status in patients with peripheral neuroblastic tumors: a report from the Children's Cancer Group. Cancer 2001; 92(10) 2699-2708.

[51] Negroni A, Scarpa S, Romeo A, Ferrari S, Modesti A, Raschella G: Decrease of proliferation rate and induction of differentiation by a MYCN antisense DNA oligomer in a human neuroblastoma cell line. Cell Growth Differ 1991; 2(10) 511-518.

[52] Kang JH, Rychahou PG, Ishola TA, Qiao J, Evers BM, Chung DH: MYCN silencing induces differentiation and apoptosis in human neuroblastoma cells. Biochem Biophys Res Commun 2006; 351(1) 192-197.

[53] Nara K, Kusafuka T, Yoneda A, Oue T, Sangkhathat S, Fukuzawa M: Silencing of MYCN by RNA interference induces growth inhibition, apoptotic activity and cell differentiation in a neuroblastoma cell line with MYCN amplification. Int J Oncol 2007; 30(5) 1189-1196.

[54] Spengler BA, Lazarova DL, Ross RA, Biedler JL: Cell lineage and differentiation state are primary determinants of MYCN gene expression and malignant potential in human neuroblastoma cells. Oncol Res 1997; 9(9) 467-476.

[55] Yan X, Kennedy CR, Tilkens SB, Wiedemeier O, Guan H, Park JI, Chan AM: Cooperative Cross-Talk between Neuroblastoma Subtypes Confers Resistance to Anaplastic Lymphoma Kinase Inhibition. Genes Cancer 2011; 2(5) 538-549.

[56] Alam G, Cui H, Shi H, Yang L, Ding J, Mao L, Maltese WA, Ding HF: MYCN promotes the expansion of Phox2B-positive neuronal progenitors to drive neuroblastoma development. Am J Pathol 2009; 175(2) 856-866.

[57] Edsjo A, Nilsson H, Vandesompele J, Karlsson J, Pattyn F, Culp LA, Speleman F, Pahlman S: Neuroblastoma cells with overexpressed MYCN retain their capacity to undergo neuronal differentiation. Lab Invest 2004; 84(4) 406-417.

[58] Dimitroulakos J, Squire J, Pawlin G, Yeger H: NUB-7: a stable I-type human neuroblastoma cell line inducible along N- and S-type cell lineages. Cell Growth Differ 1994; 5(4) 373-384.

[59] Mora J, Cheung NK, Juan G, Illei P, Cheung I, Akram M, Chi S, Ladanyi M, Cordon-Cardo C, Gerald WL: Neuroblastic and Schwannian stromal cells of neuroblastoma are derived from a tumoral progenitor cell. Cancer Res 2001; 61(18) 6892-6898.

[60] Ambros IM, Zellner A, Roald B, Amann G, Ladenstein R, Printz D, Gadner H, Ambros PF: Role of ploidy, chromosome 1p, and Schwann cells in the maturation of neuroblastoma. N Engl J Med 1996; 334(23) 1505-1511.

[61] Mora J, Akram M, Cheung NK, Chen L, Gerald WL: Laser-capture microdissected schwannian and neuroblastic cells in stage 4 neuroblastomas have the same genetic alterations. Med Pediatr Oncol 2000; 35(6) 534-537.

[62] Valent A, Benard J, Venuat AM, Silva J, Duverger A, Duarte N, Hartmann O, Spengler BA, Bernheim A: Phenotypic and genotypic diversity of human neuroblastoma studied in three IGR cell line models derived from bone marrow metastases. Cancer Genet Cytogenet 1999; 112(2) 124-129.

[63] Ciccarone V, Spengler BA, Meyers MB, Biedler JL, Ross RA: Phenotypic diversification in human neuroblastoma cells: expression of distinct neural crest lineages. Cancer Res 1989; 49(1) 219-225.

[64] Ambros IM, Attarbaschi A, Rumpler S, Luegmayr A, Turkof E, Gadner H, Ambros PF: Neuroblastoma cells provoke Schwann cell proliferation in vitro. Med Pediatr Oncol 2001; 36(1) 163-168.

[65] Kwiatkowski JL, Rutkowski JL, Yamashiro DJ, Tennekoon GI, Brodeur GM: Schwann cell-conditioned medium promotes neuroblastoma survival and differentiation. Cancer Res 1998; 58(20) 4602-4606.

[66] Wagner JA, Kostyk SK: Regulation of neural cell survival and differentiation by peptide growth factors. Curr Opin Cell Biol 1990; 2(6) 1050-1057.

[67] Huang D, Rutkowski JL, Brodeur GM, Chou PM, Kwiatkowski JL, Babbo A, Cohn SL: Schwann cell-conditioned medium inhibits angiogenesis. Cancer Res 2000; 60(21) 5966-5971.

[68] Crawford SE, Stellmach V, Ranalli M, Huang X, Huang L, Volpert O, De Vries GH, Abramson LP, Bouck N: Pigment epithelium-derived factor (PEDF) in neuroblastoma: a multifunctional mediator of Schwann cell antitumor activity. J Cell Sci 2001; 114(Pt 24) 4421-4428.

[69] Chlenski A, Liu S, Crawford SE, Volpert OV, DeVries GH, Evangelista A, Yang Q, Salwen HR, Farrer R, Bray J *et al*: SPARC is a key Schwannian-derived inhibitor controlling neuroblastoma tumor angiogenesis. Cancer Res 2002; 62(24) 7357-7363.

[70] Seo DW, Li H, Guedez L, Wingfield PT, Diaz T, Salloum R, Wei BY, Stetler-Stevenson WG: TIMP-2 mediated inhibition of angiogenesis: an MMP-independent mechanism. Cell 2003; 114(2) 171-180.

[71] Filleur S, Nelius T, de Riese W, Kennedy RC: Characterization of PEDF: a multi-functional serpin family protein. J Cell Biochem 2009; 106(5) 769-775.

[72] Notari L, Baladron V, Aroca-Aguilar JD, Balko N, Heredia R, Meyer C, Notario PM, Saravanamuthu S, Nueda ML, Sanchez-Sanchez F *et al*: Identification of a lipase-linked cell membrane receptor for pigment epithelium-derived factor. J Biol Chem 2006; 281(49) 38022-38037.

[73] Manalo KB, Choong PF, Dass CR: Pigment epithelium-derived factor as an impending therapeutic agent against vascular epithelial growth factor-driven tumor-angiogenesis. Mol Carcinog 2011; 50(2) 67-72.

[74] Nagaraju GP, Sharma D: Anti-cancer role of SPARC, an inhibitor of adipogenesis. Cancer Treat Rev 2011; 37(7) 559-566.

[75] Kzhyshkowska J, Gratchev A, Goerdt S: Stabilin-1, a homeostatic scavenger receptor with multiple functions. J Cell Mol Med 2006; 10(3) 635-649.

[76] Byzova T: Integrins in bone recognition and metastasis. J Musculoskelet Neuronal Interact 2004; 4(4) 374.

[77] Raines EW, Lane TF, Iruela-Arispe ML, Ross R, Sage EH: The extracellular glycoprotein SPARC interacts with platelet-derived growth factor (PDGF)-AB and -BB and in-

hibits the binding of PDGF to its receptors. Proc Natl Acad Sci U S A 1992; 89(4) 1281-1285.

[78] Kupprion C, Motamed K, Sage EH: SPARC (BM-40, osteonectin) inhibits the mitogenic effect of vascular endothelial growth factor on microvascular endothelial cells. J Biol Chem 1998; 273(45) 29635-29640.

[79] Liu S, Tian Y, Chlenski A, Yang Q, Salwen HR, Cohn SL: 'Cross-talk' between Schwannian stroma and neuroblasts promotes neuroblastoma tumor differentiation and inhibits angiogenesis. Cancer Lett 2005; 228(1-2) 125-131.

[80] Orimo A, Gupta PB, Sgroi DC, Arenzana-Seisdedos F, Delaunay T, Naeem R, Carey VJ, Richardson AL, Weinberg RA: Stromal fibroblasts present in invasive human breast carcinomas promote tumor growth and angiogenesis through elevated SDF-1/CXCL12 secretion. Cell 2005; 121(3) 335-348.

[81] Nyberg P, Salo T, Kalluri R: Tumor microenvironment and angiogenesis. Front Biosci 2008; 13 6537-6553.

[82] Orimo A, Weinberg RA: Stromal fibroblasts in cancer: a novel tumor-promoting cell type. Cell Cycle 2006; 5(15) 1597-1601.

[83] Zeine R, Salwen HR, Peddinti R, Tian Y, Guerrero L, Yang Q, Chlenski A, Cohn SL: Presence of cancer-associated fibroblasts inversely correlates with Schwannian stroma in neuroblastoma tumors. Mod Pathol 2009; 22(7) 950-958.

[84] Cuiffo BG, Karnoub AE: Mesenchymal stem cells in tumor development: Emerging roles and concepts. Cell Adh Migr 2012; 6(3) 220-230.

[85] Karnoub AE, Dash AB, Vo AP, Sullivan A, Brooks MW, Bell GW, Richardson AL, Polyak K, Tubo R, Weinberg RA: Mesenchymal stem cells within tumour stroma promote breast cancer metastasis. Nature 2007; 449(7162) 557-563.

[86] Du W, Hozumi N, Sakamoto M, Hata J, Yamada T: Reconstitution of Schwannian stroma in neuroblastomas using human bone marrow stromal cells. Am J Pathol 2008; 173(4) 1153-1164.

[87] Mishra PJ, Humeniuk R, Medina DJ, Alexe G, Mesirov JP, Ganesan S, Glod JW, Banerjee D: Carcinoma-associated fibroblast-like differentiation of human mesenchymal stem cells. Cancer Res 2008; 68(11) 4331-4339.

[88] Ara T, DeClerck YA: Mechanisms of invasion and metastasis in human neuroblastoma. Cancer Metastasis Rev 2006; 25(4) 645-657.

[89] Geminder H, Sagi-Assif O, Goldberg L, Meshel T, Rechavi G, Witz IP, Ben-Baruch A: A possible role for CXCR4 and its ligand, the CXC chemokine stromal cell-derived factor-1, in the development of bone marrow metastases in neuroblastoma. J Immunol 2001; 167(8) 4747-4757.

[90] Real C, Glavieux-Pardanaud C, Vaigot P, Le-Douarin N, Dupin E: The instability of the neural crest phenotypes: Schwann cells can differentiate into myofibroblasts. Int J Dev Biol 2005; 49(2-3) 151-159.

[91] Ross RA, Spengler BA, Domenech C, Porubcin M, Rettig WJ, Biedler JL: Human neuroblastoma I-type cells are malignant neural crest stem cells. Cell Growth Differ 1995; 6(4) 449-456.

[92] Sugimoto T, Kato T, Sawada T, Horii Y, Kemshead JT, Hino T, Morioka H, Hosoi H: Schwannian cell differentiation of human neuroblastoma cell lines in vitro induced by bromodeoxyuridine. Cancer Res 1988; 48(9) 2531-2537.

[93] Masetti R, Biagi C, Zama D, Vendemini F, Martoni A, Morello W, Gasperini P, Pession A: Retinoids in Pediatric Onco-Hematology: the Model of Acute Promyelocytic Leukemia and Neuroblastoma. Adv Ther 2012.

[94] Wagner LM, Danks MK: New therapeutic targets for the treatment of high-risk neuroblastoma. J Cell Biochem 2009; 107(1) 46-57.

[95] Zage PE, Kletzel M, Murray K, Marcus R, Castleberry R, Zhang Y, London WB, Kretschmar C: Outcomes of the POG 9340/9341/9342 trials for children with high-risk neuroblastoma: a report from the Children's Oncology Group. Pediatr Blood Cancer 2008; 51(6) 747-753.

[96] Dextraze ME, Wagner JR, Hunting DJ: 5-Bromodeoxyuridine radiosensitization: conformation-dependent DNA damage. Biochemistry 2007; 46(31) 9089-9097.

[97] Berry SE, Kinsella TJ: Targeting DNA mismatch repair for radiosensitization. Semin Radiat Oncol 2001; 11(4) 300-315.

[98] Dickson PV, Hamner JB, Sims TL, Fraga CH, Ng CY, Rajasekeran S, Hagedorn NL, McCarville MB, Stewart CF, Davidoff AM: Bevacizumab-induced transient remodeling of the vasculature in neuroblastoma xenografts results in improved delivery and efficacy of systemically administered chemotherapy. Clin Cancer Res 2007; 13(13) 3942-3950.

[99] de Pasquale MD, Castellano A, de Sio L, de Laurentis C, Mastronuzzi A, Serra A, Cozza R, Jenkner A, de Ioris MA: Bevacizumab in pediatric patients: how safe is it? Anticancer Res 2011; 31(11) 3953-3957.

[100] Ek ET, Dass CR, Choong PF: PEDF: a potential molecular therapeutic target with multiple anti-cancer activities. Trends Mol Med 2006; 12(10) 497-502.

[101] Hoshina D, Abe R, Yamagishi SI, Shimizu H: The role of PEDF in tumor growth and metastasis. Curr Mol Med 2010; 10(3) 292-295.

[102] Streck CJ, Zhang Y, Zhou J, Ng C, Nathwani AC, Davidoff AM: Adeno-associated virus vector-mediated delivery of pigment epithelium-derived factor restricts neuroblastoma angiogenesis and growth. J Pediatr Surg 2005; 40(1) 236-243.

[103] Napoli I, Noon LA, Ribeiro S, Kerai AP, Parrinello S, Rosenberg LH, Collins MJ, Harrisingh MC, White IJ, Woodhoo A *et al*: A central role for the ERK-signaling pathway in controlling Schwann cell plasticity and peripheral nerve regeneration in vivo. Neuron 2012; 73(4) 729-742.

[104] Dvorak HF: Tumors: wounds that do not heal. Similarities between tumor stroma generation and wound healing. The New England journal of medicine 1986; 315(26) 1650-1659.

[105] Dvorak HF, Weaver VM, Tlsty TD, Bergers G: Tumor microenvironment and progression. Journal of Surgical Oncology 2011; 103(6) 468-474.

[106] Paszek MJ, Zahir N, Johnson KR, Lakins JN, Rozenberg GI, Gefen A, Reinhart-King CA, Margulies SS, Dembo M, Boettiger D *et al*: Tensional homeostasis and the malignant phenotype. Cancer Cell 2005; 8(3) 241-254.

[107] Lam WA, Cao L, Umesh V, Keung AJ, Sen S, Kumar S: Extracellular matrix rigidity modulates neuroblastoma cell differentiation and N-myc expression. Molecular Cancer 2010; 9.

[108] Yan Q, Sage EH: SPARC, a matricellular glycoprotein with important biological functions. Journal of Histochemistry and Cytochemistry 1999; 47(12) 1495-1505.

[109] Chlenski A, Cohn SL: Modulation of matrix remodeling by SPARC in neoplastic progression. Seminars in Cell and Developmental Biology 2010; 21(1) 55-65.

[110] De S, Chen J, Narizhneva NV, Heston W, Brainard J, Sage EH, Byzova TV: Molecular Pathway for Cancer Metastasis to Bone. J Biol Chem 2003; 278(40) 39044-39050.

[111] Tai IT, Dai M, Owen DA, Chen LB: Genome-wide expression analysis of therapy-resistant tumors reveals SPARC as a novel target for cancer therapy. Journal of Clinical Investigation 2005; 115(6) 1492-1502.

[112] Bhoopathi P, Gorantla B, Sailaja GS, Gondi CS, Gujrati M, Klopfenstein JD, Rao JS: SPARC overexpression inhibits cell proliferation in neuroblastoma and is partly mediated by tumor suppressor protein PTEN and AKT. PLoS ONE 2012; 7(5).

[113] Gorantla B, Bhoopathi P, Chetty C, Gogineni VR, Sailaja GS, Gondi CS, Rao JS: Notch signaling regulates tumor-induced angiogenesis in SPARC-overexpressed neuroblastoma. Angiogenesis 2012 1-16.

[114] Perez-Moreno M, Fuchs E: Catenins: keeping cells from getting their signals crossed. Dev Cell 2006; 11(5) 601-612.

[115] Mesnil M: Connexins and cancer. Biol Cell 2002; 94(7-8) 493-500.

[116] Mariotti A, Perotti A, Sessa C, Ruegg C: N-cadherin as a therapeutic target in cancer. Expert Opin Investig Drugs 2007; 16(4) 451-465.

[117] Hirschi KK, Xu CE, Tsukamoto T, Sager R: Gap junction genes Cx26 and Cx43 individually suppress the cancer phenotype of human mammary carcinoma cells and restore differentiation potential. Cell Growth Differ 1996; 7(7) 861-870.

[118] Jimenez T, Fox WP, Naus CCG, Galipeau J, Belliveau DJ: Connexin over-expression differentially suppresses glioma growth and contributes to the bystander effect following HSV-thymidine kinase gene therapy. Cell Communication and Adhesion 2006; 13(1-2) 79-92.

[119] Yamasaki H, Omori Y, Krutovskikh V, Zhu W, Mironov N, Yamakage K, Mesnil M: Connexins in tumour suppression and cancer therapy. Novartis Foundation Symposium 1999; 219 241-260.

[120] Gumbiner BM: Cell adhesion: The molecular basis of tissue architecture and morphogenesis. Cell 1996; 84(3) 345-357.

[121] Charalabopoulos K, Binolis J, Karkabounas S: Adhesion molecules in carcinogenesis. Experimental Oncology 2002; 24(4) 249-257.

[122] Takeichi M: Cadherins: A molecular family important in selective cell-cell adhesion. Annual Review of Biochemistry 1990; 59 237-252.

[123] Mühlenhoff M, Oltmann-Norden I, Weinhold B, Hildebrandt H, Gerardy-Schahn R: Brain development needs sugar: The role of polysialic acid in controlling NCAM functions. Biological Chemistry 2009; 390(7) 567-574.

[124] Seidenfaden R, Krauter A, Hildebrandt H: The neural cell adhesion molecule NCAM regulates neuritogenesis by multiple mechanisms of interaction. Neurochemistry International 2006; 49(1) 1-11.

[125] Yoon KJ, Danks MK: Cell adhesion molecules as targets for therapy of neuroblastoma. Cancer Biology and Therapy 2009; 8(4) 306-311.

[126] Cavallaro U, Schaffhauser B, Christofori G: Cadherins and the tumour progression: Is it all in a switch? Cancer Letters 2002; 176(2) 123-128.

[127] Vleminckx K, Vakaet Jr L, Mareel M, Fiers W, Van Roy F: Genetic manipulation of E-cadherin expression by epithelial tumor cells reveals an invasion suppressor role. Cell 1991; 66(1) 107-119.

[128] Lipschutz JH, Kissil JL: Expression of β-catenin and γ-catenin in epithelial tumor cell lines and characterization of a unique cell line. Cancer Letters 1998; 126(1) 33-41.

[129] Ghadimi BM, Behrens J, Hoffmann I, Haensch W, Birchmeier W, Schlag PM: Immunohistological analysis of E-cadherin, α-, β- and γ-catenin expression in colorectal cancer: Implications for cell adhesion and signaling. European Journal of Cancer 1999; 35(1) 60-65.

[130] Mariotti A, Perotti A, Sessa C, Rüegg C: N-cadherin as a therapeutic target in cancer. Expert Opinion on Investigational Drugs 2007; 16(4) 451-465.

[131] Li G, Satyamoorthy K, Herlyn M: N-cadherin-mediated intercellular interactions promote survival and migration of melanoma cells. Cancer Research 2001; 61(9) 3819-3825.

[132] Hazan RB, Phillips GR, Qiao RF, Norton L, Aaronson SA: Exogenous expression of N-cadherin in breast cancer cells induces cell migration, invasion, and metastasis. Journal of Cell Biology 2000; 148(4) 779-790.

[133] Tran NL, Nagle RB, Cress AE, Heimark RL: N-cadherin expression in human prostate carcinoma cell lines: An epithelial-mesenchymal transformation mediating adhesion with stromal cells. American Journal of Pathology 1999; 155(3) 787-798.

[134] Lammens T, Swerts K, Derycke L, de Craemer A, de Brouwer S, de Preter K, van Roy N, Vandesompele J, Speleman F, Philippé J *et al*: N-Cadherin in neuroblastoma disease: Expression and clinical significance. PLoS ONE 2012; 7(2).

[135] Jossin Y: Neuronal migration and the role of Reelin during early development of the cerebral cortex. Molecular Neurobiology 2004; 30(3) 225-251.

[136] D'Arcangelo G, Miao GG, Chen SC, Soares HD, Morgan JI, Curran T: A protein related to extracellular matrix proteins deleted in the mouse mutant reeler. Nature 1995; 374(6524) 719-723.

[137] Benhayon D, Magdaleno S, Curran T: Binding of purified Reelin to ApoER2 and VLDLR mediates tyrosine phosphorylation of Disabled-1. Molecular Brain Research 2003; 112(1-2) 33-45.

[138] Trommsdorff M, Gotthardt M, Hiesberger T, Shelton J, Stockinger W, Nimpf J, Hammer RE, Richardson JA, Herz J: Reeler/disabled-like disruption of neuronal migration in knockout mice lacking the VLDL receptor and ApoE receptor 2. Cell 1999; 97(6) 689-701.

[139] Ballif BA, Arnaud L, Arthur WT, Guris D, Imamoto A, Cooper JA: Activation of a Dab1/CrkL/C3G/Rap1 pathway in Reelin-stimulated neurons. Current Biology 2004; 14(7) 606-610.

[140] Jossin Y, Cooper JA: Reelin, Rap1 and N-cadherin orient the migration of multipolar neurons in the developing neocortex. Nature Neuroscience 2011; 14(6) 697-U289.

[141] Taniguchi H, Kawauchi D, Nishida K, Murakami F: Classic cadherins regulate tangential migration of precerebellar neurons in the caudal hindbrain. Development 2006; 133(10) 1923-1931.

[142] Rieger S, Senghaas N, Walch A, Köster RW: Cadherin-2 controls directional chain migration of cerebellar granule neurons. PLoS biology 2009; 7(11).

[143] Yang X, Chrisman H, Weijer CJ: PDGF signalling controls the migration of mesoderm cells during chick gastrulation by regulating N-cadherin expression. Development 2008; 135(21) 3521-3530.

[144] Perrone G, Vincenzi B, Zagami M, Santini D, Panteri R, Flammia G, Verzi A, Lepanto D, Morini S, Russo A *et al*: Reelin expression in human prostate cancer: a marker of tumor aggressiveness based on correlation with grade. Mod Pathol 2007; 20(3) 344-351.

[145] Becker J, Fröhlich J, Perske C, Pavlakovic H, Wilting J: Reelin signalling in neuroblastoma: Migratory switch in metastatic stages. International Journal of Oncology 2012; 41(2) 681-689.

[146] Brodeur GM, Seeger RC, Barrett A, Castleberry RP, D'Angio G, De Bernardi B, Evans AE, Favrot M, Freeman AI, Haase G *et al*: International criteria for diagnosis, staging and response to treatment in patients with neuroblastoma. Prog Clin Biol Res 1988; 271 509-524.

[147] Söhl G, Willecke K: An update on connexin genes and their nomenclature in mouse and man. Cell Communication and Adhesion 2003; 10(4-6) 173-180.

[148] Morley M, Jones C, Sidhu M, Gupta V, Bernier SM, Rushlow WJ, Belliveau DJ: PKC inhibition increases gap junction intercellular communication and cell adhesion in human neuroblastoma. Cell and Tissue Research 2010; 340(2) 229-242.

[149] Mandlekar S, Kong ANT: Mechanisms of tamoxifen-induced apoptosis. Apoptosis 2001; 6(6) 469-477.

[150] Rohlff C, Blagosklonny MV, Kyle E, Kesari A, Kim IY, Zelner DJ, Hakim F, Trepel J, Bergan RC: Prostate cancer cell growth inhibition by tamoxifen is associated with inhibition of protein kinase C and induction of p21(waf1/cip1). Prostate 1998; 37(1) 51-59.

[151] Folkman MJ, Long DM, Jr., Becker FF: Tumor growth in organ culture. Surgical forum 1962; 13 81-83.

[152] Chung AS, Lee J, Ferrara N: Targeting the tumour vasculature: insights from physiological angiogenesis. Nature reviews Cancer 2010; 10(7) 505-514.

[153] Pistoia V, Bianchi G, Borgonovo G, Raffaghello L: Cytokines in neuroblastoma: from pathogenesis to treatment. Immunotherapy 2011; 3(7) 895-907.

[154] Nagy JA, Chang SH, Shih SC, Dvorak AM, Dvorak HF: Heterogeneity of the tumor vasculature. Semin Thromb Hemost 2010; 36(3) 321-331.

[155] Jayson GC, Hicklin DJ, Ellis LM: Antiangiogenic therapy--evolving view based on clinical trial results. Nature reviews Clinical oncology 2012; 9(5) 297-303.

[156] Albini A, Tosetti F, Li VW, Noonan DM, Li WW: Cancer prevention by targeting angiogenesis. Nature reviews Clinical oncology 2012; 9(9) 498-509.

[157] Lyons J, 3rd, Anthony CT, Woltering EA: The role of angiogenesis in neuroendocrine tumors. Endocrinology and metabolism clinics of North America 2010; 39(4) 839-852.

[158] Roy Choudhury S, Karmakar S, Banik NL, Ray SK: Targeting angiogenesis for controlling neuroblastoma. Journal of oncology 2012; 2012 782020.

[159] Rossler J, Taylor M, Geoerger B, Farace F, Lagodny J, Peschka-Suss R, Niemeyer CM, Vassal G: Angiogenesis as a target in neuroblastoma. Eur J Cancer 2008; 44(12) 1645-1656.

[160] Meitar D, Crawford SE, Rademaker AW, Cohn SL: Tumor angiogenesis correlates with metastatic disease, N-myc amplification, and poor outcome in human neuroblastoma. Journal of clinical oncology : official journal of the American Society of Clinical Oncology 1996; 14(2) 405-414.

[161] Eggert A, Ikegaki N, Kwiatkowski J, Zhao H, Brodeur GM, Himelstein BP: High-level expression of angiogenic factors is associated with advanced tumor stage in human neuroblastomas. Clinical cancer research : an official journal of the American Association for Cancer Research 2000; 6(5) 1900-1908.

[162] Ribatti D, Alessandri G, Vacca A, Iurlaro M, Ponzoni M: Human neuroblastoma cells produce extracellular matrix-degrading enzymes, induce endothelial cell proliferation and are angiogenic in vivo. International journal of cancer Journal international du cancer 1998; 77(3) 449-454.

[163] Erdreich-Epstein A, Shimada H, Groshen S, Liu M, Metelitsa LS, Kim KS, Stins MF, Seeger RC, Durden DL: Integrins alpha(v)beta3 and alpha(v)beta5 are expressed by endothelium of high-risk neuroblastoma and their inhibition is associated with increased endogenous ceramide. Cancer research 2000; 60(3) 712-721.

[164] Lagodny J, Juttner E, Kayser G, Niemeyer CM, Rossler J: Lymphangiogenesis and its regulation in human neuroblastoma. Biochemical and biophysical research communications 2007; 352(2) 571-577.

[165] Schwab M, Westermann F, Hero B, Berthold F: Neuroblastoma: biology and molecular and chromosomal pathology. The lancet oncology 2003; 4(8) 472-480.

[166] Maris JM: The biologic basis for neuroblastoma heterogeneity and risk stratification. Current opinion in pediatrics 2005; 17(1) 7-13.

[167] Westermann F, Muth D, Benner A, Bauer T, Henrich KO, Oberthuer A, Brors B, Beissbarth T, Vandesompele J, Pattyn F *et al*: Distinct transcriptional MYCN/c-MYC activities are associated with spontaneous regression or malignant progression in neuroblastomas. Genome biology 2008; 9(10) R150.

[168] Bell E, Chen L, Liu T, Marshall GM, Lunec J, Tweddle DA: MYCN oncoprotein targets and their therapeutic potential. Cancer letters 2010; 293(2) 144-157.

[169] Fotsis T, Breit S, Lutz W, Rossler J, Hatzi E, Schwab M, Schweigerer L: Down-regulation of endothelial cell growth inhibitors by enhanced MYCN oncogene expression in human neuroblastoma cells. European journal of biochemistry / FEBS 1999; 263(3) 757-764.

[170] Hatzi E, Murphy C, Zoephel A, Ahorn H, Tontsch U, Bamberger AM, Yamauchi-Takihara K, Schweigerer L, Fotsis T: N-myc oncogene overexpression down-regulates leukemia inhibitory factor in neuroblastoma. European journal of biochemistry / FEBS 2002; 269(15) 3732-3741.

[171] Breit S, Ashman K, Wilting J, Rossler J, Hatzi E, Fotsis T, Schweigerer L: The N-myc oncogene in human neuroblastoma cells: down-regulation of an angiogenesis inhibitor identified as activin A. Cancer research 2000; 60(16) 4596-4601.

[172] Hatzi E, Breit S, Zoephel A, Ashman K, Tontsch U, Ahorn H, Murphy C, Schweigerer L, Fotsis T: MYCN oncogene and angiogenesis: down-regulation of endothelial growth inhibitors in human neuroblastoma cells. Purification, structural, and functional characterization. Advances in experimental medicine and biology 2000; 476 239-248.

[173] Schramm A, von Schuetz V, Christiansen H, Havers W, Papoutsi M, Wilting J, Schweigerer L: High activin A-expression in human neuroblastoma: suppression of malignant potential and correlation with favourable clinical outcome. Oncogene 2005; 24(4) 680-687.

[174] Chanthery YH, Gustafson WC, Itsara M, Persson A, Hackett CS, Grimmer M, Charron E, Yakovenko S, Kim G, Matthay KK *et al*: Paracrine signaling through MYCN enhances tumor-vascular interactions in neuroblastoma. Science translational medicine 2012; 4(115) 115ra113.

[175] Westermark UK, Wilhelm M, Frenzel A, Henriksson MA: The MYCN oncogene and differentiation in neuroblastoma. Seminars in cancer biology 2011; 21(4) 256-266.

[176] Pinon LG, Minichiello L, Klein R, Davies AM: Timing of neuronal death in trkA, trkB and trkC mutant embryos reveals developmental changes in sensory neuron dependence on Trk signalling. Development 1996; 122(10) 3255-3261.

[177] Eggert A, Grotzer MA, Ikegaki N, Liu XG, Evans AE, Brodeur GM: Expression of the neurotrophin receptor TrkA down-regulates expression and function of angiogenic stimulators in SH-SY5Y neuroblastoma cells. Cancer research 2002; 62(6) 1802-1808.

[178] Segerstrom L, Fuchs D, Backman U, Holmquist K, Christofferson R, Azarbayjani F: The anti-VEGF antibody bevacizumab potently reduces the growth rate of high-risk neuroblastoma xenografts. Pediatric research 2006; 60(5) 576-581.

[179] Backman U, Svensson A, Christofferson R: Importance of vascular endothelial growth factor A in the progression of experimental neuroblastoma. Angiogenesis 2002; 5(4) 267-274.

[180] Gong H, Pottgen C, Stuben G, Havers W, Stuschke M, Schweigerer L: Arginine deiminase and other antiangiogenic agents inhibit unfavorable neuroblastoma growth: potentiation by irradiation. International journal of cancer Journal international du cancer 2003; 106(5) 723-728.

[181] Svensson A, Backman U, Jonsson E, Larsson R, Christofferson R: CHS 828 inhibits neuroblastoma growth in mice alone and in combination with antiangiogenic drugs. Pediatric research 2002; 51(5) 607-611.

[182] Ribatti D, Ponzoni M: Antiangiogenic strategies in neuroblastoma. Cancer treatment reviews 2005; 31(1) 27-34.

[183] Yin SQ, Wang JJ, Zhang CM, Liu ZP: The development of MetAP-2 inhibitors in cancer treatment. Curr Med Chem 2012; 19(7) 1021-1035.

[184] Wassberg E, Pahlman S, Westlin JE, Christofferson R: The angiogenesis inhibitor TNP-470 reduces the growth rate of human neuroblastoma in nude rats. Pediatric research 1997; 41(3) 327-333.

[185] Nagabuchi E, VanderKolk WE, Une Y, Ziegler MM: TNP-470 antiangiogenic therapy for advanced murine neuroblastoma. Journal of pediatric surgery 1997; 32(2) 287-293.

[186] Yoshizawa J, Mizuno R, Yoshida T, Hara A, Ashizuka S, Kanai M, Kuwashima N, Kurobe M, Yamazaki Y: Inhibitory effect of TNP-470 on hepatic metastasis of mouse neuroblastoma. The Journal of surgical research 2000; 93(1) 82-87.

[187] Katzenstein HM, Rademaker AW, Senger C, Salwen HR, Nguyen NN, Thorner PS, Litsas L, Cohn SL: Effectiveness of the angiogenesis inhibitor TNP-470 in reducing the growth of human neuroblastoma in nude mice inversely correlates with tumor burden. Clinical cancer research : an official journal of the American Association for Cancer Research 1999; 5(12) 4273-4278.

[188] Shusterman S, Grupp SA, Barr R, Carpentieri D, Zhao H, Maris JM: The angiogenesis inhibitor tnp-470 effectively inhibits human neuroblastoma xenograft growth, especially in the setting of subclinical disease. Clinical cancer research : an official journal of the American Association for Cancer Research 2001; 7(4) 977-984.

[189] Ribatti D, Alessandri G, Baronio M, Raffaghello L, Cosimo E, Marimpietri D, Montaldo PG, De Falco G, Caruso A, Vacca A *et al*: Inhibition of neuroblastoma-induced angiogenesis by fenretinide. International journal of cancer Journal international du cancer 2001; 94(3) 314-321.

[190] Castle VP, Ou X, O'Shea S, Dixit VM: Induction of thrombospondin 1 by retinoic acid is important during differentiation of neuroblastoma cells. The Journal of clinical investigation 1992; 90(5) 1857-1863.

[191] Yang QW, Liu S, Tian Y, Salwen HR, Chlenski A, Weinstein J, Cohn SL: Methylation-associated silencing of the thrombospondin-1 gene in human neuroblastoma. Cancer research 2003; 63(19) 6299-6310.

[192] Yang Q, Tian Y, Liu S, Zeine R, Chlenski A, Salwen HR, Henkin J, Cohn SL: Thrombospondin-1 peptide ABT-510 combined with valproic acid is an effective antiangiogenesis strategy in neuroblastoma. Cancer research 2007; 67(4) 1716-1724.

[193] Gurtner GC, Werner S, Barrandon Y, Longaker MT: Wound repair and regeneration. Nature 2008; 453(7193) 314-321.

[194] Motz GT, Coukos G: The parallel lives of angiogenesis and immunosuppression: cancer and other tales. Nature reviewsImmunology 2011; 11(10) 702-711.

[195] Willenborg S, Lucas T, van Loo G, Knipper JA, Krieg T, Haase I, Brachvogel B, Hammerschmidt M, Nagy A, Ferrara N *et al*: CCR2 recruits an inflammatory macrophage subpopulation critical for angiogenesis in tissue repair. Blood 2012; 120(3) 613-625.

[196] Schiffer JT, Kirby K, Sandmaier B, Storb R, Corey L, Boeckh M: Timing and severity of community acquired respiratory virus infections after myeloablative versus non-myeloablative hematopoietic stem cell transplantation. Haematologica 2009; 94(8) 1101-1108.

[197] Gale DP, Maxwell PH: The role of HIF in immunity. The international journal of biochemistry & cell biology 2010; 42(4) 486-494.

[198] Pietras A, Hansford LM, Johnsson AS, Bridges E, Sjolund J, Gisselsson D, Rehn M, Beckman S, Noguera R, Navarro S *et al*: HIF-2alpha maintains an undifferentiated state in neural crest-like human neuroblastoma tumor-initiating cells. Proceedings of the National Academy of Sciences of the United States of America 2009; 106(39) 16805-16810.

[199] Murdoch C, Muthana M, Coffelt SB, Lewis CE: The role of myeloid cells in the promotion of tumour angiogenesis. Nature reviewsCancer 2008; 8(8) 618-631.

[200] Mosser DM, Edwards JP: Exploring the full spectrum of macrophage activation. Nature reviewsImmunology 2008; 8(12) 958-969.

[201] Gordon S: Alternative activation of macrophages. Nature reviewsImmunology 2003; 3(1) 23-35.

[202] Gordon S, Martinez FO: Alternative activation of macrophages: mechanism and functions. Immunity 2010; 32(5) 593-604.

[203] Hao NB, Lu MH, Fan YH, Cao YL, Zhang ZR, Yang SM: Macrophages in tumor microenvironments and the progression of tumors. Clinical & developmental immunology 2012; 2012(Journal Article) 948098.

[204] Nucera S, Biziato D, De Palma M: The interplay between macrophages and angiogenesis in development, tissue injury and regeneration. The International journal of developmental biology 2011; 55(4-5) 495-503.

[205] De Palma M, Venneri MA, Galli R, Sergi Sergi L, Politi LS, Sampaolesi M, Naldini L: Tie2 identifies a hematopoietic lineage of proangiogenic monocytes required for tumor vessel formation and a mesenchymal population of pericyte progenitors. Cancer cell 2005; 8(3) 211-226.

http://dx.doi.org/10.5772/55486

[206] Venneri MA, De Palma M, Ponzoni M, Pucci F, Scielzo C, Zonari E, Mazzieri R, Doglioni C, Naldini L: Identification of proangiogenic TIE2-expressing monocytes (TEMs) in human peripheral blood and cancer. Blood 2007; 109(12) 5276-5285.

[207] Biswas SK, Sica A, Lewis CE: Plasticity of macrophage function during tumor progression: regulation by distinct molecular mechanisms. Journal of immunology (Baltimore, Md: 1950) 2008; 180(4) 2011-2017.

[208] van Golen KL, Wu ZF, Qiao XT, Bao L, Merajver SD: RhoC GTPase overexpression modulates induction of angiogenic factors in breast cells. Neoplasia (New York, NY) 2000; 2(5) 418-425.

[209] Sidky YA, Borden EC: Inhibition of angiogenesis by interferons: effects on tumor- and lymphocyte-induced vascular responses. Cancer research 1987; 47(19) 5155-5161.

[210] Dikov MM, Ohm JE, Ray N, Tchekneva EE, Burlison J, Moghanaki D, Nadaf S, Carbone DP: Differential roles of vascular endothelial growth factor receptors 1 and 2 in dendritic cell differentiation. Journal of immunology (Baltimore, Md: 1950) 2005; 174(1) 215-222.

[211] Gabrilovich DI, Chen HL, Girgis KR, Cunningham HT, Meny GM, Nadaf S, Kavanaugh D, Carbone DP: Production of vascular endothelial growth factor by human tumors inhibits the functional maturation of dendritic cells. Nature medicine 1996; 2(10) 1096-1103.

[212] Oyama T, Ran S, Ishida T, Nadaf S, Kerr L, Carbone DP, Gabrilovich DI: Vascular endothelial growth factor affects dendritic cell maturation through the inhibition of nuclear factor-kappa B activation in hemopoietic progenitor cells. Journal of immunology (Baltimore, Md: 1950) 1998; 160(3) 1224-1232.

[213] Gabrilovich DI, Ishida T, Nadaf S, Ohm JE, Carbone DP: Antibodies to vascular endothelial growth factor enhance the efficacy of cancer immunotherapy by improving endogenous dendritic cell function. Clinical cancer research : an official journal of the American Association for Cancer Research 1999; 5(10) 2963-2970.

[214] Curiel TJ, Cheng P, Mottram P, Alvarez X, Moons L, Evdemon-Hogan M, Wei S, Zou L, Kryczek I, Hoyle G *et al*: Dendritic cell subsets differentially regulate angiogenesis in human ovarian cancer. Cancer research 2004; 64(16) 5535-5538.

[215] Fainaru O, Almog N, Yung CW, Nakai K, Montoya-Zavala M, Abdollahi A, D'Amato R, Ingber DE: Tumor growth and angiogenesis are dependent on the presence of immature dendritic cells. FASEB journal : official publication of the Federation of American Societies for Experimental Biology 2010; 24(5) 1411-1418.

[216] Conejo-Garcia JR, Buckanovich RJ, Benencia F, Courreges MC, Rubin SC, Carroll RG, Coukos G: Vascular leukocytes contribute to tumor vascularization. Blood 2005; 105(2) 679-681.

[217] Coussens LM, Tinkle CL, Hanahan D, Werb Z: MMP-9 supplied by bone marrow-derived cells contributes to skin carcinogenesis. Cell 2000; 103(3) 481-490.

[218] Mentzel T, Brown LF, Dvorak HF, Kuhnen C, Stiller KJ, Katenkamp D, Fletcher CD: The association between tumour progression and vascularity in myxofibrosarcoma and myxoid/round cell liposarcoma. Virchows Archiv : an international journal of pathology 2001; 438(1) 13-22.

[219] Starkey JR, Crowle PK, Taubenberger S: Mast-cell-deficient W/Wv mice exhibit a decreased rate of tumor angiogenesis. International journal of cancerJournal international du cancer 1988; 42(1) 48-52.

[220] Coussens LM, Raymond WW, Bergers G, Laig-Webster M, Behrendtsen O, Werb Z, Caughey GH, Hanahan D: Inflammatory mast cells up-regulate angiogenesis during squamous epithelial carcinogenesis. Genes & development 1999; 13(11) 1382-1397.

[221] Soucek L, Lawlor ER, Soto D, Shchors K, Swigart LB, Evan GI: Mast cells are required for angiogenesis and macroscopic expansion of Myc-induced pancreatic islet tumors. Nature medicine 2007; 13(10) 1211-1218.

[222] Ho KL: Ultrastructure of cerebellar capillary hemangioblastoma. II. Mast cells and angiogenesis. Acta Neuropathologica 1984; 64(4) 308-318.

[223] Zhang W, Stoica G, Tasca SI, Kelly KA, Meininger CJ: Modulation of tumor angiogenesis by stem cell factor. Cancer research 2000; 60(23) 6757-6762.

[224] Munitz A, Levi-Schaffer F: Eosinophils: 'new' roles for 'old' cells. Allergy 2004; 59(3) 268-275.

[225] Shojaei F, Wu X, Zhong C, Yu L, Liang XH, Yao J, Blanchard D, Bais C, Peale FV, van Bruggen N *et al*: Bv8 regulates myeloid-cell-dependent tumour angiogenesis. Nature 2007; 450(7171) 825-831.

[226] Yang L, DeBusk LM, Fukuda K, Fingleton B, Green-Jarvis B, Shyr Y, Matrisian LM, Carbone DP, Lin PC: Expansion of myeloid immune suppressor Gr+CD11b+ cells in tumor-bearing host directly promotes tumor angiogenesis. Cancer cell 2004; 6(4) 409-421.

[227] Fridman WH, Pages F, Sautes-Fridman C, Galon J: The immune contexture in human tumours: impact on clinical outcome. Nature reviewsCancer 2012; 12(4) 298-306.

[228] Ohm JE, Gabrilovich DI, Sempowski GD, Kisseleva E, Parman KS, Nadaf S, Carbone DP: VEGF inhibits T-cell development and may contribute to tumor-induced immune suppression. Blood 2003; 101(12) 4878-4886.

[229] Zou W: Regulatory T cells, tumour immunity and immunotherapy. Nature reviewsImmunology 2006; 6(4) 295-307.

[230] Facciabene A, Peng X, Hagemann IS, Balint K, Barchetti A, Wang LP, Gimotty PA, Gilks CB, Lal P, Zhang L *et al*: Tumour hypoxia promotes tolerance and angiogenesis via CCL28 and T(reg) cells. Nature 2011; 475(7355) 226-230.

[231] Facciabene A, Santoro S, Coukos G: Know thy enemy: Why are tumor-infiltrating regulatory T cells so deleterious? Oncoimmunology 2012; 1(4) 575-577.

[232] Yu AL, Gilman AL, Ozkaynak MF, London WB, Kreissman SG, Chen HX, Smith M, Anderson B, Villablanca JG, Matthay KK *et al*: Anti-GD2 antibody with GM-CSF, interleukin-2, and isotretinoin for neuroblastoma. The New England journal of medicine 2010; 363(14) 1324-1334.

[233] Rossler J, Taylor M, Geoerger B, Farace F, Lagodny J, Peschka-Suss R, Niemeyer CM, Vassal G: Angiogenesis as a target in neuroblastoma. European journal of cancer (Oxford, England : 1990) 2008; 44(12) 1645-1656.

[234] Song L, Asgharzadeh S, Salo J, Engell K, Wu HW, Sposto R, Ara T, Silverman AM, DeClerck YA, Seeger RC *et al*: Valpha24-invariant NKT cells mediate antitumor activity via killing of tumor-associated macrophages. The Journal of clinical investigation 2009; 119(6) 1524-1536.

[235] Asgharzadeh S, Pique-Regi R, Sposto R, Wang H, Yang Y, Shimada H, Matthay K, Buckley J, Ortega A, Seeger RC: Prognostic significance of gene expression profiles of metastatic neuroblastomas lacking MYCN gene amplification. Journal of the National Cancer Institute 2006; 98(17) 1193-1203.

[236] Mellman I, Coukos G, Dranoff G: Cancer immunotherapy comes of age. Nature 2011; 480(7378) 480-489.

[237] Sabzevari H, Gillies SD, Mueller BM, Pancook JD, Reisfeld RA: A recombinant antibody-interleukin 2 fusion protein suppresses growth of hepatic human neuroblastoma metastases in severe combined immunodeficiency mice. Proceedings of the National Academy of Sciences of the United States of America 1994; 91(20) 9626-9630.

[238] Katsanis E, Orchard PJ, Bausero MA, Gorden KB, McIvor RS, Blazar BR: Interleukin-2 gene transfer into murine neuroblastoma decreases tumorigenicity and enhances systemic immunity causing regression of preestablished retroperitoneal tumors. Journal of immunotherapy with emphasis on tumor immunology : official journal of the Society for Biological Therapy 1994; 15(2) 81-90.

[239] Bausero MA, Panoskaltsis-Mortari A, Blazar BR, Katsanis E: Effective immunization against neuroblastoma using double-transduced tumor cells secreting GM-CSF and interferon-gamma. Journal of immunotherapy with emphasis on tumor immunology : official journal of the Society for Biological Therapy 1996; 19(2) 113-124.

[240] Johnson BD, Gershan JA, Natalia N, Zujewski H, Weber JJ, Yan X, Orentas RJ: Neuroblastoma cells transiently transfected to simultaneously express the co-stimulatory

molecules CD54, CD80, CD86, and CD137L generate antitumor immunity in mice. Journal of Immunotherapy 2005; 28(5) 449-460.

[241] Johnson BD, Jing W, Orentas RJ: CD25+ regulatory T cell inhibition enhances vaccine-induced immunity to neuroblastoma. Journal of Immunotherapy 2007; 30(2) 203-214.

[242] Croce M, Corrias MV, Orengo AM, Brizzolara A, Carlini B, Borghi M, Rigo V, Pistoia V, Ferrini S: Transient depletion of CD4(+) T cells augments IL-21-based immunotherapy of disseminated neuroblastoma in syngeneic mice. International journal of cancerJournal international du cancer 2010; 127(5) 1141-1150.

[243] Fest S, Huebener N, Bleeke M, Durmus T, Stermann A, Woehler A, Baykan B, Zenclussen AC, Michalsky E, Jaeger IS *et al*: Survivin minigene DNA vaccination is effective against neuroblastoma. International journal of cancerJournal international du cancer 2009; 125(1) 104-114.

[244] Huebener N, Fest S, Hilt K, Schramm A, Eggert A, Durmus T, Woehler A, Stermann A, Bleeke M, Baykan B *et al*: Xenogeneic immunization with human tyrosine hydroxylase DNA vaccines suppresses growth of established neuroblastoma. Molecular cancer therapeutics 2009; 8(8) 2392-2401.

[245] Craddock JA, Lu A, Bear A, Pule M, Brenner MK, Rooney CM, Foster AE: Enhanced tumor trafficking of GD2 chimeric antigen receptor T cells by expression of the chemokine receptor CCR2b. Journal of immunotherapy (Hagerstown, Md: 1997) 2010; 33(8) 780-788.

[246] Jing W, Yan X, Hallett WH, Gershan JA, Johnson BD: Depletion of CD25(+) T cells from hematopoietic stem cell grafts increases posttransplantation vaccine-induced immunity to neuroblastoma. Blood 2011; 117(25) 6952-6962.

[247] Truitt RL, Piaskowski V, Kirchner P, McOlash L, Camitta BM, Casper JT: Immunological evaluation of pediatric cancer patients receiving recombinant interleukin-2 in a phase I trial. Journal of immunotherapy : official journal of the Society for Biological Therapy 1992; 11(4) 274-285.

[248] Bowman L, Grossmann M, Rill D, Brown M, Zhong WY, Alexander B, Leimig T, Coustan-Smith E, Campana D, Jenkins J *et al*: IL-2 adenovector-transduced autologous tumor cells induce antitumor immune responses in patients with neuroblastoma. Blood 1998; 92(6) 1941-1949.

[249] Rousseau RF, Haight AE, Hirschmann-Jax C, Yvon ES, Rill DR, Mei Z, Smith SC, Inman S, Cooper K, Alcoser P *et al*: Local and systemic effects of an allogeneic tumor cell vaccine combining transgenic human lymphotactin with interleukin-2 in patients with advanced or refractory neuroblastoma. Blood 2003; 101(5) 1718-1726.

[250] Osenga KL, Hank JA, Albertini MR, Gan J, Sternberg AG, Eickhoff J, Seeger RC, Matthay KK, Reynolds CP, Twist C *et al*: A phase I clinical trial of the hu14.18-IL2 (EMD 273063) as a treatment for children with refractory or recurrent neuroblastoma and

melanoma: a study of the Children's Oncology Group. Clinical cancer research : an official journal of the American Association for Cancer Research 2006; 12(6) 1750-1759.

[251] Park JR, Digiusto DL, Slovak M, Wright C, Naranjo A, Wagner J, Meechoovet HB, Bautista C, Chang WC, Ostberg JR *et al*: Adoptive transfer of chimeric antigen receptor re-directed cytolytic T lymphocyte clones in patients with neuroblastoma. Molecular therapy : the journal of the American Society of Gene Therapy 2007; 15(4) 825-833.

[252] Russell HV, Strother D, Mei Z, Rill D, Popek E, Biagi E, Yvon E, Brenner M, Rousseau R: A phase 1/2 study of autologous neuroblastoma tumor cells genetically modified to secrete IL-2 in patients with high-risk neuroblastoma. Journal of immunotherapy (Hagerstown, Md: 1997) 2008; 31(9) 812-819.

[253] Pule MA, Savoldo B, Myers GD, Rossig C, Russell HV, Dotti G, Huls MH, Liu E, Gee AP, Mei Z *et al*: Virus-specific T cells engineered to coexpress tumor-specific receptors: persistence and antitumor activity in individuals with neuroblastoma. Nature medicine 2008; 14(11) 1264-1270.

[254] Shusterman S, London WB, Gillies SD, Hank JA, Voss SD, Seeger RC, Reynolds CP, Kimball J, Albertini MR, Wagner B *et al*: Antitumor activity of hu14.18-IL2 in patients with relapsed/refractory neuroblastoma: a Children's Oncology Group (COG) phase II study. Journal of clinical oncology : official journal of the American Society of Clinical Oncology 2010; 28(33) 4969-4975.

[255] Meitar D, Crawford SE, Rademaker AW, Cohn SL: Tumor angiogenesis correlates with metastatic disease, N-myc amplification, and poor outcome in human neuroblastoma. Journal of clinical oncology : official journal of the American Society of Clinical Oncology 1996; 14(2) 405-414.

[256] Breit S, Ashman K, Wilting J, Rossler J, Hatzi E, Fotsis T, Schweigerer L: The N-myc oncogene in human neuroblastoma cells: down-regulation of an angiogenesis inhibitor identified as activin A. Cancer research 2000; 60(16) 4596-4601.

[257] Eggert A, Ikegaki N, Kwiatkowski J, Zhao H, Brodeur GM, Himelstein BP: High-level expression of angiogenic factors is associated with advanced tumor stage in human neuroblastomas. Clinical cancer research : an official journal of the American Association for Cancer Research 2000; 6(5) 1900-1908.

[258] Fotsis T, Breit S, Lutz W, Rossler J, Hatzi E, Schwab M, Schweigerer L: Down-regulation of endothelial cell growth inhibitors by enhanced MYCN oncogene expression in human neuroblastoma cells. European journal of biochemistry / FEBS 1999; 263(3) 757-764.

[259] Holmquist-Mengelbier L, Fredlund E, Lofstedt T, Noguera R, Navarro S, Nilsson H, Pietras A, Vallon-Christersson J, Borg A, Gradin K *et al*: Recruitment of HIF-1alpha

and HIF-2alpha to common target genes is differentially regulated in neuroblastoma: HIF-2alpha promotes an aggressive phenotype. Cancer cell 2006; 10(5) 413-423.

[260] Ribatti D, Alessandri G, Vacca A, Iurlaro M, Ponzoni M: Human neuroblastoma cells produce extracellular matrix-degrading enzymes, induce endothelial cell proliferation and are angiogenic in vivo. International journal of cancerJournal international du cancer 1998; 77(3) 449-454.

[261] Yasuda C, Sakata S, Kakinoki S, Takeyama Y, Ohyanagi H, Shiozaki H: In vivo evaluation of microspheres containing the angiogenesis inhibitor, TNP-470, and the metastasis suppression with liver metastatic model implanted neuroblastoma. Pathophysiology : the official journal of the International Society for Pathophysiology / ISP 2010; 17(2) 149-155.

[262] Ribatti D, Raffaghello L, Marimpietri D, Cosimo E, Montaldo PG, Nico B, Vacca A, Ponzoni M: Fenretinide as an anti-angiogenic agent in neuroblastoma. Cancer letters 2003; 197(1-2) 181-184.

[263] Guo Y, Pino-Lagos K, Ahonen CA, Bennett KA, Wang J, Napoli JL, Blomhoff R, Sockanathan S, Chandraratna RA, Dmitrovsky E *et al*: A retinoic acid-rich tumor microenvironment provides clonal survival cues for tumor-specific CD8+ T cells. Cancer research 2012(Journal Article).

[264] Kim ES, Serur A, Huang J, Manley CA, McCrudden KW, Frischer JS, Soffer SZ, Ring L, New T, Zabski S *et al*: Potent VEGF blockade causes regression of coopted vessels in a model of neuroblastoma. Proceedings of the National Academy of Sciences of the United States of America 2002; 99(17) 11399-11404.

[265] Backman U, Christofferson R: The selective class III/V receptor tyrosine kinase inhibitor SU11657 inhibits tumor growth and angiogenesis in experimental neuroblastomas grown in mice. Pediatric research 2005; 57(5 Pt 1) 690-695.

[266] Beaudry P, Nilsson M, Rioth M, Prox D, Poon D, Xu L, Zweidler-Mckay P, Ryan A, Folkman J, Ryeom S *et al*: Potent antitumor effects of ZD6474 on neuroblastoma via dual targeting of tumor cells and tumor endothelium. Molecular cancer therapeutics 2008; 7(2) 418-424.

[267] Katzenstein HM, Rademaker AW, Senger C, Salwen HR, Nguyen NN, Thorner PS, Litsas L, Cohn SL: Effectiveness of the angiogenesis inhibitor TNP-470 in reducing the growth of human neuroblastoma in nude mice inversely correlates with tumor burden. Clinical cancer research : an official journal of the American Association for Cancer Research 1999; 5(12) 4273-4278.

[268] Ribatti D, Alessandri G, Baronio M, Raffaghello L, Cosimo E, Marimpietri D, Montaldo PG, De Falco G, Caruso A, Vacca A *et al*: Inhibition of neuroblastoma-induced angiogenesis by fenretinide. International journal of cancerJournal international du cancer 2001; 94(3) 314-321.

[269] Beppu K, Jaboine J, Merchant MS, Mackall CL, Thiele CJ: Effect of imatinib mesylate on neuroblastoma tumorigenesis and vascular endothelial growth factor expression. Journal of the National Cancer Institute 2004; 96(1) 46-55.

[270] Dickson PV, Hamner JB, Sims TL, Fraga CH, Ng CY, Rajasekeran S, Hagedorn NL, McCarville MB, Stewart CF, Davidoff AM: Bevacizumab-induced transient remodeling of the vasculature in neuroblastoma xenografts results in improved delivery and efficacy of systemically administered chemotherapy. Clinical cancer research : an official journal of the American Association for Cancer Research 2007; 13(13) 3942-3950.

[271] Segerstrom L, Fuchs D, Backman U, Holmquist K, Christofferson R, Azarbayjani F: The anti-VEGF antibody bevacizumab potently reduces the growth rate of high-risk neuroblastoma xenografts. Pediatric research 2006; 60(5) 576-581.

[272] Yang D, Chen Q, Yang H, Tracey KJ, Bustin M, Oppenheim JJ: High mobility group box-1 protein induces the migration and activation of human dendritic cells and acts as an alarmin. Journal of leukocyte biology 2007; 81(1) 59-66.

[273] Nilsson MB, Zage PE, Zeng L, Xu L, Cascone T, Wu HK, Saigal B, Zweidler-McKay PA, Heymach JV: Multiple receptor tyrosine kinases regulate HIF-1alpha and HIF-2alpha in normoxia and hypoxia in neuroblastoma: implications for antiangiogenic mechanisms of multikinase inhibitors. Oncogene 2010; 29(20) 2938-2949.

[274] Zhen Z, Sun X, He Y, Cai Y, Wang J, Guan Z: The sequence of drug administration influences the antitumor effects of bevacizumab and cyclophosphamide in a neuroblastoma model. Medical oncology (Northwood, London, England) 2011; 28 Suppl 1(Journal Article) S619-625.

[275] Rossler J, Monnet Y, Farace F, Opolon P, Daudigeos-Dubus E, Bourredjem A, Vassal G, Geoerger B: The selective VEGFR1-3 inhibitor axitinib (AG-013736) shows antitumor activity in human neuroblastoma xenografts. International journal of cancerJournal international du cancer 2011; 128(11) 2748-2758.

[276] Clinicaltrials.gov. In.

[277] Twardowski P, Figlin RA: Bevacizumab plus interferon alpha in patients with metastatic renal cell carcinoma. Nature clinical practiceOncology 2008; 5(8) 436-437.

[278] Garcia JA, Mekhail T, Elson P, Triozzi P, Nemec C, Dreicer R, Bukowski RM, Rini BI: Clinical and immunomodulatory effects of bevacizumab and low-dose interleukin-2 in patients with metastatic renal cell carcinoma: results from a phase II trial. BJU international 2011; 107(4) 562-570.

[279] Li B, Lalani AS, Harding TC, Luan B, Koprivnikar K, Huan Tu G, Prell R, VanRoey MJ, Simmons AD, Jooss K: Vascular endothelial growth factor blockade reduces intratumoral regulatory T cells and enhances the efficacy of a GM-CSF-secreting cancer immunotherapy. Clinical cancer research : an official journal of the American Association for Cancer Research 2006; 12(22) 6808-6816.

[280] Manning EA, Ullman JG, Leatherman JM, Asquith JM, Hansen TR, Armstrong TD, Hicklin DJ, Jaffee EM, Emens LA: A vascular endothelial growth factor receptor-2 inhibitor enhances antitumor immunity through an immune-based mechanism. Clinical cancer research : an official journal of the American Association for Cancer Research 2007; 13(13) 3951-3959.

[281] Huang KW, Wu HL, Lin HL, Liang PC, Chen PJ, Chen SH, Lee HI, Su PY, Wu WH, Lee PH et al: Combining antiangiogenic therapy with immunotherapy exerts better therapeutical effects on large tumors in a woodchuck hepatoma model. Proceedings of the National Academy of Sciences of the United States of America 2010; 107(33) 14769-14774.

[282] Chinnasamy D, Yu Z, Kerkar SP, Zhang L, Morgan RA, Restifo NP, Rosenberg SA: Local delivery of interleukin-12 using T cells targeting VEGF receptor-2 eradicates multiple vascularized tumors in mice. Clinical cancer research : an official journal of the American Association for Cancer Research 2012; 18(6) 1672-1683.

[283] Farsaci B, Higgins JP, Hodge JW: Consequence of dose scheduling of sunitinib on host immune response elements and vaccine combination therapy. International journal of cancerJournal international du cancer 2012; 130(8) 1948-1959.

Chapter 6

T-Cadherin Stimulates Melanoma Cell Proliferation and Mesenchymal Stromal Cell Recruitment, but Inhibits Angiogenesis in a Mouse Melanoma Model

K. A. Rubina, E. I. Yurlova, V. Yu. Sysoeva, E. V. Semina, N. I. Kalinina, A. A. Poliakov, I. N. Mikhaylova, N. V. Andronova and H. M. Treshalina

Additional information is available at the end of the chapter

http://dx.doi.org/10.5772/53350

1. Introduction

Melanocytes are special pigment cells that reside predominantly in the skin and eyes. In the skin, melanocytes are located in the bottom layer (the stratum basale) of the skin's epidermis and in the hair follicles (Gray-Schopfer et al., 2001). Melanocytes produce melanins responsible for skin and hair color and perform protection function of the basal keratinocytes from ultraviolet light through synthesis and donation of melanin (Gray-Schopfer et al., 2001). Melanocytes maintain constant contact with the basal layer of the epidermis through direct interaction with basal keratinocytes and via secretion of soluble factors. Upon ultraviolet radiation, keratinocytes produce factors that control melanocyte proliferation, differentiation and motility (Gray-Schopfer et al., 2007). Melanocytes maintain during a lifetime a stable-ratio of 1:5 with basal keratinocytes (Fitzpatrick et al., 1979).

Initially, cutaneous melanocytes originate from neural crest cells and migrate into the skin during embryonic development. Neural crest cells start their migration from the neural tube shortly after the closure of the neural tube. These cells migrate along several well-defined pathways in a ventral direction from the neural tube through the somites. As the epithelial somites undergo a transition to form the dermatome (presumptive dermis), myotome (presumptive muscle), and sclerotome (presumptive vertebrae), most ventrally migrating neural crest cells invade the rostral half of each sclerotome and avoid the caudal (posterior) part of

INTECH
open science | open minds

© 2013 The Author(s). Licensee InTech. This chapter is distributed under the terms of the Creative Commons Attribution License http://creativecommons.org/licenses/by/3.0), which permits unrestricted use, distribution, and reproduction in any medium, provided the original work is properly cited.

each sclerotome (Rickmann et. al., 1985; Teillet et al., 1987; Serbedzua et al., 1989; Ranscht and Bronner, 1991).

Originated from a population of highly motile neural crest progenitors, melanocytes protect basal keratinocytes, in the skin. At the same time, they could become precursors of the most dangerous form of cancer - melanoma. Skin cancer including the most frequently occurring forms such as basal cell carcinoma, squamous cell carcinoma and melanoma, is one of the most common human malignancies. Today melanoma is one the fastest growing malignancies. The high propensity of melanoma to form metastasis is the most important feature that distinguishes melanoma from other types of skin cancers. According to the World Health Organization, melanoma accounts for only 25% of skin cancers. However, it is the most dangerous form of skin cancer leading to high mortality. If diagnosed early it can be successfully removed by surgical resection and about 80% of cases are cured this way (Gray-Schopfer et al., 2001). However, at progressed metastatic stages melanoma is highly resistant to currently existing therapies and has a very poor prognosis. This area requires future research to understand melanoma biology and develop new therapeutic solutions.

Melanoma begins as a benign naevus but can quickly progress to the malignant stage (Bar-Eli., 1997; Luca and Bar-Eli., 1998). Herewith melanocytes start to proliferate and spread, which can be limited to the epidermis (junctional naevus), or the dermis (dermal naevus) or both (compound naevus) (Gray-Schopfer et al., 2001). Naevi can progress to the radial-growth-phase (RGP) melanoma which is an intra-epidermal lesion with sporadic local microinvasion into the underlying derma. However, RGP melanoma can transform into the vertical-growth phase (VGP) melanoma with a higher invasive potential in which melanoma cells from tumor nodules or nests invade the underlying derma. Finally, melanoma can develop metastases after the vertical growth phase (Clark et al., 1984). Not all melanomas pass through each of these phases and can progress from isolated melanocytes or naevi, while both, RGP or VGP, can develop directly into metastatic malignant melanoma (Miller et al., 2006). Four main clinical subtypes of melanoma are described (Clark et al., 1984). Superficial spreading melanoma (SSM) is the most common form and it is associated with severe sunburns, especially at an early age (Ishihara et al., 2001; Gilchrest et al., 1999). In most cases, SSM is flat, with intra-epidermal microinvasion, particularly at the edges of the lesion. Nodular melanoma comprises raised nodules and has almost no flat parts. Acral lentiginous melanoma (ALM) is not linked to UV exposure and is usually found on the palms of the hands, soles of the feet and in the nail bed (Kuchelmeister et al., 2000). Lentigo maligna appears to be flat and is associated with chronic sun exposure in elderly people.

2. Cadherin-mediated adhesion in melanoma progression

Tumor progression is characterized by uncontrolled cell proliferation, high invasive potential into surrounding tissue and metastasis to distant organs. It is believed that this is largely due to disruption or dysfunction of intercellular contacts (Hanahan and Weinberg, 2000). Cadherins comprise a large family of Ca^{2+}-dependent adhesion molecules (Angst et al., 2001; Gumbiner, 2005) and are involved in tissue and organ development durig embryogenesis and maintainance of the normal cell arrangement in the adult organism. The regulation of cadherin expression patterns and their activity at the neural crest-forming area plays a critical role in emigration of melanocyte precursors - neural crest cells from the neural tube (Nakagawa and Takeichi, 1998).

Cadherins play an important role in specific cell-cell adhesion, cell recognition and signaling (Angst et al., 2001; Gumbiner, 2005; Wheelock and Johnson, 2003). Cadherins are transmembrane glycoproteins with their extracellular part responsible for homotypic binding between the neighboring cells, while intracellular part is involved in anchoring cadherins to the cytoskeleton. Cadherins interact with the cytoskeleton via catenins (alfa and beta catenins and p120) and form a multicomponent complex which also comprises a number of regulatory molecules such as protein tyrosine kinase, protein tyrosine phosphatase and small GTPases (Perez-Moreno et al., 2003; Sallee et al., 2006; Gumbiner, 2005; Vincent et al., 2004; Rubina et al., 2007).

Disruption of cadherin adherent junctions and their dysfunction has been associated with tumor cell invasion and metastasis (Takeichi, 1993). In human carcinoma the loss of E-cadherin expression leads to dedifferentiation and increased invasiveness of carcinoma cells (Frixen et al., 1991). The change in the expression pattern of cadherins in melanocytes from E-cadherin, P-cadherin and desmoglein to N-cadherin is associated with melanocyte transformation and metastasis (Bonitsis et al., 2006). In normal skin, melanocytes project multiple extensions to keratinocytes and form cadherin adhesive contacts with the basal keratinocytes, which control maintain proliferation and correct positioning of melanocytes (Haas and Herlyng, 2005; Haass et al., 2005). E-cadherin is mainly responsible fot these cell-cell interaction. The loss of functional E-cadherin or its downregulation let melanocytes escape form keratinocyte control and correlates with high invasiveness and metastasis of the overlying melanoma cells (Hsu et al., 1996; Silye et al., 1998).

Downregulation of E-cadherin and/or its dysfunction is one of the earliest steps in the development of metastases in cutaneous melanoma (Johnson, 1999). E-cadherin expression is detected in cultured melanocytes and naevus cells, while its expression is often lost in cultured melanoma cells from the primary tumors or metastasis (Danen et al., 1996). In the radial growth phase melanoma cells could retain expression of membrane E-cadherin (Sanders et al., 1999). It was even noted that there is a correlation between E-cadherin expression and the depth of the primary tumor (Andersen et al., 2004). Experiments on re-expression of E-cadherin using adenoviral transfer of full length E-cadherin cDNA showed the reduction in tumorigenicity and decrease in proliferation rate of melanoma cells (Hsu et al., 2000). The mechanism of E-cadherin transcriptional downregulation in melanomas involves gene silencing by methylation or transrepression by the Snail protein from a superfamily of zinc-finger transcription factors (Tsutsumida et al., 2004). Thus it was suggested that E-cadherin could play an important role in the preventing the melanocytes transformation and limiting their proliferation (cited in Bonitsis et al., 2006).

Catenins are a group of cadherin-associated molecules and they were also suggested to be involved in malignant transformation of melanocytes. The change in catenin expression pattern was found in melanocytic naevus and melanomas, where the expression of alfa and beta catenins was reduced or altered, while beta catenin was often overexpressed (Zhang and Hersey., 1999). The loss of E-cadherin in melanocytes may also indirectly influence the β-catenin cytoplasmic content and affects the β-catenin/wnt signaling pathways. Namely, the reduction in the membranous E-cadherin resulted in the accumulation of free cytoplasmic β-catenin which did not degrade in proteasomes and was translocated to the nucleus. Nuclear β-catenin could be involved in regulation of gene expression responsible for growth and metastasis control via β-catenin/wnt signaling pathways (McGary et al., 2002). Also the presence of the functional E-cadherin in melanocytes ensured their correct adhesion to keratinocytes and limited their motility and proliferation (Gruss et al., 2001; Tang et al., 1994).

Despite the majority of studies showed a correlation between the decreased E-cadherin expression and tumorigenicity of melanoma cells, there were data suggestintg that in some cases E-cadherin expression could be retained or even elevated in melanoma (Ruiter and van Muijen, 1998; Nishizawa et al., 2005). It was reported that membranous E-cadherin was present in the metastasizing melanomas and their corresponding lymph node metastasis (Silye et al., 1998).

The loss of E-cadherin expression in melanomas correlates with the increase in N-cadherin expression. This change contributed to the survival advantage of melanoma cells and their invasive and migratory properties (McGary et al., 2002). The shift in cadherin expression pattern was found both in vivo and in vitro (Hsu et al., 1996; Hsu et al., 2000). It was suggested that melanoma cells form N-cadherin adhesion contacts with fibroblasts, vascular endothelial cells, and adjacent melanoma cells (Li and Herlyn, 2000). The N-cadherin-mediated adhesion facilitated migration of melanoma cells over dermal fibroblasts and their transmigration into the vascular system (Haass and Herlyn, 2005; Li et al., 2002) and induced formation of communication gap junction between melanoma cells and the surrounding stroma (McGary et al., 2002). Anti-N-cadherin antibodies retarded the transendothelial migration of melanoma cells and induced their apoptosis, which linked the N-cadherin in the ability of melanoma cells for diapedesis (Li et al., 2002; Sandig et al., 1997; Voura et al., 1998). Surprisingly, adenoviral gene transfer of E-cadherin inhibited N-cadherin expression in melanoma cells and their survival and migration (Hsu et al., 2000). At the same time N-cadherin overexpression did not affect the endogenous E-cadherin expression (Li et al., 2001).

Little is known about the role of P-cadherin in the progression of malignant melanomas. P-cadherin is expressed in basal keratinocytes, melanocytes, in the cells of the basal and outer layers of skin appendages (Klymkowsky and Parr, 1995). As Similarly to E-cadherin, P-cadherin was thought to be involved in the regulation of melanocyte proliferation and migration (Klymkowsky and Parr, 1995). It was found that the soluble form of P-cadherin missing the transmembrane and the cytoplasmic part was expressed in melanoma cells (Bauer et al., 2005) and was associated with increasing tumor thickness and metastasis and reduced patient survival (Bachmann et al., 2005).

VE-cadherin is another member of the cadherin superfamily, which was shown to be involved in melanoma progression. VE-cadherin was found to be exclusively expressed on endothelial cells in normal vessels and mediated homophilic contacts between neighboring cells regulating endothelial barrier function (Dejana, 1996). VE-cadherin is essential for both the development and the maintenance of blood vessels in the adult organism. In the embryo, VE-cadherin appeared at a very early stage of vascular development in mesodermal cells of yolk sac mesenchyme; it was also expressed in progenitor cells during the early angioblast differentiation and endocardial development (Dejana et al., 2000; Cavallaro et al., 2006). At the later stages, VE-cadherin expression was restricted to the peripheral layer of blood islands that give rise to endothelial cells (Dejana et al., 2000).

VE-cadherin was also shown to be important for melanoma cell invasion and metastasis. At the beginning of diapedesis, endothelial cells located below the attached melanoma cells disassemble their VE-cadherin-mediated adhesion contacts. This allowed melanoma cell to penetrate through the VE-cadherin-negative regions in the endothelial cell monolayer and intercalate between endothelial cells. Subsequently, the endothelial cells surrounding the melanoma cells extended processes and spread over melanoma. The leading edges of the projections of endothelial cell expressed high levels of N-cadherin but not VE-cadherin. VE-cadherin expression was restored when the endothelial cells met and reformed cell-cell contacts above the melanoma cell (Voura et al., 1998). Highly aggressive human cutaneous and uveal melanoma cells were also found to express VE-cadherin in contrast to less aggressive cells (Hendrix et al., 2001). This expression contributed to the ability of melanoma cells to mimic endothelial cells and form patterned networks of vascular channels (Hendrix et al., 2001; Hendrix et al., 2003). These data indicated that melanoma cells cooperate with the endothelial cells in the process of invasion and that the regulated changes in the expression of cadherins played an essential role in melanoma growth and metastasis.

Thus, further studies are required to elucidate the biochemical and cellular mechanism of melanoma transformation and progression and the role of cadherins in this process. Lately, an atypical member of the cadherin superfamily – T-cadherin was was shown to be involved in melanoma progression. However, its role and mechanism of action were not completely understood.

3. T-cadherin in cancer

T-cadherin is a unique member of cadherin superfamily because it lacks the transmembrane and cytoplasmic domains and is anchored to the cell membrane via a glycosyl-phosphatidylinositol (GPI) moiety (Fredette and Ranscht, 1994; Fredette et al., 1996; Ranscht and Dours-Zimmermann 1991). Although T-cadherin contains five Ca^{2+}–binding domains on its N-terminal end it does not have the His-Ala-Val motif responsible for the recognition and binding of the classical cadherins. It was shown that T-cadherin can mediate week homophilic adhesion in aggregation assays *in vitro* (Vestal and Ranscht, 1992; Resink et al., 1999) but the lack of intracellular domain strongly suggested that T-cadherin is not involved in stable cell-cell adhesion. Moreover, T-cadherin was show to be absent from the adherent junctions and was located within lipid rafts in the plasma membrane (Philippova et al., 1998); was redistributed to the leading edge in migrating cells (Philippova et al., 2003). These imply T-cadherin as a navigation receptor involved in transduction of extracellular cues in migrating cells rather than an adhesion molecule.

Little is known about the biological role and underlying mechanisms of T-cadherin in malignant transformation and tumor progression. In some reports, T-cadherin was regarded as a tumor suppressor and its downregulation was associated with tumor progression. Downregulation of T-cadherin was shown to be associated also with tumorogenicity in breast (Riener et al., 2008), lung (Sato et al., 1998), and gallbladder cancers (Adachi et al., 2009). However, in other cancers such as ovarian, endometrial (Widschwendter et al., 2004; Suehiro et al., 2008) and osteosarcoma (Zucchini et al., 2004), decreased expression of T-cadherin positively correlated with patient survival. T-cadherin was upregulated in human invasive hepatocellular carcinomas (Riou et al., 2006) and astrocytomas (Gutmann et al., 2001).

T-cadherin is expressed in the basal layer of keratinocytes, in melanocytes and in vascular cells of the dermal blood vessels in the normal skin (Zhou et al., 2002; Kuphal et al., 2009; Rubina et al., 2012). However, its expression was consequently lost upon cell transformation and tumor progression in pre-malignant skin lesions and in non-melanoma skin cancer. In skin lesions, such as actinic keratosis T-cadherin was abundantly expressed in the atypical keratinocytes, while its expression varied in Bowen disease and was weaker than in the normal skin (Pfaff et al., 2010). Expression of T-cadherin was reduced in psoriatic samples (Zhou et al., 2003) and was down-regulated or completely absent in invasive cutaneous squamous cell carcinoma (Takeuchi et al., 2002a) and in basal cell carcinoma of the skin (Takeuchi et al., 2002b). Data obtained in our lab supported these findings and confirmed that T-cadherin expression was not changed if cells maintained the attachment to the basal membrane in the lesions characterized by slow or controlled keratinocytes growth (keratoacanthoma, psoriasis, actinic keratosis and superficial basalioma) (Rubina et al., 2012). However, T-cadherin expression in keratinocytes was downregulated upon tumor progression in basosquamous cell carcinoma, squamous cell carcinoma and in some cases of basal cell carcinoma, i.e. tumors with high proliferative, invasive, and metastatic potential (Rubina et al., 2012).

Apart from regulation of keratinocyte proliferation, T-cadherin may affect tumor progression through its direct involvement in neovascularization. While in the normal blood vessels T-cadherin was abundantly expressed in endothelial and mural cells (Ivanov et al., 2001), its expression was altered in tumor vessels in Lewis carcinoma lung metastasis and F9 endodermal teratocarcinoma and in human xenografts PC-3 prostate cancer or A673 rhabdomyosarcoma (Riou et al., 2006; Wyder et al., 2000). Inactivation of T-cadherin gene limited mammary tumor vascularization and reduced tumor growth in the mouse mammary tumor virus (MMTV)-polyoma virus middle T (PyV-mT) transgenic model (Hebbard et al., 2008). In human hepatocellular carcinoma (HCC) T-cadherin was also upregulated in intratumoral capillary endothelial cells and this increase correlated with tumor growth and metastasis (Adachi et al., 2006). Data obtained in our lab indicated that in pre-malignant skin lesions all blood vessels uniformly expressed T-cadherin (Rubina et al., 2012). The aberrant expression of T-cadherin and vascular markers was detected in aggressively developing skin tumors such as basosquamous cell carcinoma, squamous cell carcinoma and in some cases of basal cell carcinoma. We suggested that the high level of expression of T-cadherin in the normal keratinocytes and in benign tumors regulates the growth of blood vessels. Upon malignant transformation expression of T-cadherin was lost in tumor cells and altered on vascular cells. This caused the abnormality and excessive vascularization of the tumors (Rubina et al., 2012).

The role of T-cadherin in melanoma progression and vascularization was addressed in a few studies and the results were contradictory. T-cadherin was expressed in normal human skin melanocytes (Kuphal et al., 2009; Bosserhoff et al., 2011). However, it was shown that the precursors of melanocytes did not express T-cadherin and invaded T-cadherin negative rostral parts of sclerotomes avoiding T-cadherin positive caudal parts of sclerotomes during neural crest cell migration (Ranscht and Bronner-Fraser, 1991). These results led to a hypothesis that T-cadherin is a navigating receptor that provides topographic guidance for migrating melanocyte precursors, and that de-differentiated or transformed melanocytes may loose T-cadherin expression. Indeed, T-cadherin expression was found to be diminished in melanocytes induced to de-differentiate to melanoblast-related cells and T-cadherin expression was undetectable in about 80% of human melanoma cell lines (Kuphal et al., 2009; Bosserhoff et al., 2011). While T-cadherin was expressed in benign naevus nests, its expression was lost in most tissue samples of human primary melanoma, lymph and visceral melanoma metastasis indicating the potential role of T-cadherin in melanoma progression (Kuphal et al., 2009). In addition, T-cadherin re-expression by stable transfection in human melanoma cells reduced the rate of tumor growth in the *nu/nu* mouse tumor model, decreased cell capacity for anchorage-independent growth, and for migration and invasion *in vitro* (Kuphal et al., 2009). However, it was shown in other studies that T-cadherin overexpression in endothelial cells stimulated intratumoral angiogenesis in tumor co-culture spheroid model with melanoma cells *in vitro* (Ghosh et al., 2007). Despite T-cadherin expression is lost in the majority of melanoma cell lines, 20% of melanomas still express T-cadherin (Kuphal et al., 2009; Bosserhoff et al., 2011) and possess invasive and metastatic potential.

To gain insights into the function of T-cadherin in melanoma progression and growth we first examined T-cadherin expression in the normal human skin melanocytes, melanoma cells and the blood vessels of the primary melanomas and melanoma metastasis in human samples and in the experimental models.

4. T-cadherin expression in human melanoma

We performed a comparative study of T-cadherin expression in normal skin and in melanoma samples. Tissue samples of primary human melanoma and metastasis obtained from patients undergoing surgical treatment were immediately frozen with liquid nitrogen and stored at -80°C. Human skin biopsies from healthy donors and melanoma samples of patients were immunostained with antibodies against T-cadherin and vascular cell markers and analyzed using fluorescent microscope.

Human skin biopsies from 6 healthy donors, 10 tissue samples of primary human melanoma and 12 samples of visceral melanoma metastasis were obtained from Blokhin Russian Cancer Research Center of Russian Academy of Medical Sciences. Consequent cryosections of the samples (7μm thick) were fixed in 4% paraformaldehyde (PRS Panreac, Spain), whashed and then incubated in a mixture of primary antibodies against T-cadherin (rabbit anti-human, ProSci, USA) or endothelial cells marker vWF (Von Willebrand factor, mouse anti-human, BD

Biosciences, USA), or melanoma (gp100) Ab-3 (Ab-3 is a mixture of Ab-1 (HMB45) and Ab-2 (HMB50) antibodies which are extremely sensitive and recognize differentiating melanocytes and melanomas, Lab Vision- Neomarkers, USA) – for 1 hour and subsequent extensive washing in PBS. Then sections were incubated in a mixture of secondary antibodies Alexa488-conjugated donkey anti-mouse and Alexa594-conjugated donkey anti-rabbit or Alexa488-conjugated donkey anti-rabbit and Alexa594-conjugated donkey anti-mouse (Molecular Probes, USA) (1μg/ml in PBS). Cell nuclei were counterstained with DAPI (Molecular Probes, USA). Images were obtained using Zeiss Axiovert 200M microscope equipped with CCD camera AxioCam HRc and Axiovision software (Zeiss, Germany) and further processed using Adobe PhotoShop software (Adobe Systems, USA).

We assessed the areas occupied by the T-cadherin-positive melanoma cells using MetaMorph 5.0 (Universal Imaging) and Adobe PhotoShop software (Adobe Systems). In a field of view, we determined the T-cadherin-positive areas and normalized to the DAPI-stained area unit of each section. For the quantification, T-cadherin-positive areas were counted in 4-5 fields of view (1.107 mm^2) on 10 random sections for each sample at 100x total magnification (10x objective).

In the normal skin T-cadherin was abundantly expressed in basal keratinocytes, in differentiating keratinocytes, in the stromal cells and in all blood vessels located in the underlying derma (Fig.1).

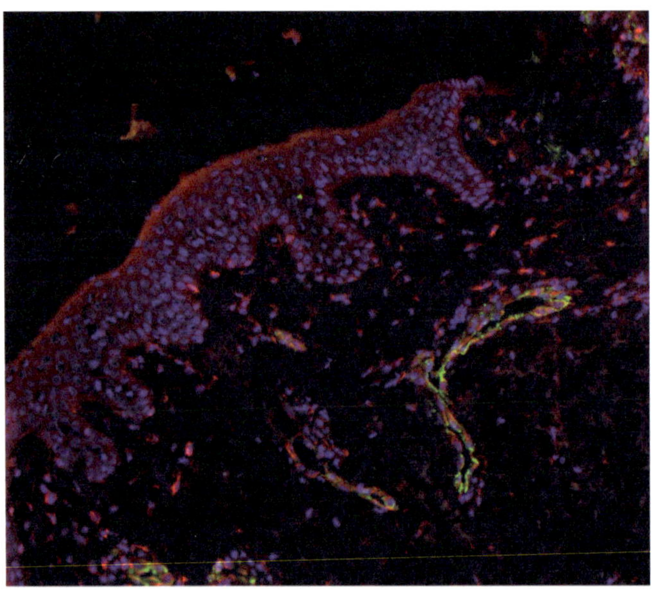

Figure 1. Double immunofluorescent staining of normal skin samples with antibodies against T-cadherin (red) and vWF (green). T-cadherin expression was detected in the basal keratinocytes, suprabasal layers, stromal cells and in the blood vessels (colocalization of T-cadherin and vWF is showed by the arrow). Nuclei were counterstained with DAPI (blue). Bars, 100 μm.

The immunofluorescent staining with gp 100 antibodies demonstrated that differentiating melanocytes were located beneath the layer of epidermal basal keratinocytes and extended their processes over keratinocytes (Fig. 2A). We were able to show the expression of T-cadherin in differentiating melanocytes by the overlay of green and red fluorescence (Fig. 2A, B and C) and in mature melanocytes by mapping the red fluorescence that revealed T-cadherin expression (Fig. 2C) with a phase-contrast image where the dark cells corresponded to mature melanocytes (Fig. 2C and D).

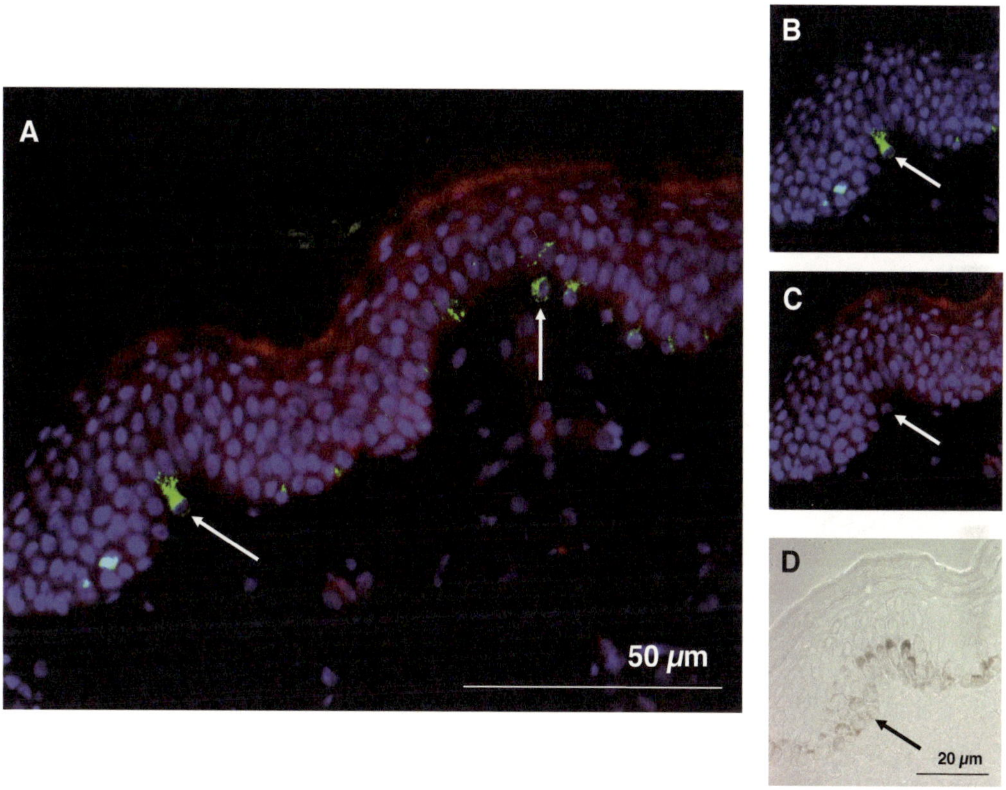

Figure 2. Double immunofluorescent staining of normal skin samples with antibodies against T-cadherin (red) (A, B, C) and gp 100 (green) (A, B). Figure D depicts phase contrast image. Figures B, C, D represent parallel frozen sections of the same sample. Differentiating melanocytes (green fluorescence in A, B) and mature melanocytes (phase contrast image with dark cells in D and corresponding immunofluorescent staining against T-cadherin – red fluorescence in C) all express T-cadherin. Nuclei were counterstained with DAPI (blue). Colocalization of T-cadherin and gp 100 is showed by the arrow. Bars, 100 μm.

Previous studies demonstrated that T-cadherin expression is reduced during cancer progression. Thus, we examined T-cadherin expression in melanoma samples of patients undergoing surgical treatment. Consequent cryosections of 10 tissue samples of the primary human melanoma and 12 samples of visceral metastasis, including two cases of primary melanoma that developed metastasis within a year were double immunostained with antibodies against melanoma cell marker gp 100, T-cadherin, endothelial cell marker vWF and analyzed using fluorescent microscope.

The tissue staining with subsequent image analysis showed that in the primary melanoma 60% of the sections was occupied by melanoma cells uniformly expressing T-cadherin (Fig.3A), while 30% of the sections contained areas with heterogeneous, mosaic pattern of T-cadherin expression where some melanoma cells were T-cadherin positive and some cells - T-cadherin negative (Fig.3B and 3C), and the rest 10% exhibited no T-cadherin expression.

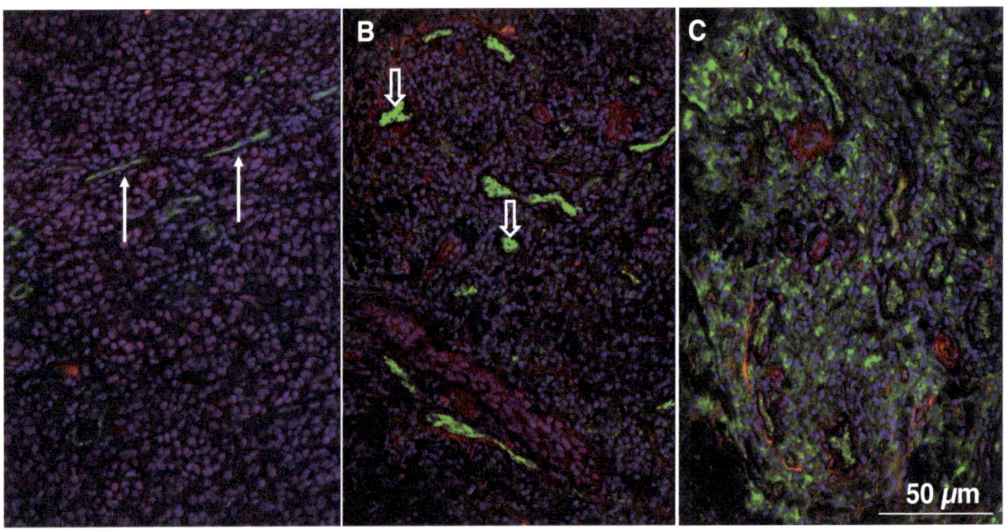

Figure 3. Double immunofluorescent staining of the primary melanoma sample with antibodies against T-cadherin (red) (A, B, C) and vWF (green) (A, B) or gp 100 (green) (C). Nuclei were counterstained with DAPI (blue). Blood vessels that expressed T-cadherin are showed by the arrow in A, blood vessels with no T-cdherin are marked by an empty arrow in B. Bars, 50 μm.

Tumor growth and progression require blood supply. There are three mechanisms by which solid tumors acquire their blood supply. First, tumor and the surrounding stromal cells secrete angiogenic factors that stimulate vessel growth and recruitment into the tumor from the preexisting vessels in a well described process of angiogenesis (Folkman et al., 1971; Folkman et al., 1992, Folkman 1995). Asahara and colleagues demonstrated the incorporation of circulating endothelial progenitors form the peripheral blood into sites of ischemia-induced angiogenesis (Asahara et al., 1997). Beyond these two mechanisms, aggressive primary and metastatic melanomas are capable of generating microcirculatory channels composed of extracellular matrix and lined by tumor cells that express VE-cadherin (Hendrix et al., 2001; Maniotis et al., 1999). These vascular channels (lacunas) allow blood flow. However, lacunas are not strictly vasculogenic or angiogenic because they are formed by melanoma cells (Folberg et al., 2002; Maniotis et al., 1999). Therefore the name "vasculogenic mimicry" was assigned to the process by which melanoma cells generate non-endothelial cell-lined channels (Maniotis et al., 1999). This vasculogenic mimicry adds challenges to the practical surgery and requires new cancer diagnostic and treatment strategies.

Our data indicate that the areas devoid of T-cadherin in the primary melanomas were more intensively vascularized than the areas with high level of T-cadherin expression. 80% of vWF-positive blood vessels also expressed T-cadherin (arrows in Fig.3A), while no T-cadherin could be detected in the rest of the blood vessels (arrows in Fig.3A, 4A). Besides vWF-positive blood vessels in the primary melanomas (Fig.4A) and in the visceral metastasis, vascular channels devoid of endothelial cells were found. Interestingly, vascular channels were lined up by the cells expressing T-cadherin (Fig.4A, C).

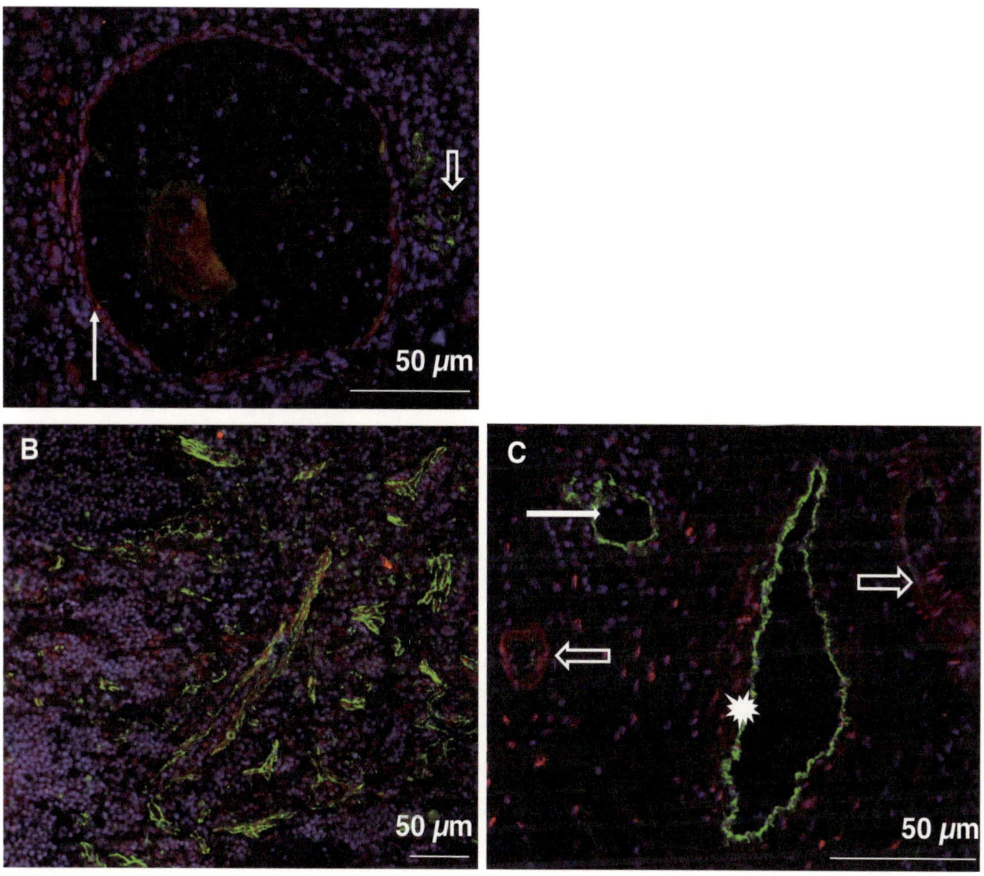

Figure 4. Double immunofluorescent staining of the primary melanoma (A) and visceral metastasis samples (B, C) with antibodies against T-cadherin (red) and vWF (green). (A) Large lacuna can be seen in the center of the image of the primary melanoma (showed by an arrow). The walls of the lacunas in the primary melanomas (A) and metastasis (B, C) were lined up by T-cadherin positive melanoma cells (red). Blood vessels of the primary melanomas and metastasis were heterogeneous. In (A) vWF-positive blood vessels with no T-cadherin expression could be seen located in the immediate vicinity of the lacuna (green) fluorescence, marked by an empty arrow in A): in (B and asterisk in C) both variants of vWF-positive blood vessels are presented: T-cadherin positive and T-cadherin negative (arrows in A and C, respectively). Nuclei were counterstained with DAPI (blue). Bars, 50 μm.

Our data indicated that T-cadherin expression in human melanoma was gradually reduced upon melanoma progression. While nearly 60% of melanoma cells in the primary melanomas expressed T-cadherin, 30% of the sections exhibited a mosaic pattern of T-cadherin expression in melanoma cells and 10% of the sections were T-cadherin negative. In metastasis, 60% of the sections were occupied by melanoma cells with heterogeneous T-cadherin expression (mosaic pattern) and the number of T-cadherin-positive cells was reduced to 30% (Fig. 5). These results were in agreement with the data obtained by Kuphal (Kuphal et al., 2009) who detected T-cadherin expression in melanocytes in the healthy skin and intratumoral capillaries of the primary melanoma samples while T-cadherin expression was lost in melanoma cells.

The same pattern was previously described for pre-cancer skin lesions and non-melanoma skin cancer: T-cadherin expression was gradually lost upon malignization. The aberrant expression of T-cadherin was also detected in the blood vessels and correlated with the histological features and invasive behavior of more aggressive tumors (Rubina et al., 2012).

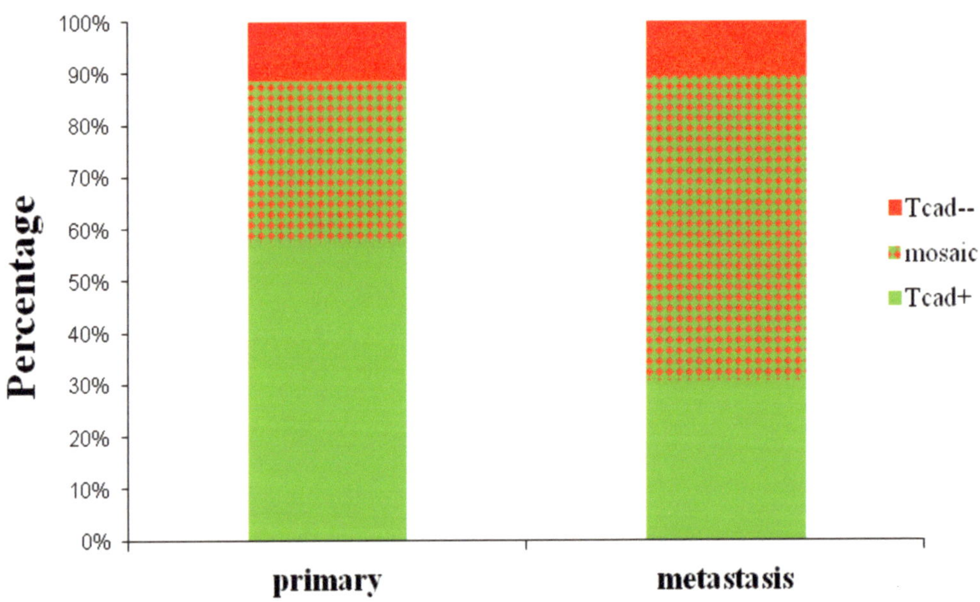

Figure 5. Loss of the expression of T-cadherin in melanocytes during metastasis.

To elucidate the potential role of T-cadherin in melanoma progression and growth, we used an established model of highly aggressive murine melanoma B16F10 in BDF1 mice. The murine melanoma B16F10 with lung metastases is considered as an adequate model for testing the efficacy of new anticancer therapies in preclinical evaluations and the forecasting model of human disseminated melanoma in anticancer screening (Teicher and Andrews, 2004).

http://dx.doi.org/10.5772/53350

5. The effect of T-cadherin expression on melanoma cell proliferation and apoptosis

To assess the effect of T-cadherin expression on melanoma cell proliferation we generated stable cell lines of murine malignant melanoma B16F10 cells (ATCC® №CRL-6475™) by transfecting the cells with pcDNA-Tcad using Lipofectamine™ 2000 reagent (Invitrogen, USA. As a control, luciferase cDNA fragment in the antisense orientation was cloned into the pcDNA 3.1 vector. The cells were cultured and transfected as described before (Yurlova et al., 2010). For stable cell line generation transfected cells were cloned and selected by incubation with 2 mg/ml G418 (Invitrogen, USA). For some experiments we also used the polyclonal mouse melanoma B16F10 cell cultures obtained after transfection and subsequent selection with G418 without cloning. Expression of T-cadherin in polyclonal mouse melanoma cell cultures and melanoma cell clones was examined by Western blotting. Three clones of B16F10 melanoma cells with different level of T-cadherin expression was chosen: a control clone with no T-cadherin (T-), clone with low T-cadherin expression (T+) and clone with high T-cadherin expression (T++) (Yurlova et al., in press).

To investigate the effect of T-cadherin expression on melanoma cell proliferation, cells were seeded on 6-well plates and harvested by trypsinization after 24, 48 and 72 h in culture and counted with the Countess® (Invitrogen, USA). After 3 days, the number of T-cadherin-expressing cells (T+ and T++) was 44-48% higher compared to the control (Fig. 6A). We obtained similar results using the impedance measurement with xCELLigence system: the cell index was continuously monitored with 1 min interval for 5 hrs and with 10 min interval for 96 hrs. (Fig. 6B). The xCELLigence system (Roche, USA) monitors cellular events in real time and measures electrical impedance across microelectrodes integrated on the bottom of E-Plates. Thus, our data indicated that T-cadherin expression in mouse B16F10 melanoma cells increased their proliferation *in vitro*.

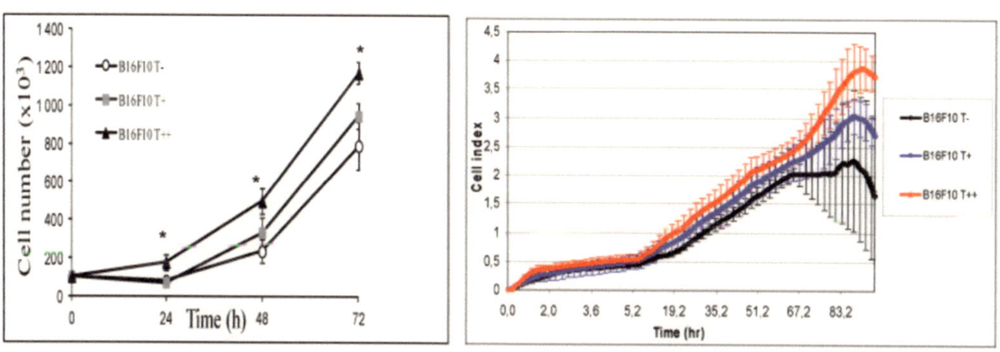

Figure 6. T-cadherin expression stimulated proliferation of B16F10 cells *in vitro*. (A) Cells were incubated in RPMI 1640 medium containing 10% FBS for indicated periods of time, harvested and counted using CellCounter. (B) The cell proliferation assay was performed with xCELLigence system. Attachment of 5000 cells per chamber was monitored with the impedance measurement of the xCELLigence System for 96 hrs. The cell indexes of B16F10 T- (control cells, black), T+ (cells with low level of T-cadherin, blue) and T++ (cells with high level of T-cadherin, red) are shown. Results are presented as the means ± SEM of three independent experiments.

To evaluate the effect of T-cadherin expression on apoptosis of B16F10 cells we performed staining with Annexin V. The B16F10 cell clones were resuspended in 200 μl of Annexin V binding buffer (BD Biosciences, USA), incubated with 5 μl of Annexin V-Phycoerythrin (BD Biosciences, USA) and 10 μl of 7-AAD (BD Biosciences, USA) for 15 min in the dark. The percentage of apoptotic cells was evaluated by flow cytometry (FACSCanto II™, BD Biosciences, USA). The fraction and absolute number (data not shown) of apoptotic and dead cells in T-cadherin-expressing clones were not significantly different from the control.

Thus, in contrast to the earlier study by Kuphal (Kuphal et al., 2009) who found no effect of T-cadherin expression on human melanoma cell proliferation, the current study showed that the expression of T-cadherin in mouse melanoma cells stimulated their proliferation *in vitro* and had no effect on the apoptosis.

6. Effect of T-cadherin expression on tumor growth and metastatic potentials of B16F10 clones in vivo

Animal studies were conducted according to the guidelines of the Institutional Animal Care and Use committee of Cardiology Research Center (permit number 385.06.2009). In order to establish a relationship between T-cadherin expression level and increased proliferation of melanoma cells and melanoma growth in vivo, we injected the clones of B16F10 cells with different level of T-cadherin expression into BDF1 mice. $1x10^6$ B16F10 cells (T-, T+, or T++ clones) in 0.3 ml of serum-free media were injected subcutaneously in BDF1 mice (n=11 in each group). 28 days after the injection, animals were sacrificed and primary tumors and lungs were collected. The measurement of the tumors was performed 4 times a week over 28 days. The tissue samples were embedded in Tissue-Tek (Sakura, USA), frozen in liquid nitrogen and stored at -80°C. The cryosections (6 μm) were fixed in 4% formaldehyde. To analyze the necrosis areas, cryosections were stained with Mayer's hematoxylin. Vascularization and stroma content was analyzed using the following primary antibodies: anti-T-cadherin, anti-CD31 to visualize endothelial cells (1:100, BD Biosciences, USA), anti-NG2 to visualize pericytes (1:100, Abcam, USA), anti-CD90 to visualize MSCs (1:100, BD Biosciences, USA). For negative controls, non-specific IgGs were used in similar concentration. Cell nuclei were counterstained with DAPI (Sigma-Aldrich, USA). The sections were analyzed using Leica AF6000 microscope and MetaMorph 5.0 (Universal Imaging, USA). For statistics, five view fields on five random sections for each tumor sample were used. The blood vessels were separated into three groups: capillaries (CD31-positive vessels without lumen and with length <20 μm); medium vessels (CD31-positive vessels with length 20-40 μm), and large vessels (with diameter >40 μm). The contribution of the stroma into the growth of primary tumor was determined as the area of CD90-positive cells in a field normalized to the DAPI-stained area of each cryosection. To evaluate the necrosis area we calculated the number of cryosections containing necrosis foci and normalized it to the total number of assessed sections.

The growth kinetic of tumors was compared within the next 4 weeks and then the histopathology was studied. The T+ and T++ B16F10 cells generated tumors 2.5 and 3 times larger than

http://dx.doi.org/10.5772/53350

control B16F10 cells, correspondingly (Fig. 7A). Difference between the control and T-cadherin-expressing tumor volumes was statistically significant. The histological analysis showed that tumors formed by the control and T-cadherin-expressing B16F10 clones had different morphology. The tumors generated by the T-cadherin-expressing melanoma clones contained wider areas of necrosis (Fig. 7B).

We also compared the spontaneous metastatic potential of the B16F10 clones. 28 days after injection, tumor-bearing mice were sacrificed and their lungs were analyzed. We found that T-cadherin overexpression enhanced spontaneous metastatic activity of B16F10 cells. The B16F10 clones with high level of T-cadherin (T++) formed metastasis in 54.5% cases in comparison to 18.2% and 9.1% formed by T+ and T- cells, respectively. Taken together, these results suggested that the expression of T-cadherin stimulated growth of the primary tumors *in vivo* and enhanced their invasion and metastatic potential.

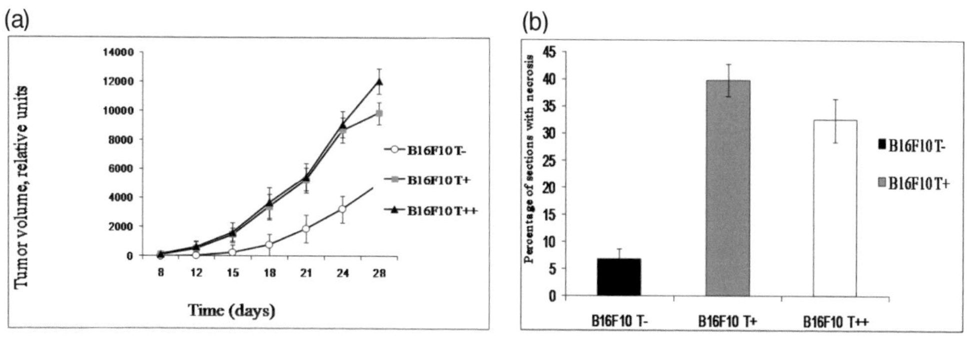

Figure 7. T-cadherin expression in B16F10 cells stimulates tumor growth *in vivo*. (A) $1x10^6$ of B16F10 cells (T-, T+, or T++) were injected subcutaneously in BDF1 mice (n=11). The tumor volume was measured every 3 day after the tumor cell inoculation. Data represent the mean ± SEM. (B) The necrosis area was calculated as the number of cryosections containing necrosis foci normalized to the total number of sections. Results are the means ± SEM, $p<0.05$.

7. Effect of T-cadherin expression on tumor vascularization

Because T-cadherin was shown to inhibit angiogenesis in some models (Rubina et al., 2007) we examined the effect of T-cadherin on the neovascularization of B16F10 primary melanoma sites. For that, cryosections of primary melanomas were stained with anti-CD31 antibody to visualize endothelial cells in the blood vessels penetrating the tumor. The quantitative evaluation revealed a 1.3-1.5-fold decrease in the number of medium size vessels and 1.5-2-fold reduction in capillaries in T-cadherin-expressing primary melanomas compared to the control (Fig. 8). There was no detected difference in the amount of large or stable vessels using double immunofluorescent staining with anti-CD31 and anti-NG2 (marker of pericytes and smooth muscle cells) antibodies (data not shown).

Similar results were obtained using melanoma primary tumors formed by polyclonal mouse melanoma cell culture (data not shown). We concluded that the effects of T-cadherin were not related to the individual features of the selected clones.

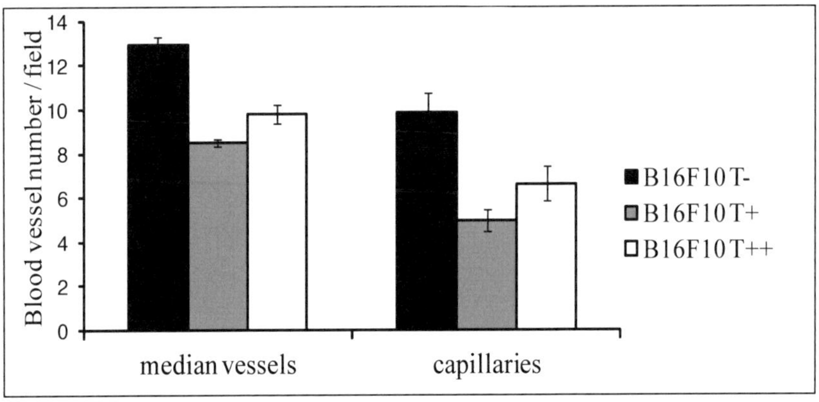

Figure 8. T-cadherin expression in B16F10 cells caused the reduction in tumor vascularization. 28 days after the melanoma cell inoculation, sections of primary tumors formed by the B16F10 T-, T+ or T++ cells were stained with anti-CD31 and anti-T-cadherin antibodies. The quantitative assessment of the blood vessels from 30 random fields of five independent tumors is presented. The results are the means ± SEM of three independent experiments, $p<0.05$.

These results suggested that T-cadherin overexpression in B16F10 melanoma cells suppresses tumor neovascularization by limiting tumor neoangiogenesis.

8. Effect of T-cadherin expression on host stroma

Over the past decade it was discovered that heterogeneous population of progenitor cells known as multipotent stromal cells or mesenchymal stem cells (MSCs) derived from the bone marrow or adipose tissue exhibited a marked tropism for tumors (Klopp et al., 2011). Circulating in the blood stream, MSC from the bone marrow or resident mesenchymal stromal cells could engraft within the tumor microenvironment and incorporate into the stroma of solid tumors as tumor-associated fibroblasts and contribute to the growth of the primary tumor sites (Mishra et al., 2008; Spaeth et al., 2008). MSCs can also act as pericytes-like cells and potentiate tumor growth, vascularization and metastasis. The mechanism by which MSCs support the tumor growth and progression is in the intercellular interactions with tumor cells and the release of the paracrine signals (Spaeth et al., 2009). MSCs themselves are likely to respond to chemoattractants similar to many immune cells that migrate to injury or inflammation site (Spaeth et al., 2008).

To examine whether T-cadherin expression influences the recruitment/proliferation of stromal cells in the model of mouse melanoma growth and progression, cryosections of primary tumor sites were stained with anti-CD90 antibody to visualize the activated stroma (Campioni et al., 2008) (Fig. 9A). Immunofluorescent analysis revealed a 2.4–2.9-fold increase in the CD90 positive areas in the T-cadherin-expressing tumor samples compared to the controls (Fig. 9B). CD90-positive cells were arranged in a form of cell aggregates among the tumor cells or located perivascular around CD31-positive vessels structures. Thus, for the first time we revealed that the expression of T-cadherin stimulated the recruitment of CD90-positive cells to the primary tumor site. The CD90-positive cells were represented mainly by MSCs. However, some populations of neutrophils, T cells and monocytes could also express CD90 and be recruited to the tumors (Rege and Hagood, 2006).

To support the *in vivo* data on the T-cadherin-mediated recruitment of the stromal cells to the growing tumor, we established a transwell assay in which MSCs were co-cultured with the melanoma clones with different T-cadherin expression. The transwell system allowed exchange of the medium in the absence of direct interaction between cells in the lower and upper chambers. The MSCs were isolated from subcutaneous adipose tissue of the inguinal region of CBA/C57BL male mice and cultured until the 2nd passage as described before (Rubina et al., 2009). To assess the effect of T-cadherin expression in melanoma cells on their ability to induce MSC migration, MSCs were seeded in the upper chamber and melanoma cell clones were seeded in the lower chamber. The MSCs were allowed to migrate across the collagene-covered membrane and the conditioned medium from the B16F10 clones served as a chemoattractant. We found that migration of MSCs towards the conditioned medium from the T++ B16F10 cells was at least 1.5-fold higher than towards the T+ or T- B16F10 cells (Fig. 10).

We did not detect the shedding of T-cadherin into the conditioned medium from the T-cadherin expressing B16F10 clones using Western blotting (data not shown). Thus, we suggested that the observed effects on MSCs migration were mediated by secretion of chemoattractants and growth factors into the conditioned medium by the T-cadherin expressing melanoma cells. To prove that we studied the expression of angiogenec factors, extracellular matrix proteins, adhesion molecules and chemokines using the PCR Array assay (SABiosciences, USA) and quantitative PCR.

9. T-cadherin expression changes the gene expression pattern in B16F10 melanoma cells

For PCR Array assay, total RNA was isolated from B16F10 clones using RNeasy Mini kit. 1 μg of total RNA was treated with DNase, cDNA was prepared using RT2 First Strand kit (SABiosciences, USA). For each experiment, cDNA sample was mixed with RT2 qPCR Master mix and distributed across the PCR array 96-well plates. After cycling with real-time PCR (IQ5 PCR platform, Bio Rad, USA), obtained amplification data (fold-changes in Ct values) was analyzed with SABiosciences software. RNA expression of each gene was normalized using 5 housekeeping genes. The relative expression of each gene, compared to expression in the control B16F10 clone was calculated on the website using $\Delta\Delta$Ct method. A gene was considered as differentially regulated if the difference was >2-fold compared with the control clone.

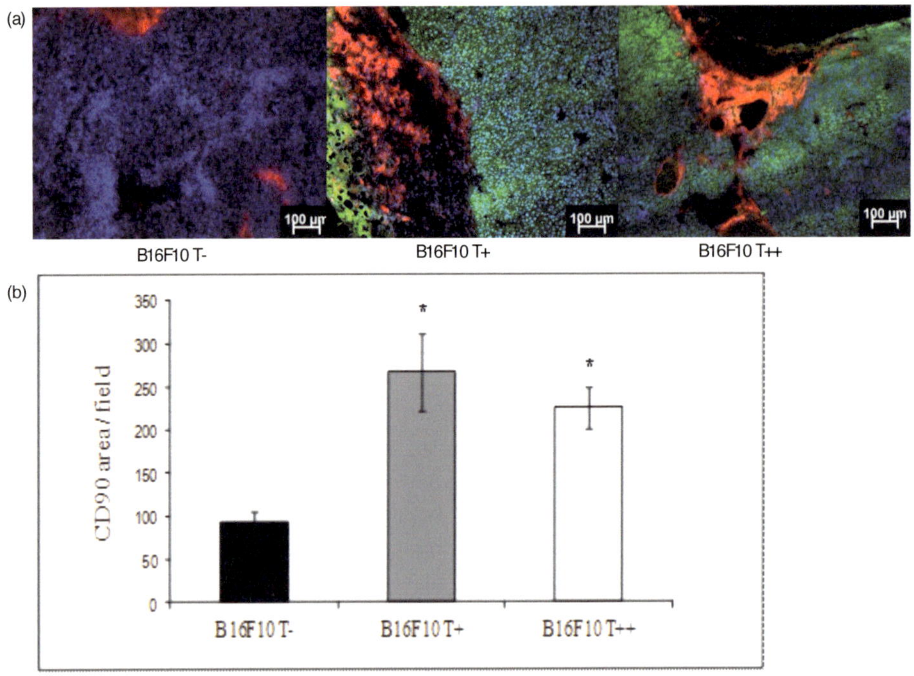

Figure 9. The effect of T-cadherin expression in B16F10 cells on MSC recruitment. (A) 28 days after melanoma cell inoculation, sections of the primary tumor formed by the B16F10 T- (left), T+ (middle), or T++ (right) cells were stained with anti-CD90 (red) and with anti-T-cadherin (green) antibody. Bars - 100 µm. (B) The contribution of the stroma into the growth of primary tumor was determined as an area of CD90-positive cells in a field normalized to the DAPI-stained area unit of each cryosection using program MetaMorph 5.0. Results are the means ± SEM of three independent experiments, $p<0.05$.

For quantitative PCR the RNeasy Mini Kit (Qiagen, Germany) was used to extract the total RNA. cDNA were prepared using the RevertAid H Minus First Strand cDNA Synthesis Kit (Fermentas, USA). The primers were obtained from Sintol (Russia). Real-time qPCR analysis was performed with SYBR Green I on Rotor – Gene™ 3000 (Corbett Research, UK). The gene expression was normalized to the expression of β-actin and GAPDH. The primer specificity was confirmed by melting curve analysis. The qRT-PCR was repeated five times.

We performed quantitative PCR and PCR Array Assay of melanoma cells and revealed that T-cadherin expression in B16F10 melanoma cells resulted the increase in expression of chemokines CXCL10, CCL5, CXCL11 and CCL7, which were earlier implicated in the growth and metastasis of different neuroectodermal tumors (Somasundaram and Herlyn, 2009). In a screen of several human and mouse melanoma cell lines, it was detected that the expression of chemokine receptors CCR7, CCR10, CXCR1, CXCR2 and CXCR4 could dramatically increase the rate of metastases (Longo-Imedio et al., 2005; Simonetti et al., 2006; Singh et al., 2009; Wiley et al., 2001). In the present study, the up-regulation of CXCL10, CCL5, CXCL11 and CCL7 genes was found to be correlated with the increase in spontaneous metastatic activity in the B16F10 mouse melanoma model.

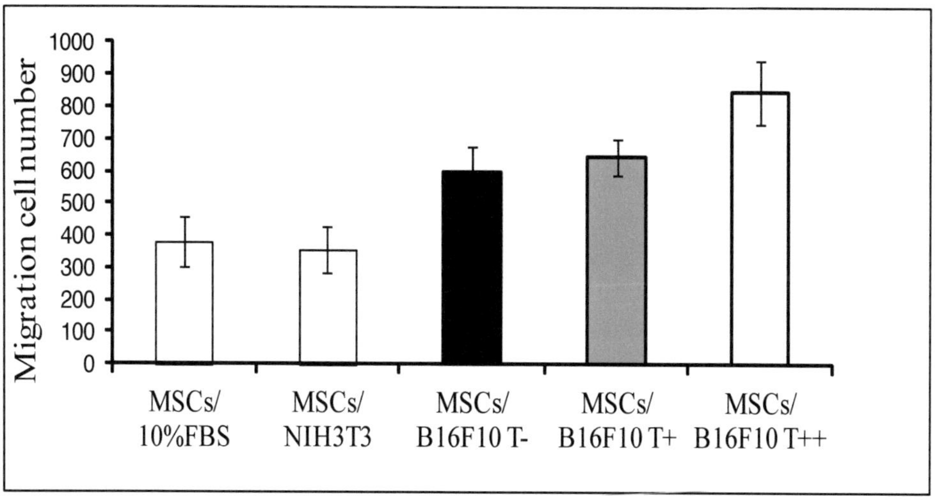

Figure 10. The effect of conditioned medium from the B16F10 cell clones with different T-cadherin expression on migration of MSCs. Migrated MSCs were quantified after fixation and hematoxylin staining of the membrane. The results are the means ± SEM of three independent experiments performed in duplicates, $p<0.05$.

Gene	Annealing temperature	Forward 5'-3'	Reverse 5'-3'
GAPDH	60	GACCCCTTCATTGACCTCAACTAC	TGGTGGTGCAGGATGCATTGCTGA
β-actin	61	AGTGTGACGTTGACATCCGTA	GCCAGAGCAGTAATCTCCTTCT
VEGF A	60	AGAGCAGAAGTCCCATGAAGTGA	TCAATCGGACGGCAGTAGCT
PDGF B	58,5	TCTCTGCTGCTACCTGCGTCTGG	GTGTGCTCGGGTCATGTTCAAGTC
HGF	60	TCATTGGTAAAGGAGGCAGCTATA	CTGGCATTTGATGCCACTCTTA
MMP2	53	AGTTCCCGTTCCGCTTCC	GACACATGGGGCACCTTCTG
EGF	60	CCTGCCCCCTTCCTAGTTTTC	CTCCGTTCTGTTGGTCTACCC
uPAR	60	CGTTACCTCGAGTGTGCGTCCTG	AGCCTCGGGTGTAGTCCTCATCCT
c-Met	60	CAACGAGAGCTGTACCTTGACCTTA	GCGGGACCAACTGTGCAT
uPA	53	GAATGCGCCTGCTGTC	AGGGTCGCTTCTGGTTGTC
MMP9	61	GCGGTGTGGGGCGAGGTG	CCAGGGGGAAAGGCGTGTG

Table 1. Sequences of primers used in qRT-PCR.

In normal conditions, the blood vessel growth is strictly controlled by the balance between pro-angiogenic and and anti-angiogenic factors. At the same time, tumor progression is accompanied by neoangiogenesis due to enhanced production of pro-angiogenic molecules by tumor and stromal cells (Hanahan and Folkman, 1996). To elucidate the mechanisms responsible for T-cadherin-mediated suppression of angiogenesis in primary melanoma we performed qRT PCR and PCR Arrays. No difference in the mRNA expression level of the main angiogenic growth factors such as VEGF A, HGF, bFGF, EGF, PDGF B, TGFβ between control and T-cadherin-expressing clones was revealed. However, PCR Array analysis revealed that T-cadherin expression in B16F10 cells resulted in upregulation of mRNA of such antiangiogenic molecules as CXCL 10 (Strieter et al., 1995); angiopoietin 2 (Cao et al., 2007); procollagen type XVIIIα1 - a precursor of the angiogenesis inhibitor endostatin (O'Reilly et al., 1997) and chromogranin A - a precursor of angiogenesis inhibitor vasostatin-1 (Belloni et al., 2007). Angiopoietin 2 acts together with VEGF A in initiating blood vessel growth through inhibition of the interactions between endothelial and perivascular cells and destabiliziation of blood vessels. However, in the absence of VEGF A, angiopoietin 2 suppresses angiogenesis and promotes vessel regression (Holash et al., 1999). Since in the present study VEGF A level was not changed after the expression of T-cadherin, the elevated angiopoietin 2 expression could act in reducing the number of newly formed vessels. We also found that the T-cadherin-expressing B16F10 cells demonstrated decreased expression of angiogenic molecules TGFα (Leker et al., 2009) and Tie 1 (Sato et al., 1995). Thus, the PCR Array analysis indicated that the balance between the pro-angiogenic and anti-angiogenic factors was shifted towards the latter, which could reduce the number of medium size vessels and capillaries in vivo.

It is well known that MSCs secrete many growth factors and cytokines and their production increases in hypoxic conditions (Rubina et al., 2009; Martin-Rendon 2007). Among them is HGF/SF, which is a potent stimulator of DNA synthesis and growth in normal human melanocytes and melanoma cells (Halaban et al., 1993). Thus, it was shown that overexpression of the proto-oncogene c-Met (HGFR - HGF receptor) is tightly correlated with human melanoma progression from the radial to the vertical stage (Natali et al., 1993). In the present study we found that control B16F10 melanoma cells expressed low levels of c-Met and no HGF. Our quantitative PCR analysis demonstrated that T-cadherin overexpression resulted in 6-fold increase in the content of c-Met mRNA in melanoma cells. This data suggested that one of the mechanisms by which T-cadherin could be able to affect the growth of B16F10 melanoma cells is the regulation of c-Met/HGF signaling pathway. We speculated that the melanoma cells expressing T-cadherin could secrete the high levels of chemokines resulting in MSCs recruitment to the primary tumor site. MSCs in hypoxic conditions are known to increase the production of HGF (Rubina et al., 2009). Thus, in hypoxic conditions of the primary tumor the recruited MSCs could produce the high levels of HGF, which upon binding to c-Met on melanoma cells could cause their increased proliferation and invasion

Apparently, invasive and metastasizing cancers are characterized by the change in integrin expression pattern (Makrilia et al., 2009). Thus, the overexpressions of integrins such as α3, α5 and α1 or their single subunits were shown to be involved in melanoma growth and progression (Kuphal et al., 2005). So we compared the expression level of certain integrins in the control and T-cadherin expressing melanoma cells using PCR Array. We revealed the upregulation of mRNA expression of α5, αV, αE, and β3 integrins upon T-cadherinsion. This correlated with the increase in the metastatic activity of those cells and possibly contributed to melanoma progression.

http://dx.doi.org/10.5772/53350

It was shown that the overexpression of some integrins can induce matrix metalloproteinases (MMPs) expression in melanoma cells or their activation (Khatib et al., 2001; Sil et al., 2011). Several MMPs including MMP-1, -2, -3, -7, -9, -13, -14, -15, -16 as well as uPA were implicated in human melanoma progression, invasion and metastasis (Bianchini et al., 2006; Ria et al., 2010). Using qRT-PCR we examined the expression of mRNA of MMPs with gelatinase activity and uPA. No differences in MMP2, MMP9 and uPA expression in the control and T-cadhering positive B16F10 cell clones were revealed. Further PCR The array analysis established that MMP14 was the only protease with enhanced expression detected in the T-cadherin expressing clone T++.

Melanoma cells express multiple isoforms of laminin that were shown to mediate cell attachment and invasion via integrin receptors using laminin as a substrate (Oikawa et al., 2011). In addition, expression of fibronectin was correlated with the acquisition of invasive and metastatic behavior of human melanoma (Gaggioli et al., 2007). Using PCR Array analysis we found that T-cadherin overexpressing melanoma cells exhibited the elevated level of fibronectin 1 and laminin $\alpha3$ expression suggesting their role in the increased metastatic potential of these cells. The obtained data indicated that T-cadherin expression affects the expression of certain genes involved in regulation of melanoma growth and progression.

In contrast to the results obtained in the present study, the re-expression of T-cadherin by stable transfection in human melanoma cells reduced the rate of tumor growth in the nu/nu mouse tumor model, decreased cell capacity for anchorage-independent growth, migration and invasion in vitro, while cell proliferation was not affected (Kuphal et al., 2009).This discrepancy could be due to the differences in the experimental conditions of the models (highly aggressive murine melanoma B16F10 in the BDF1 mice versus human melanoma cells injected into immunodeficient nu/nu mice). The difference could also be explained by the distinct signaling pathways and spectrum growth factors and receptors expressed by mouse and human melanoma.

10. Conclusions

In the present study, we found that T-cadherin is expressed in normal epidermal keratinocytes, vascular cells of the dermal blood vessels and melanocytes in the human skin. However, upon malignant transformation we observed mosaic pattern of T-cadherin expression in primary melanomas and partial or complete loss of T-cadherin in melanoma metastasis. These data are in accordance with the earlier published results and confirmed the correlation between tumor progression and the loss of T-cadherin expression. It was previously reported that 80% of the human melanoma cell lines did not express T-cadherin and re-expression of T-cadherin reduced the tumorigenicity of these cell lines in nu/nu mouse model. However, 20% of human melanoma cell lines abundantly expressed T-cadherin and possessed invasive and metastatic potential. This prompted us to use a well-described model of highly aggressive murine melanoma B16F10 in BDF1 mice and examine the effect of T-cadherin expression in melanoma cells on their proliferation, tumor growth, invasive and metastatic potential and neovascularization. We showed that overexpression of T-cadherin in melanoma B16F10 cells resulted in the increased tumor growth and metastasi as well as the recruitment of MSC into the primary site. We suggested that in response to the chemoattractants (chemokines) produced by the T-cadherin-expressing tumors, the stromal cells migrated into the primary site and produced HGF. In return, HGF triggered the HGF/c-Met signaling cascade in T-cadherin-expressing melanoma cells that could lead to their increased proliferation and metastasis. The elevated expression level of prooncogenic integrins, the extracellular matrix components and MMP14 in these cells could be contributing factors to enhanced metastatic and invasive potential. However, T-cadherin expression in melanoma cells exerted inhibitory effect on vascularization of the primary tumors, which is likely to be due to the switch in the balance of pro- and antiangiogenic molecules. The established link between the expression of T-cadherin and pathological processes that trigger neovascularization and tumor progression are particularly important in search for new approaches for inhibiting metastasis of the less curable tumors such as disseminated melanoma of the skin. Further investigations studies are needed to identify the role of T-cadherin in the initiation of tumor progression associated with the regulation of neoangiogenesis. Our studies provided new evidence on the role of tumor microenvironment and will help to identify the critical points for suppressing the blood supply at the early stages of tumor progression. We concluded that the expression of T-cadherin in melanoma cells underlies a novel mechanism of stem cell tropism to malignant solid tumors, which may be important for the development of the optimal stem cell-based therapy. Investigation of such mechanisms is an important task in finding new targets for cancer treatment.

Grant support

This work was supported by a grant (№ 16.512.12.2005) of the Ministry for Education and Science of Russian Federation and grant (№ 08-04-01024-a) of Russian Foundation for Basic Research.

Author details

K. A. Rubina[1*], E. I. Yurlova[1], V. Yu. Sysoeva[1], E. V. Semina[2], N. I. Kalinina[1], A. A. Poliakov[4], I. N. Mikhaylova[3], N. V. Andronova[3] and H. M. Treshalina[3]

*Address all correspondence to: rkseniya@mail.ru

1 Faculty of Basic Medicine, M.V. Lomonosov Moscow State University, Moscow, Russian Federation

2 Institute of Experimental Cardiology, Cardiology Research Center of Russia, Moscow, Russian Federation

http://dx.doi.org/10.5772/53350

3 N.N. Blokhin Russian Cancer Research Center of Russian Academy of Medical Sciences, Moscow, Russian Federation

4 Division of Developmental Neurobiology, MRC National Institute for Medical Research, London, UK

References

[1] Adachi Y, Takeuchi T, Nagayama T, Ohtsuki Y, & Furihata M (2009) Zeb1-mediated T-cadherin repression increases the invasive potential of gallbladder cancer. FEBS Letters, 583(2):430-436.

[2] Adachi Y, Takeuchi T, Sonobe H & Ohtsuki Y (2006) An adiponectin receptor, T-cadherin, was selectively expressed in intratumoral capillary endothelial cells in hepatocellular carcinoma: possible cross talk between T-cadherin and FGF-2 pathways. Virchows Arch, 448(3):311-18.

[3] Andersen K, Nesland JM, Holm R, Florenes VA, Fodstad O & Maelandsmo GM (2004) Expression of S100A4 combined with reduced E-cadherin expression predicts patient outcome in malignant melanoma. Mod Pathol, 17:990–997.

[4] Asahara T, Murohara T, Sullivan A, Silver M, van der ZR, Li T, Wit-zenbichler B, Schatteman G & Isner JM (1997) Isolation of putative progenitor endothelial cells for angiogenesis. Science, 275:964 –967.

[5] Bachmann IM, Straume O, Puntervoll HE, Kalvenes MB & Akslen LA (2005) Importance of P-cadherin, beta-catenin, and Wnt5a/frizzled for progression of melanocytic tumors and prognosis in cutaneous melanoma. Clin Cancer Res, 11:8606–8614.

[6] Bar-Eli M (1997) Molecular mechanisms of melanoma metastasis. J Cell Physiol, 173:275–278.

[7] Bauer R, Hein R & Bosserhoff AK (2005) A secreted form of P-cadherin is expressed in malignant melanoma. Exp Cell Res, 305:418–426.

[8] Belloni D, Scabini S, Foglieni C, Veschini L, Giazzon A, Colombo B, et al. (2007) The vasostatin-I fragment of chromogranin A inhibits VEGF-induced endothelial cell proliferation and migration. FASEB J, 21(12):3052–3062.

[9] Bianchini F, D'Alessio S, Fibbi G, Del Rosso M & Calorini L (2006) Cytokine-dependent invasiveness in B16 murine melanoma cells: role of uPA system and MMP-9. Oncol Rep, 15(3):709-14.

[10] Bonitsis N, Batistatou A, Karantima S, Charalabopoulos K (2006) The role of cadherin/catenin complex in malignant melanoma. Oncol, 28(3):187–193.

[11] Bosserhoff AK, Ellmann L, Kuphal S (2011) Melanoblasts in culture as an in vitro system to determine molecular changes in melanoma. Exp Dermatol, 20(5):435-40.

[12] Cao Y, Sonveaux P, Liu S, Zhao Y, Mi J, Clary BM, et al. (2007) Systemic overexpression of angiopoietin-2 promotes tumor microvessel regression and inhibits angiogenesis and tumor growth. Cancer Res, 67(8):3835–3844.

[13] Campioni D, Lanza F, Moretti S, Ferrari L, Cuneo A. (2008) Loss of Thy-1 (CD90) antigen expression on mesenchymal stromal cells from hematologic malignancies is induced by in vitro angiogenic stimuli and is associated with peculiar functional and phenotypic characteristics. Cytotherapy, 10(1):69-82.

[14] Cavallaro U, Leibner S, Dejana E (2006) Endothelial cadherins and tumor angiogenesis. Exp Cell Res, 312(5):659-667.

[15] Clark WH, Elder DE, Guerry D, Epstein MN, Greene MH & Van Horn M (1984) A study of tumor progression: the precursor lesions of superficial spreading and nodular melanoma. Hum Pathol, 15:1147–1165.

[16] Danen EH, de Vries TJ, Morandini R, Ghanem GG,Ruiter DJ & van Muijen GN (1996) E-cadherin expression in humanmelanoma. Melanoma Res, 6:127–131.

[17] Dejana E (1996) Endothelial adherens junctions: implications in the control of vascular permeability and angiogenesis. J Clin Invest, 98:1949–1953.

[18] Dejana E, Lampugnani MG, Martinez-Estrada O & Bazzoni G (2000) The molecular organization of endothelial junctions and their functional role in vascular morphogenesis and permeability. Int J Dev Biol, 44:743-748.

[19] Fitzpatrick TB, Szabo G, Seizi M & Quevedo WC (1979) Biology of the melanoma pigmentary system. In: Dermatology in General Medicine. Fitzpatrick TB, Eisen A, Wolf K, Freedberg I, Austen KC. New York: Mc Graw-Hill, 131–145.

[20] Folberg R, Hendrix MJC & Maniotis AJ (2002) Vasculogenic Mimicry and Tumor Angiogenesis. American Journal of Pathology, 156(2):361-381.

[21] Folkman J (1971) Tumor angiogenesis: therapeutic implication. N Engl J Med, 285(21):1182-6.

[22] Folkman J (1992) The role of angiogenesis in tumor growth. Seminars in Cancer Biology, 3(2):65-71

[23] Folkman J (1995) Angiogenesis in cancer, vascular, rheumatoid and other diseases. Nature Medicine, 1(1):37–31.

[24] Fredette BJ & Ranscht B (1994) T-cadherin expression delineates specific regions of the developing motoraxon-hindlimb projection pathway. J Neurosci, 14(12):7331-46.

[25] Fredette BJ, Miller J & Ranscht B (1996) Inhibition of motor axon growth by T-cadherin substrata. Development, 122(10):3163-71.

[26] Frixen UH, Behrens J, Sachs M, Eberle G, Voss B, Warda A, Lochner D & Birchmeier W (1991) E-cadherin-mediated cell-cell adhesion prevents invasiveness of human carcinoma cells. J Cell Biol, 113:173–185.

[27] Gaggioli C, Robert G, Bertolotto C, Bailet O, Abbe P, Spadafora A, et al. (2007) Tumor-derived fibronectin is involved in melanoma cell invasion and regulated by V600E B-Raf signaling pathway. J Invest Dermatol, 127(2):400-410.

[28] Ghosh S, Joshi MB, Ivanov D, Feder-Mengus C, Spagnoli GC, Martin I, Erne P & Resink TJ (2007) Use of multicellular tumor spheroids to dissect endothelial cell-tumor cell interactions: a role for T-cadherin in tumor angiogenesis. FEBS Letters, 581(23): 4523-4528.

[29] Gilchrest BA, Eller MS, Geller AC & Yaar M (1999) The pathogenesis of melanoma induced by ultraviolet radiation. N Engl J Med, 340:1341–1348.

[30] Gray-Schopfer V, Wellbrock C, Marais R (2001) Melanoma biology and new targeted therapy. Nature, 445(7130):851-857.

[31] Gruss C & Herlyn M (2001) Role of cadherins and matrixins in melanoma. Curr Opin Oncol, 13:117–123.

[32] Gumbiner BM (2005) Regulation of cadherin-mediated adhesion in morphogenesis. Nature Rev Mol Cell Biol, 6(8):622-634.

[33] Haass NK & Herlyn M (2005) Normal human melanocyte homeostasis as a paradigm for understanding melanoma. J Investig Dermatol Symp Proc, 10:153–163.

[34] Haass NK, Smalley KS, Li L & Herlyn M (2005) Adhesion, migration and communication in melanocytes and melanoma. Pigment Cell Res, 18:150–159.

[35] Halaban R, Rubin JS & White W (1993) Met and HGF-SF in normal melanocytes and melanoma cells. EXS, 65:329-339.

[36] Hanahan D & Folkman J (1996) Patterns and emerging mechanisms of the angiogenic switch during tumorigenesis. Cell, 86(3):353-364.

[37] Hanahan D & Weinberg RA (2000) The hallmarks of cancer. Cell, 100:57–70.

[38] Hebbard LW, Garlatti M, Young LJ, Cardiff RD, Oshima RG & Ranscht B (2008) T-cadherin supports angiogenesis and adiponectin association with the vasculature in a mouse mammary tumor model. Cancer Res, 68(5):1407-1416.

[39] Hendrix MJ, Seftor EA, Hess AR & Seftor RE (2003) Molecular plasticity of human melanoma cells. Oncogene, 22:3070–3075.

[40] Hendrix MJ, Seftor EA, Meltzer PS Gardner LM, Hess AR, Kirschmann DA, Schatteman GC & Seftor RE (2001) Expression and functional significance of VE-cadherin in aggressive human melanoma cells: Role in vasculogenic mimicry. Proc Natl Acad Sci USA, 98:8018–8023.

[41] Holash J, Maisonpierre PC, Compton D, Boland P, Alexander CR, Zagzag D, Yancopolous GD & Wiegand SJ (1999) Vessel cooption, regression, and growth in tumors mediated by angiopoietins and VEGF. Science, 284(5422):1994-1998.

[42] Hsu MY, Meier FE, Nesbit M, Hsu JY, Van Belle P, Elder DE & Herlyn M (2000) E-cadherin expression in melanoma cells restores keratinocyte-mediated growth control and downregulates expression of invasion-related adhesion receptors. Am J Pathol, 156:1515–1525.

[43] Hsu MY, Wheelock MJ, Johnson KR & Herlyn M (1996) Shifts in cadherin profiles between human normal melanocytes and melanomas. J Investig Dermatol Symp Proc, 1:188–194.

[44] Ishihara K, Saida T & Yamamoto A (2001) Updated statistical data for malignant melanoma in Japan. Int J Clin Oncol, 6:109–116.

[45] Ivanov D, Philippova M, Antropova, J, Gubaeva F, Iljinskaya O, Tararak E, Bochkov V, Erne P, Resink T & Tkachuk V (2001) Expression of cell adhesion molecule T-cadherin in the human vasculature. Histochemistry and Cell Biology, 115(3):231–242.

[46] Johnson JP (1999) Cell adhesion molecules in the development and progression of malignant melanoma. Cancer Metastasis Rev, 18:345–357.

[47] Khatib AM, Nip J, Fallavollita L, Lehmann M, Jensen G & Brodt P (2001) Regulation of urokinase plasminogen activator/plasmin-mediated invasion of melanoma cells by the integrin vitronectin receptor alphaVbeta3. Int J Cancer, 91(3):300-308.

[48] Klopp AH, Gupta A, Spaeth E, Andreeff M & Marini F (2011) Concise Review: Dissecting a Discrepancy in the Literature: Do Mesenchymal Stem Cells Support or Suppress Tumor Growth? Stem Cells, 29(1):11–19.

[49] Kuchelmeister C, Schaumburg LG & Garbe C (2000) Acral cutaneous melanoma in caucasians: clinical features, histopathology and prognosis in 112 patients. Br J Dermatol, 143:275–280.

[50] Kuphal S, Bauer R & Bosserhoff AK (2005) Integrin signaling in malignant melanoma. Cancer Metastasis Rev, 24(2):195-222.

[51] Kuphal S, Martyn AC, Pedley J, Crowther LM, Bonazzi VF, Parsons PG, Bosserhoff AK, Hayward NK & Boyle GM (2009) H-cadherin expression reduces invasion of malignant melanoma. Pigment Cell and Melanoma Research, 22(3):296-306.

[52] Leker RR, Toth ZE, Shahar T, Cassiani-Ingoni R, Szalayova I, Key S, Bratincsák A & Mezey E (2009) Transforming growth factor alpha induces angiogenesis and neurogenesis following stroke. Neuroscience, 163(1):233-243.

[53] Li G & Herlyn M (2000) Dynamics of intercellular communication during melanoma development. Mol Med Today, 6:163–169.

[54] Longo-Imedio MI, Longo N, Treviño I, Lázaro P & Sánchez-Mateos P (2005) Clinical significance of CXCR3 and CXCR4 expression in primary melanoma. Int J Cancer, 117(5):861-865.

[55] Luca MR & Bar-Eli M (1998) Molecular changes in human melanoma metastasis. Histol Histopathol, 13:1225–1231.

[56] Makrilia N, Kollias A, Manolopoulos L & Syrigos K (2009) Cell adhesion molecules: role and clinical significance in cancer. Cancer Invest, 27(10):1023-1037.

[57] Maniotis AJ, Folberg R, Hess A, Seftor EA, Gardner LM, Pe'er J, Trent JM, Meltzer PS & Hendrix MJ (1999) Vascular channel formation by human melanoma cells in vivo and in vitro: Vasculogenic mimicry. Am J Pathol, 155:739–752.

[58] Martin-Rendon E, Hale SJ, Ryan D, Baban D, Forde SP, Roubelakis M, Sweeney D, Moukayed M, Harris AL, Davies K & Watt SM (2007) Transcriptional profiling of human cord blood CD133+ and cultured bone marrow mesenchymal stem cells in response to hypoxia. Stem Cells, 25(4):1003-1012.

[59] McGary EC, Lev DC & Bar-Eli M (2002) Cellular adhesion pathways and metastatic potential of human melanoma.Cancer Biol Ther, 1:459–465.

[60] Miller A J & Mihm MC (2006) Melanoma. N. Engl. J. Med, 355:51–65.

[61] Mishra PJ, Humeniuk R, Medina DJ, Alexe G, Mesirov JP, Ganesan S, Glod JW & Banerjee D (2008) Carcinoma-associated fibroblast-like differentiation of human mesenchymal stem cells. Cancer Res, 68(11):4331–4339.

[62] Nakagawa S & Takeichi M (1998) Neural crest emigration from the neural tube depends on regulated cadherin expression. Development, 125:2963–2967.

[63] Natali PG, Nicotra MR, Di Renzo MF, Prat M, Bigotti A, Cavaliere R & Comoglio PM (1993) Expression of the c-Met/HGF receptor in human melanocytic neoplasms: demonstration of the relationship to malignant melanoma tumour progression. Br J Cancer, 68(4):746-750.

[64] Nishizawa A, Nakanishi Y, Yoshimura K, Sasajima Y, Yamazaki N, Yamamoto A, Hanada K, Kanai Y & Hirohashi S (2005) Clinicopathologic significance of dysadherin expression in cutaneous malignant melanoma: immunohistochemical analysis of 115 patients. Cancer, 103:1693–1700.

[65] Oikawa Y, Hansson J, Sasaki T, Rousselle P, Domogatskaya A, Rodin S, Tryggvason K & Patarroyo M (2011) Melanoma cells produce multiple laminin isoforms and strongly migrate on α5 laminin(s) via several integrin receptors. Exp Cell Res, 317(8): 1119-1133.

[66] O'Reilly MS, Boehm T, Shing Y, Fukai N, Vasios G, Lane WS Flynn E, Birkhead JR, Olsen BR & Folkman J (1997) Endostatin: an endogenous inhibitor of angiogenesis and tumor growth. Cell, 88(2):277-285.

[67] Perez-Moreno M, Jamora C, Fuchs E (2003) Sticky business: orchestrating cellular signals at adherens junctions. Cell, 112: 535-548.

[68] Pfaff D, Philippova M, Buechner SA, Maslova K, Mathys T, Erne P & Resink TJ (2010) T-cadherin loss induces an invasive phenotype in human keratinocytes and squamous cell carcinoma (SCC) cells in vitro and is associated with malignant transformation of cutaneous SCC in vivo. Brit J Dermat, 163(2):353-363.

[69] Philippova M, Ivanov D, Tkachuk V, Erne P & Resink TJ (2003) Polarisation of T-cadherin to the leading edge of migrating vascular cells in vitro: a function in vascular cell motility? Histochem Cell Biol, 120(5):353-360.

[70] Philippova MP, Bochkov VN, Stambolsky DV, Tkachuk VA & Resink TJ (1998) T-cadherin and signal-transducing molecules co-localize in caveolin-rich membrane domain of vascular smooth muscle cells. FEBS Lett, 429(2):207-210.

[71] Ranscht B & Bronner-Fraser M (1991) T-cadherin expression alternates with migrating neural crest cells in the trunk of the avian embryo. Development, 111:15-22.

[72] Ranscht B & Dours-Zimmermann MT (1991) T-cadherin, a novel cadherin cell adhesion molecule in the nervous system lacks the conserved cytoplasmic region. Neuron, 7(3):391-402.

[73] Rege TA & Hagood JS (2006) Thy-1 as a regulator of cell-cell and cell-matrix interactions in axon regeneration, apoptosis, adhesion, migration, cancer, and fibrosis. FASEB J., 20(8):1045-54. Review.

[74] Resink TJ, Kuzmenko YS, Kern F, Stambosly D, Bochkov VN, Tkachuk VA, Erne P & Niermann T (1999) LDL binds to surface expressed human T-cadherin in transfected HEK293 cells and influences homophilic adhesive interactions. FEBS Letters, 463:29-34.

[75] Ria R, Reale A, Castrovilli A, Mangialardi G, Dammacco F, Ribatti D & Vacca A (2010) Angiogenesis and progression in human melanoma. Dermatol Res Pract, 2010:185-191.

[76] Riener MO, Nikolopoulos E, Herr A, Wild PJ, Hausmann M, Wiech T, Orlowska-Volk M, Lassmann S, Walch A & Werner M (2008) Microarray comparative genomic hybridization analysis of tubular breast carcinoma shows recurrent loss of the CDH13 locus on 16q. Human Pathology, 39(11):1621-1629.

[77] Riou P, Saffroy R, Chenailler C, Franc B, Gentile C, Rubinstein E, Resink T, Debuire B, Piatier-Tonneau D & Lemoine A (2006) Expression of T-cadherin in tumor cells influences invasive potential of human hepatocellular carcinoma. FASEB Journal, 20(13):2291-2301.

[78] Rubina K, Kalinina N, Efimenko A, Lopatina T, Melikhova V Tsokolaeva Z, Sysoeva V, Tkachuk V & Parfyonova Y (2009) Adipose stromal cells stimulate angiogenesis

via promoting progenitor cell differentiation, secretion of angiogenic factors, and enhancing vessel maturation. Tissue Eng Part A, 15(8):2039–2050.

[79] Rubina K, Kalinina N, Potekhina A, Efimenko A, Semina E, Poliakov A, Wilkinson DG, Parfyonova Y & Tkachuk V (2007) T-cadherin suppresses angiogenesis in vivo by inhibiting migration of endothelial cells. Angiogenesis, 10(3):183-195

[80] Rubina K, Sysoeva V, Semina E, Yurlova E, Khlebnikova A, Molochkov V & Tkachuk V (2012) Malignant transformation in skin is associated with the loss of T-cadherin expression in human keratinocytes and heterogeneity in T-cadherin expression in tumor vasculature. Tumor Angiogenesis, edited by Sophia Ran, 135-166.

[81] Rubina KA, Kalinina NI, Parfyonova YeV & Tkachuk VA (2007) Signal Transduction Research Trends. Cadhernin Signaling in Vascular Cells: T-Cadherin is a New Player. Editors: Nickolas O. Grachevsky, 95-129.

[82] Ruiter DJ & van Muijen GN (1998) Markers of melanocytic tumour progression. J Pathol, 186: 340–342.

[83] Sallee JL, Wittchen ES, Burridge K (2006) Regulation of cell adhesion by protein tyrosine phosphatases. Cell-cell adhesion. J. Biol. Chem, 281(24):16189-16192.

[84] Sanders DS, Blessing K, Hassan GA, Bruton R, Marsden JR, Jankowski J (1999) Alterations in cadherin and catenin expression during the biological progression of melanocytic tumours. Mol Pathol, 52:151–157.

[85] Sandig M, Voura EB, Kalnins VI & Siu CH (1997) Role of cadherins in the transendothelial migration of melanoma cells in culture. Cell Motil Cytoskeleton, 38:351-364.

[86] Sato M, Mori Y, Sakurada A, Fujimura S & Horii A (1998) The H-cadherin (CDH13) gene is inactivated in human lung cancer. Human Genetics, 103(1):96-101.

[87] Sato TN, Tozawa Y, Deutsch U, Wolburg-Buchholz K, Fujiwara Y, Gendron-Maguire M, Gridley T, Wolburg H, Risau W & Qin Y (1995) Distinct roles of the receptor tyrosine kinases Tie-1 and Tie-2 in blood vessel formation. Nature, 376(6535):70-74.

[88] Sil H, Sen T & Chatterjee A (2011) Fibronectin-integrin (alpha5beta1) modulates migration and invasion of murine melanoma cell line B16F10 by involving MMP-9. Oncol Res, 19(7):335-348.

[89] Silye R, Karayiannakis AJ, Syrigos KN, Poole S, van Noorden S, Batchelor W, Regele H, Sega W, Boesmueller H, Krausz T & Pignatelli M (1998) E-cadherin/catenin complex in benign and malignant melanocytic lesions. J Pathol, 186: 350–355.

[90] Simonetti O, Goteri G, Lucarini G, Filosa A, Pieramici T, Rubini C, Biagini G & Offidani A (2006) Potential role of CCL27 and CCR10 expression in melanoma progression and immune escape. Eur J Cancer, 42(8):1181-1187.

[91] Singh S, Nannuru KC, Sadanandam A, Varney ML & Singh RK (2009) CXCR1 and CXCR2 enhances human melanoma tumourigenesis, growth and invasion. Br J Cancer, 100(10):1638-1646.

[92] Somasundaram R & Herlyn D (2009) Chemokines and the environment in neuroectodermal tumor-host interaction. Semin Cancer Biol, 19(2):92-96.

[93] Spaeth E, Klopp A, Dembinski J, Andreeff M & Marini F (2008) Inflammation and tumor microenvironments: defining the migratory itinerary of mesenchymal stem cells. Gene Ther, 15(10):730-738.

[94] Spaeth EL, Dembinski JL, Sasser AK, Watson K, Klopp A, Hall B, Andreeff M & Marini F (2009) Mesenchymal stem cell transition to tumor-associated fibroblasts contributes to fibrovascular network expansion and tumor progression. PLoS One, 4(4):e4992.

[95] Strieter RM, Kunkel SL, Arenberg DA, Burdick MD & Polverini PJ (1995) Interferon gamma-inducible protein 10 (IP-10), a member of the C-X-C chemokine family, is an inhibitor of angiogenesis. Biochem Biophys Res Commun, 210(1):51-57.

[96] Suehiro Y, Okada T, Anno K, Okayama N, Ueno K, Hiura M, Nakamura M, Kondo T, Oga A, Kawauchi S, Hirabayashi K, Numa F, Ito T, Saito T, Sasaki K & Hinoda Y (2008) Aneuploidy predicts outcome in patients with endometrial carcinoma and is related to lack of CDH13 hypermethylation. Clin Cancer Res, 14(11):3354-3361.

[97] Takeichi M (1993) Cadherins in cancer: implications for invasion and metastasis. Curr Opin Cell Biol, 5(5):806–811.

[98] Takeuchi T, Liang SB & Ohtsuki Y (2002b) Downregulation of expression of a novel cadherin molecule, T-cadherin, in basal cell carcinoma of the skin. Molecular Carcinogenesis, 35(4):173-179.

[99] Takeuchi T, Liang SB, Matsuyoshi N, Zhou S, Miyachi Y, Sonobe H & Ohtsuki Y (2002a) Loss of T-cadherin (CDH13, H-cadherin) expression in cutaneous squamous cell carcinoma. Laboratory Investigation, 82(8):1023-1029.

[100] Tang A, Eller MS, Hara M, Yaar M, Hirohashi S & Gilchrest BA (1994) E-cadherin is the major mediator of human melanocyte adhesion to keratinocytes in vitro. J Cell Sci, 107:983–992.

[101] Teicher BA & Andrews PA (2004) Preclinical screening, clinical trials, and approval. Anticancer Drug Development Guide by B.A.Teicher and P.A.Andrews. Humana Press, Totowa, p.450.

[102] Teillet M, Kalcheim C & Le Douarin NM (1987) Formation of the dorsal root ganglia in the avian embryo: segmental origin and migratory behavior of the neural crest progenitor cells. Devl Biol, 120:329-347.

[103] Tsutsumida A, Hamada J, Tada M, Aoyama T, Furuuchi K, Kawai Y, Yamamoto Y, Sugihara T & Moriuchi T (2004) Epigenetic silencing of E- and P-cadherin gene expression in human melanoma cell lines. Int J Oncol, 25:1415–1421.

[104] Vestal DJ & Ranscht B (1992) Glycosyl phosphatidylinositol-anchored T-cadherin mediates calcium-dependent, homophilic cell adhesion. J Cell Biol, 119:451-461.

[105] Vincent PA, Xiao K, Buckley KM & Kowalczyk AP (2004) VE-cadherin: adhesion at arm's length. Am.J. Physiol. Cell Physiol, 286:987-997.

[106] Voura EB, Sandig M & Siu CH (1998) Cell-cell interactions during transendothelial migration of tumor cells. Microsc Res Tech, 43: 265–275.

[107] Wheelock MJ & Johnson KR (2003) Cadherins as modulators of cellular phenotype. Annu Rev Cell Dev Biol, 19:207–235.

[108] Widschwendter A, Ivarsson L, Blassnig A, Müller HM, Fiegl H, Wiedemair A, Müller-Holzner E, Goebel G, Marth C & Widschwendter M (2004) CDH1 and CDH13 methylation in serum is an independent prognostic marker in cervical cancer patients. International Journal of Cancer, 109(2):163-166.

[109] Wiley H, Gonzalez EB, Maki W, Wu M & Hwang ST (2001) Expression of CC chemokine receptor-7 (CCR7) and regional lymph node metastasis of B16 murine melanoma. J Natl Cancer Inst, 93(21):1638-1643.

[110] Wyder L, Vitality A, Schneider H, Hebbard LW, Moritz DR, Wittmer M, Ajmo M & Klemenz R (2000) Increased expression of H/T-cadherin in tumor-penetrating blood vessels. Cancer Research, 60(17):4682-4688.

[111] Yurlova EI, Rubina KA, Sysoeva VYu, Semina EV, Kalinina NI, Sharonov GV, Suzdaltseva YG, Andronova NV, Treshalina HM & Tkachuk VA. T-cadherin inhibits neoangiogenesis but stimulates primary tumor growth and invasion of murine melanoma B16F10. Scientific Reports. (in press).

[112] Yurlova EI, Rubina KA, Sysoeva VYu, Sharonov GV, Semina EV, Parfenova YeV & Tkachuk VA (2010) T-cadherin suppresses the cell proliferation of mouse melanoma B16F10 and tumor angiogenesis in the model of chorioallantoic membrane. Cell Differentiation and Proliferation, 41(4): 217-226.

[113] Zhang XD & Hersey P (1999) Expression of catenins and p120cas in melanocytic nevi and cutaneous melanoma: deficient alpha-catenin expression is associated with melanoma progression. Pathology, 31:239–246.

[114] Zhou S, Matsuyoshi N, Liang SB, Takeuchi T, Ohtsuki Y & Miyachi Y (2002) Expression of T-cadherin in basal keratinocytes of skin. J Invest Dermatol, 118(6):1080-1084.

[115] Zhou S, Matsuyoshi N, Takeuchi T, Ohtsuki Y & Miyachi Y (2003) Reciprocal altered expression of T-cadherin and P-cadherin in psoriasis vulgaris. British Journal of Dermatology, 149(2):268-273.

[116] Zucchini C, Bianchini M, Valvassori L, Perdichizzi S, Benini S, Manara MC, Solmi R, Strippoli P, Picci P, Carinci P & Scotlandi K (2004) Identification of candidate genes involved in the reversal of malignant phenotype of osteosarcoma cells transfected with the liver/bone/kidney alkaline phosphatase gene. Bone, 34(4):672-679.

Chapter 7

The Use of Artemisinin Compounds as Angiogenesis Inhibitors to Treat Cancer

Qigui Li, Peter Weina and Mark Hickman

Additional information is available at the end of the chapter

http://dx.doi.org/10.5772/54109

1. Introduction

Angiogenesis takes place during development, and vascular remodeling is a controlled series of events leading to neovascularization, which supports changing tissue requirements. Blood vessels and stromal components are responsive to pro- and anti-angiogenic factors that allow vascular remodeling during development, wound healing and pregnancy. In pathological situations such as cancer, however, the same angiogenic signaling pathways are induced and exploited. Cancer angiogenesis is a requirement for the development and growth of solid tumors beyond 2–3 mm^3 (Cao et al., 2011). Several angiogenic activators including members of the vascular endothelial growth factor (VEGF) and fibroblast growth factor (FGF) gene families and various inhibitors of angiogenesis have been described. In steady-state conditions, the balance between angiogenic activators and inhibitors results in very limited new blood vessel growth in the majority of tissues. The balance tilts in favor of the angiogenic stimulators, however, in a variety of proliferative processes. It is now generally accepted that angiogenesis is a rate-limiting process in tumor growth. Without new blood vessels to supply nutrients and dispose of catabolic products, tumor cells cannot sustain proliferation and thus are likely to remain dormant (Ferrara, 2010; Daniele et al., 2012).

Survival and proliferation of cancer depends on angiogenesis, which could be a target of cancer therapy. Angiogenesis is a complex physiological process. One example of this is found in the signaling pathways associated with the stimulus of various pro-angiogenic factors, VEGF and its receptors (VEGFR) which represents one of the best-validated signaling pathways in angiogenesis. A number of drugs approved by the FDA on market have been shown to inhibit anti-angiogenic pathway of VEGF. These agents include bevacizumab, a humanized anti-VEGF-A monoclonal antibody (Ferrara 2010), and two small molecule inhibitors targeting VEGFR2, sorafenib and sunitinib (Bergers and Hanahan 2008; Ellis and Hicklin 2008; Escudier

INTECH
open science | open minds

© 2013 The Author(s). Licensee InTech. This chapter is distributed under the terms of the Creative Commons Attribution License http://creativecommons.org/licenses/by/3.0), which permits unrestricted use, distribution, and reproduction in any medium, provided the original work is properly cited.

et al., 2007; Motzer et al., 2007). Not all cancer patients, however, benefit from such anti-angiogenic therapies, and some that do benefit initially have been shown to become less responsive during the treatment as well as show some adverse effects over time (Bergers and Hanahan 2008; Chen and Cleck, 2009; Ellis and Hicklin 2008). Over the last few decades, numerous anti-angiogenic agents have been developed, and some of them have been tested in clinical settings. Angiogenesis includes a complex and multistep process, however, that has not been sufficiently elucidated. Hence, there is an urgent need to investigate the mechanisms that mediate resistance to anti-angiogenic agents. Recent advances have been made in identifying a number of novel alternate processes involved in angiogenesis. If these new findings of alternate mechanisms are confirmed, cancer therapy strategies may also be affected.

Artemisinin (ART) is a natural product of the plant *Artemisia annua L.* Reduction of ART yields the more active dihydroartemisinin (DHA), a compound which can be further converted to different derivatives, including, artesunate (AS) and artemether (AM), which are generally referred to as artemisinins (ARTs). ARTs are widely known for their potent antimalarial activity, but also been potential anti-cancer activity both *in vitro* and *in vivo* over the past few years. ARTs have inhibitory effects on cancer cell growth and also inhibit angiogenesis. Several studies have revealed that ART inhibits the growth of many transformed cell lines and has a selective cytotoxic effect. In one study, ART was shown to be more toxic to cancer than normal cells. In most of the systems, preloading of cancer cells with iron or iron-saturated holotransferrin triggers ART cytotoxicity with an increase in the activity of ARTs by 100-fold in some cell lines. It has been hypothesized that iron-activated ARTs induce damage by release of highly alkylating carbon-centered radicals and radical oxygen species (ROS). Radicals may play a role in the cell alterations reported in ARTs-treated cancer cells such as enhanced apoptosis, arrest of growth, inhibition of angiogenesis, and DNA damage. More studies have demonstrated that ART and its derivatives possess an anti-angiogenic activity (Li and Hickman, 2011).

ARTs inhibit angiogenesis which is a vital process in metastasis. AS and DHA inhibit chorioallantoic membrane angiogenesis at low concentrations and decrease the levels of two major VEGF receptors on human umbilical vein endothelial cells (ECs). AS inhibits proliferation and differentiation of human microvascular dermal ECs in a dose-dependent manner and reduces Flt-1 and KDR/flk-1 expression. Conditioned media from K562 cells pretreated with AS and DHA inhibits VEGF expression and secretion in chronic myeloid leukemia K562 cells, leading to a decrease in genetic activity associated with angiogenesis. ARTs inhibit cell migration and concomitantly decrease the expression of matrix metalloproteinase proteins such as MMP2 and the avß3 integrins in human melanoma cells. ARTs also regulate the levels of urokinase plasminogen activator (u-PA), and the matrix metalloproteinases MMP2, MMP7 and MMP9 all of which are related to metastasis. Also, ARTs have been shown to increase production of reactive oxygen species and also inhibits the hypoxia induced production of a transcription factor, hypoxia inducible factor-1α (HIF1α). The HIF1α transcription factor increases tumor angiogenesis to support the survival of poorly nourished cancer cells. ARTs have shown pleiotropic effects through different experimental studies.

Definitely, ART compounds exhibit a wide spectrum of biological activities, including, for example, anti-angiogenic, anti-tumorigenic and even anti-viral, all of which are medi-

http://dx.doi.org/10.5772/54109

cally relevant. In particular, cancer angiogenesis plays a key role in the growth, invasion, and metastasis of cancers. After more than 30 years of intensive study, many agents, including novel candidate of ARTs, that target angiogenesis as cancer therapy and prevention of metastasis of existing tumors have been translated from the laboratory to the bedside. Therefore, ARTs-induced inhibition of angiogenesis could be a promising therapeutic strategy for treatment of cancer and prevention of metastasis. Various clinical trials using ARTs for anti-cancer therapy have been guided by the anti-angiogenesis research of ARTs that has been conducted anti-cancer. Since new and alternative angiogenesis mechanisms have been found, further research on the mechanism of anti-angiogenesis could lead us to understand more deeply the possibilities inherent in the development of ARTs for cancer therapy (Li and Hickman, 2011).

The new strategies for the development of ARTs for cancer therapy and metastasis prevention should include a plan for increasing their anti-angiogenic activity through a variety of approaches ranging from medicinal chemistry approaches to develop more potent ART-analogues to changes in formulation and/or dosing. The real potential and benefits of the ART drug class for cancer treatment and metastasis prevention remain yet to be discovered. Given the interest in using ARTs for cancer therapy, the door has been opened for challenging research in this area, which is likely to yield new cancer therapies that now do not exist. The aim of this chapter is to provide an overview of the recent advances and new development of this class of drugs as potential anti-angiogenic agents.

2. Activities of artemisinins (ARTs) as anti-cancer agents

Significant antitumor activity of ART and licensed semisynthetic its derivatives has been documented *in vitro, in vivo* and through clinical trials considerable research has been focused on the most active compounds, namely, artesunate (AS) and dihydroartemisinin (DHA).

2.1. ART and its derivatives

ART and its derivatives are lactonic sesquiterpenoid compounds first discovered in China. A crude extract of the wormwood plant *Artemisia annua* (qinghao) was first used as an antipyretic 2000 years ago. The antipyretic therapy dates back to the third century B.C. in the "Handbook of Prescriptions for Emergency Treatment" edited by Ge Hong (281-340 B.C.) where he recommended tea-brewed leaves of the wormwood plant to treat fever and chills. The specific effect of ART on the fever of malaria was reported in the 16th century in the "Compendium of *Materia Medica*" published by Li Shizen in 1596 cited Ge Hong's prescription (Li and Weina, 2011). The active constituent of the extract was identified and purified in the 1970s, and named qinghaosu, or artemisinin (ART). Although ART proved effective in clinical trials in the 1980s, a number of semi-synthetic derivatives were developed to improve the drug's pharmacological properties and antimalarial potency (Li et al., 2007). The structure of ART, which includes an endoperoxide bridge (C-O-O-C), is unique among antimalarial drugs. Semisynthetic ARTs are obtained from dihydroartemisinin (DHA), which is the reduced lactol derivative of ART, the main active metabolite of ARTs (Li et al., 1998). The first generation of semisynthetic ARTs includes the lipophilic arts, arteether (AE) and artemether (AM), while artesunate (AS) is the water soluble derivative (Li and Weina, 2011).

AS and its bioactive metabolite, DHA, have been the topic of considerable research attention in recent years for both anti-cancer and antimalarial indications. The key structural feature in all of the ART-related molecules that mediates their antimalarial activity, and some of their anti-cancer activities, is an endoperoxide bridge. The endoperoxides are a promising class of antimalarial drugs which may meet the dual challenges posed by drug-resistant parasites and the rapid progression of malarial illness. Of the available derivatives, AS has the most favorable pharmacological profile for use in ART-based combination therapy treatment of uncomplicated malaria and intravenous therapy of severe malaria (Li and Weina, 2010a). The effectiveness of AS has been mostly attributed to its rapid and extensive hydrolysis to DHA (Batty et al., 1998b; Davis et al., 2001; Li et al., 2009; Navaratnam et al., 2000).

Artemisone, a second-generation ART which is not metabolized to DHA, has shown improved pharmacokinetic properties including a longer half-life and lower toxicity (D'Alessandro et al., 2007; Schmuck et al., 2009) (Figure 1). Fully synthetic ART derivatives have also been designed by preserving the peroxide moiety which confers potent drug activity. These compounds are easily synthesized from simple starting materials; accordingly, these compounds are currently under intense development (Creek et al., 2008; Jefford 2007; Ramirez et al., 2009; Taylor et al., 2004). Hundreds of these compounds have been made; many resemble ART, but only one of these compounds, arteflene, has been taken beyond preclinical development (Radloff et al., 1996).

ART and its active derivatives have been widely used as antimalarial drugs for more than 30 years, and they have also been shown recently to be effective in killing cancer cells (Li et al., 2011). A number of studies demonstrated that ART and its bioactive derivatives exhibit potent anti-cancer effects in a variety of human cancer cell model systems. Recently, the anti-angiogenic activity of ARTs has been demonstrated, and these compounds have been shown to be potential anti-cancer agents (Crespo-Ortiz and Wei, 2012).

2.2. ARTs as first-line therapies for treatments of malaria

Global malaria control is being threatened on an unprecedented scale by rapidly growing resistance of *P. falciparum* to conventional monotherapies such as chloroquine, sulfadoxine-pyrimethamine (SP) and amodiaquine. Multi-drug resistant *falciparum* malaria is widely prevalent in South-East Asia and South America. Now Africa, the continent with highest burden of malaria is also being seriously affected by drug resistance. A significant advantage of ART and its derivatives in malaria treatment shows early evidence of cross-resistance to other antimalarial drugs. As a response to the rising tide of antimalarial drug resistance, WHO issued new Guideline for the Treatment of Malaria (WHO 2006; 2008) and recommends that treatment policies for *falciparum* malaria in all countries experiencing resistance to monotherapies should be combination therapies, preferably those containing an ART derivative.

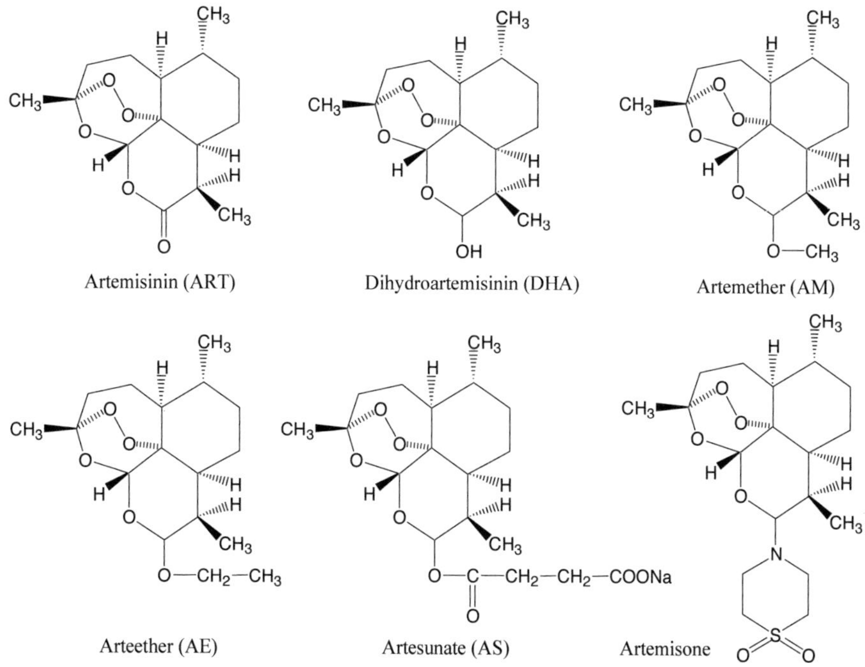

Figure 1. Chemical structures of artemisinin (ART) and its five derivatives, dihydroartemisinin (DHA), artemether (AM), arteether (AE), artesunate (AS) and artemisone

2.2.1. WHO policies in malaria treatments

The pharmacological and clinical evaluations of ART group of drugs have been taken place for 30 years and four advantages have been evaluated.

1. Rapid action and high efficacy against multi-drug resistant *P. falciparum*
2. Evidence of ART drug resistance confirmed on the Cambodia-Thailand border
3. Low toxicity (excellent safety profile)
4. Gametocidal effect (prevents the transmission of malaria from person to person)

To treat uncomplicated malaria, the objective is to cure the infection. This is important as it will help prevent progression to severe disease and prevent additional morbidity associated with treatment failure. Cure of the infection translates to eradication of the parasite from the body. In treatment evaluations in all settings, emerging evidence indicates that it is necessary to follow patients for enough time to document a clinical cure. In assessing drug efficacy in high-transmission settings, temporary suppression of infection for 14 days has not been considered sufficient. The public health goal of treatment is to reduce transmission of the infection to others, i.e. to reduce the infectious reservoir. A secondary but equally important objective of treatment is to prevent the emergence and spread of resistance to antimalarials. Tolerability, the adverse effect profile and the speed of therapeutic response are also important considerations. A brief summary of the WHO policies (WHO, 2010) for treatment of uncomplicated *falciparum* malaria is listed below:

Artemisinin-based combination therapies (ACTs) are the treatment recommended by WHO in 2010 for all cases of uncomplicated *falciparum* malaria as first-line treatment including:

- artemether plus lumefantrine,
- artesunate plus amodiaquine,
- artesunate plus mefloquine,
- artesunate plus sulfadoxine-pyrimethamine,
- dihydroartemisinin plus piperaquine.

Second-line treatment:

- an effective alternative ACT (efficacy of ACTs depend on efficacy of the partner medicine, therefore it is possible to use two different ACTs as 1st and 2nd line options)
- quinine + tetracycline or doxycycline or clindamycin

Note: The ART derivatives (oral, rectal, or parenteral formulations) and partner medicines of ACTs are not recommended as monotherapy for uncomplicated malaria due to high rates of recrudescence associated with ART monotherapy.

To treat severe malaria, the primary objective of antimalarial treatment is to prevent death. Prevention of recrudescence and avoidance of minor adverse effects are secondary. In treating cerebral malaria, prevention of neurological deficit is also an important objective. In the treatment of severe malaria in pregnancy, saving the life of the mother is the primary objective. The following WHO policies are recommended for treatment of severe and complicated *falciparum* malaria as first-line treatment (WHO 2010):

Any of the following antimalarial medicines have been recommended by the WHO in 2010 for initial treatment.

- artesunate (i.v. or i.m.)
- artemether (i.m.)
- quinine (i.v. infusion or i.m. injection).

Follow-on treatment: once the patient recovers enough and can tolerate oral treatment, the following options can be used to complete treatment:

- full course of an ACT or
- quinine + clindamycin or doxycycline

Consistent with WHO recommendations (2006; 2010), malaria endemic countries which are experiencing resistance to currently used antimalarial drug monotherapies (chloroquine, sulphadoxine/pyrimethamine or amodiaquine) should change treatment policies to the highly effective ART-based combination treatments (ACTs).

2.2.2. *ACT is a "policy standard" for first line malaria treatment*

Antimalarial combination therapies can improve treatment efficacies of failing individual components and provide some protection for individual components against the development of higher levels of resistance. ACTs have been advocated as the best available option, and are the most commonly adopted regimen in countries changing antimalarial policy in the last decade. ACTs are most preferred for their enhancement of efficacy (Price 2000; White and Olliaro, 1998; White 1999a), lower malaria incidence and their potential to lower the rate at which resistance emerges and spreads (Nosten et al., 2000; White 1999b). Five ACTs recommended by a WHO Expert Consultative Group in 2010 include AM-lumefantrine (Coartem), AS-mefloquine (Artequin), AS-amodiaquine, and AS-sulfadoxine/pyrimethamine. Recently, WHO has endorsed ACTs as the "policy standard" for all malaria infections in areas where *P. falciparum* is the predominant infecting species (WHO 2006; 2007).

ARTs rapidly reduce parasitemia, but have poor efficacy as short course monotherapy. When used in combination with another agent, the rapid reduction in parasite numbers results in relatively few parasites being exposed to the second drug (to which significant resistance may already exist), theoretically preventing emergence of additional resistance mutations (White 2004). Furthermore, since ARTs themselves are not required to mediate final cure, there should also be little opportunity for ART resistance to develop. In addition, rapid reduction of the parasite burden in vivo by ACT drug combinations reduces the frequency of gametocyte generation, increases the rates of cure and may also reduce transmission of resistant parasites (Price, 2000). Most currently recommended drug combinations for *falciparum* malaria are variants of ACT where a rapidly acting ART compound is combined with a longer half-life drug of a different class. ARTs used include DHA, AS, AM and companion drugs include mefloquine, amodiaquine, sulfadoxine/pyrimethamine, lumefantrine, piperaquine, pyronaridine, and chlorproguanil/dapsone. The standard of care must be to cure malaria by killing the last parasite. Combination antimalarial treatment is vital not only to the successful treatment of individual patients but also for public health control of malaria.

ACTs continue to be the mainstay treatment of uncomplicated falciparum malaria. For the next 8–10 years, no alternative medicines to the ART derivatives able to offer similar high levels of therapeutic efficacy are expected to enter the market. For this reason, WHO has focused its efforts not only to increase access to quality ACTs, but also to contain the risk of development of *falciparum* resistance, associated with the large-scale use of oral monotherapies for treatment of uncomplicated malaria (WHO 2006; 2007).

In January 2006, WHO appealed to manufacturers to stop marketing oral ART monotherapies and instead to promote quality ACTs in line with WHO policy. This position has been widely disseminated via WHO Offices, WHO briefings to hospital staff and in regional and inter-country briefings to representatives of national health. Major procurement and funding agencies and international suppliers have accepted the WHO recommendation and agreed not to fund or procure oral ART monotherapies. In April 2006, the Global Malaria Programme of WHO provided a technical briefing to 25 pharmaceutical companies involved in the production and marketing of ART monotherapies. Out of these, 15 declared their willingness to stop marketing ART monotherapies over a short period of time, but 10 companies did not disclose their marketing plans for the future (meeting report available at: www.who.int/malaria/docs/ Meeting_briefing19April.pdf). In addition, some countries, like China and Pakistan, have been visited by WHO delegations to address multiple domestic manufacturers involved in this sector. The evolving position of manufacturers and of National Drug Regulatory Authorities (NDRA) in malaria endemic countries is monitored and displayed on the WHO Global Malaria Programme website front-page: http://malaria.who.int/.

In May 2007, the 60th World Health Assembly resolved to take strong action against oral monotherapies and approved the resolution WHA60.18, which:

1. urges Member States to progressively cease the provision, in both the public and private sectors, of oral ART monotherapies, to promote the use of ART-combination therapies, and to implement policies that prohibit the production, marketing, distribution and the use of counterfeit antimalarial medicines;
2. requests international organizations and financing bodies to adjust their policies so as progressively cease to fund the provision and distribution of oral ART monotherapies, and to join in campaigns to prohibit the production, marketing, distribution and use of counterfeit antimalarial medicines;

The above-mentioned benefits of ACTs make them an important tool for malaria treatment and control that has led to their increased use by 2010, most countries (89 countries), adopted ACTs as their first-line treatment of uncomplicated *falciparum* malaria. Only two countries adopted ACTs exclusively as second-line treatment (Bosman and Mendis, 2007).

2.3. Anti-cancer activities of ARTs

ART and its bioactive derivatives (AS, DHA, and AM) exhibit potent anti-cancer effects in a variety of human cancer cell model systems. The pleiotropic response in cancer cells to ART includes: 1) growth inhibition by cell cycle arrest, 2) apoptosis, 3) inhibition of angiogenesis, 4) disruption of cell migration, and 5) modulation of nuclear receptor responsiveness. These effects of ARTs result from perturbations of many cellular signaling pathways *in vitro* and in animal models. Considerable research has been focused on the most active ART compounds, namely, DHA and AS.

Molecular, cellular and physiological studies have demonstrated that, depending on the tissue type and experimental system, ART and its derivatives arrest cell growth, induce an apoptotic response, alter hormone responsive properties and/or inhibit angiogenesis of human cancer cells. The Developmental Therapeutics Program of the National Cancer Institute (NCI), USA, which analyzed the activity of AS on 55 human cancer cell lines (IC_{50} values shown between nano- to micro-molar range, depending on the cancer cell line), showed that AS displays inhibitory activity against leukemia, colon, melanoma, breast, ovarian, prostate, central nervous system (CNS), and renal cancer cells (Efferth et al., 2001; 2003; Efferth, 2006). DHA also has remarkable anti-neoplastic activity against pancreatic, leukemic, osteosarcoma, and lung cancer cells (Lu et al., 2009). Moreover, artemisone (second generation ART compound) has shown better activity than ART and considerable synergistic interactions with other anti-cancer agents (Gravett et al., 2010).

ART has been found to act either directly by inducing DNA damage (genotoxicity) or indirectly by interfering with a range of signaling pathways involved in several hallmarks of malignancy. Direct DNA damage is only described in specific systems, however, while indirect effects are more commonly noted in the literature. In pancreatic cells (Panc-1), artesunate was shown to cause DNA fragmentation and membrane damage. Interestingly, low doses of artesunate were associated with oncosis-like cell death, whereas higher concentrations were shown to induce apoptosis (Du et al., 2010). The extent and type of cellular damage seems to depend on the phenotype and the origin of cell line, and it may also vary in a time- and dose-dependent manner (Crespo-Ortiz and Wei, 2012). Notably, higher sensitivity to AS was observed in rapidly growing cell lines when compared with slow growing cancer cells (Efferth et al., 2003).

Moreover, the highly stable ARTs and ART-derived trioxane dimers were shown to inhibit growth and selectively kill several human cancer cell lines without inducing cytotoxic effects on normal neighboring cells. One proposed mechanism by which ART targets cancer cells involves cleavage of the endoperoxide bridge by the relatively high concentrations of iron in cancer cells, resulting in iron depletion in those cells coupled with generation of free radicals such as reactive oxygen species (ROS) capable of inducing subsequent oxidative damage. This mechanism resembles the known mechanism of action of ART in malarial parasites. In addition to possessing higher iron influx via transferrin receptors, cancer cells are also sensitive to oxygen radicals because of a relative deficiency in antioxidant enzymes. A significant positive correlation can be made between AS sensitivity and transferrin receptor levels as well as between AS sensitivity and expression of ATP binding cassette transporters (Efferth, 2006).

Expression profiling of several classes of tumor cells has shown that ART treatment caused selective expression changes of many oncogenes and tumor suppressor genes than genes responsible for iron metabolism, which suggests that the anti-cancer properties of ARTs cannot be explained simply by the global toxic effects of oxidative damage. Alternatively, DHA, AS, and AM may well be to modulating genes and proteins coordinating growth signals, apoptosis, proliferation capacity, angiogenesis and tissue invasion, and metastasis. A complex network of interactions through different pathways may enhance the anti-cancer effect of these endoperoxide drugs leading to cancer control and cell death (Crespo-Ortiz and Wei, 2012).

ARTs have also been observed to attenuate multidrug resistance in cancer patients, an effect due in part to the inhibition of glutathione S-transferase activity. ART and its bioactive derivatives elicit their anti-cancer effects by concurrently activating, inhibiting and/or attenuating multiple complementary cell signaling pathways, which have been described in a variety of human cancer cell systems as well as in athymic mouse xenograft models. The ART compounds exert common as well as distinct cellular effects depending on the phenotype and tissue origin of the human cancer cells tested. (Firestone and Sundar 2009)

2.4. Anti-cancer mechanism of ART and its derivatives

The anti-cancer potential of ARTs has been demonstrated in various cancer cells including those of leukemia and other cancer cells of breast, ovary, liver, lung, pancreas and colon (Tan et al., 2011).The mechanisms of action of ARTs in cancer cells are associated with: 1) anti-angiogenic effects, 2) induction of apoptosis, 3) oxidative stress response, 4) oncogenes and tumor suppressor genes, and 5) multidrug resistance (Figure 2) (Efferth 2006; 2007).

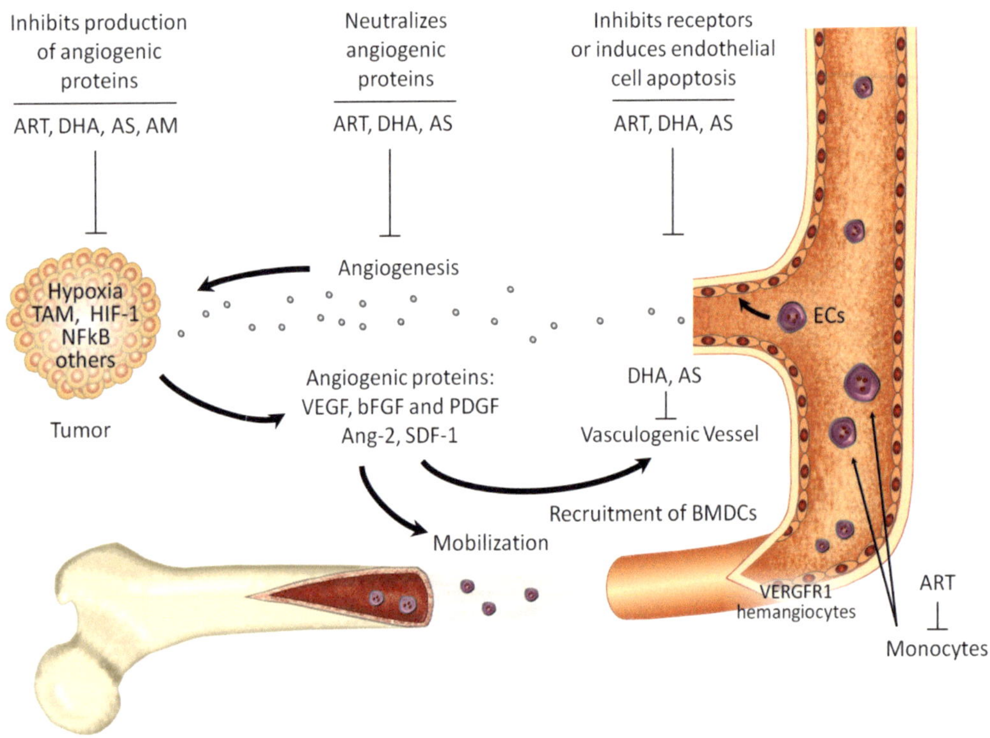

Figure 2. Schema of tumor angiogenesis induced by hypoxia and the inhibitions of tumor growth by antiangiogenic artemisinins (ART) and its derivatives of dihydroartemisinin (DHA), artesunate (AS) and artemether (AM) follows three directions, including the inhibition of tumor cell synthesis of angiogenic proteins, the neutralization of angiogenic proteins by antibodies or traps, and the inhibition of endothelial cell binding to angiogenic proteins or direct induction of endothelial cell apoptosis.

2.4.1. Anti-cancer mechanism of ARTs based on antimalarial actions

The endoperoxide moiety of ART has been shown to be pharmacologically important and responsible for antimalarial activity against the malaria parasites. The potent anti-cancer action of ARTs can be also attributed to the endoperoxide bond. In most of the *in vitro* cancer cell lines tested, preloading of cancer cells with iron or iron-saturated holo-transferrin triggers ART cytotoxicity with an increase in ARTs activity up to 100-fold against some cell lines. It has been hypothesized that iron-activated ARTs induce damage by release of highly alkylating carbon-centered radicals and ROS. Radicals may play a role in the cell alterations reported in ARTs-treated cancer cells such as enhanced apoptosis, arrest of growth, inhibition of angiogenesis, and DNA damage. Microarray analyses found that the action of ARTs seems to be modulated by the expression of oxidative stress enzymes including catalase, thioredoxin reductase, superoxide dismutase and the glutathione S-transferase family. ARTs-sensitive cells demonstrate down-regulated oxidation enzymes whereas over-expression of these enzymes renders cancer cells less sensitive to chemotherapeutic agents. The antineoplastic toxicity of ARTs appears to be also modulated by calcium metabolism, endoplasmic reticulum (ER) stress, and the expression of the translationally controlled tumor protein, TCTP, a calcium binding protein which has been also postulated as a parasite target. Although the expression of the TCTP gen, *tctp,* was initially correlated with cancer cell response to ARTs, a functional role for TCTP in the action of ARTs has yet to be found. As for malaria parasites, the role of sarcoendoplasmic $Ca^{2}+$ ATPase (SERCA) as a target of ARTs in cancer cells has also been explored (Crespo-Ortiz and Wei, 2012).

Expression profiling of several classes of tumor cells has shown that ART treatment causes selective expression changes of many more oncogenes and tumor suppressor genes than genes responsible for iron metabolism, which suggests that the anti-cancer properties of ART cannot be explained simply by the global toxic effects of oxidative damage. ART has also been observed to attenuate multidrug resistance in cancer patients, an effect due in part to the inhibition of glutathione S-transferase activity. ART and its bioactive derivatives elicit their anti-cancer effects by concurrently activating, inhibiting and/or attenuating multiple complementary cell signaling pathways, which have been described in a variety of human cancer cell systems as well as in athymic mouse xenograft models. The ART compounds exert common as well as distinct cellular effects depending on the phenotype and tissue origin of the human cancer cells tested. (Firestone and Sundar, 2009).

2.4.2. Potential general mechanisms of ART and its derivatives

Studies have identified potential general anti-cancer mechanisms of anti-cancer ARTs such as normalization of the upregulated Wnt/β-catenin pathway in colorectal cancer. Other pathways for anti-cancer activity include inhibition of enhanced angiogenesis associated with tumors. ARTs have been shown to inhibit proliferation, migration and tube formation of human umbilical vein endothelial cells (HUVEC), inhibit VEGF binding to surface receptors on HUVEC and reduce expression of VEGF receptors Flt-1 and KDR/flk-1 on HUVECs. In cancer cells, artemisinins reduce expression of the VEGF receptor KDR/flk-1 in tumor and endothelial cells and slow the growth of human ovarian cancer HO-8910 xenografts in nude mice. HUVEC apoptosis by artesunate is associated with downregulation of Bcl-2 (B-cell leukemia/lymphoma 2) and upregulation of BAX (Bcl-2-associated X protein). In addition, mRNA expression of 30 out of 90 angiogenesis-related genes correlated significantly with the cellular response to ARTs, supporting the hypothesis that ARTs exert their anti-tumor effects by inhibition of tumor angiogenesis (Krishna et al., 2008).

2.4.3. Anti-angiogenesis of ARTs including Anti-proliferation

In the process of angiogenesis, the formation of new blood vessels from pre-existing ones is essential for the supply of tumors with oxygen and nutrients. If cancers reach a size for which diffusion alone cannot supply enough oxygen and nutrients angiogenesis is promoted by numerous pro-angiogenic or anti-angiogenic factors. The anti-angiogenic activities of ARTs were shown using various models of angiogenesis, namely, proliferation, migration and tube formation of endothelial cells. As a consequence, inhibitors of angiogenesis were considered as interesting possibilities for cancer therapy. As shown by several groups around the world, ART and its derivatives inhibit angiogenesis, and a detailed description of the ART-induced anti-angiogenic mechanisms will be described in Section 3.

2.4.4. Induction of apoptosis

ARTs induce cell cycle arrest in various cell types (Efferth, 2006). For example, DHA and AS effectively mediate G1 phase arrest in HepG2 and Hep3B cells (Hou et al., 2008), and DHA treatment has been shown to reduce cell numbers of HCT116 colon cancer cells in S phase (Lu et al., 2011). Interestingly, DHA treatment has also been shown to trigger G2 phase arrest in OVCA-420 ovarian cancer cells (Jiao et al., 2007). Thus, ART-mediated cell cycle arrest is possibly cell type dependent. ARTs have also been shown to induce apoptotic cell death in a number of cell types, in which the mitochondrial-mediated apoptotic pathway plays a decisive role (Lu et al., 2011). For instance, DHA has been shown to enhance Bax and reduces Bcl-2 expression in cancer cells (Hou et al., 2008; Chen et al., 2009). DHA-induced apoptosis is abrogated by the loss of Bak and is largely reduced in cells with siRNA-mediated down-regulation of Bak or NOXA (Handrick et al., 2010). DHA has been shown to activate caspase-8, however, which is related to the death receptor-mediated apoptotic pathway in HL-60 cells (Liu et al., 2008). DHA has also been shown to enhance Fas expression and activates caspase-8 in ovarian cancer cells (Chen et al., 2009). In addition, DHA enhances death receptor 5 and activates both mitochondrial- and death receptor-mediated apoptotic pathways in prostate cancer cells (He et al., 2010). ARTs-induced apoptosis in cancer cells may involve p38 MAPK, however, rather than p53 (Hou et al., 2008; Lu et al., 2008).

Since most anti-cancer drugs kill tumor cells by the induction of apoptosis, the same may be true for ART and its derivatives. AS was first shown to promote apoptosis in tumor cells (Efferth *et al.*, 1996). This has been subsequently confirmed by other groups (Li et al., 2001; Sadava et al., 2002; Singh and Lai, 2004; Wang et al., 2002; Yamachika et al., 2004). By microarray and hierarchical cluster analyses, several apoptosis-regulating genes were identified, whose mRNA expression correlated significantly with the IC_{50} values for AS in the NCI cancer cell lines (Efferth et al., 2003).

2.4.5. Oxidative stress response

ART is first activated in malaria parasites by intra-parasitic heme-iron, which catalyzes the cleavage of the endoperoxide bond. The *Plasmodium* trophozoites and schizonts live within red blood cells, where hemoglobin serves as an amino acid source. It is taken up by the para-

http://dx.doi.org/10.5772/54109

sites into food vacuoles, where enzymatic degradation takes place (Semenov et al., 1998; Shenai et al., 2000). The release of heme-iron during hemoglobin digestion facilitates the cleavage of the endoperoxide moiety by a Fe (II) Fenton reaction. Breaking the endoperoxide bridge of ART results in the generation of reactive oxygen species, such as hydroxyl radicals and superoxide anions, which damage the food vacuole membranes and leads to subsequent auto-digestion (Krishna et al., 2004; O'Neill and Posner, 2004). In addition, the heme iron (II)-mediated decomposition of ART leads to the generation of carbon-centered radical species (Butler et al., 1998). The cleavage of the endoperoxide bond of ART and its derivatives also leads to the alkylation of heme and some *Plasmodium*-specific proteins, including the *Plasmodium falciparum* translationally controlled tumor protein (TCTP) and the sarco/endoplasmic reticulum Ca^{2+} ATPase (SERCA) ortholog of *Plasmodium falciparum* (Eckstein-Ludwig et al., 2003). Recent observations indicate, however, that heme iron (II) and oxidative stress are not the only mechanisms of ART's anti-malarial activity (Parapini et al., 2004).

By comparing the baseline antioxidant mRNA gene expression in the NCI cell line panel with the IC_{50} values for AS, oxidative stress was found to play a role in the anti-tumor activity of AS (Efferth, 2006). The expression of thioredoxin reductase and catalase correlated significantly with the IC_{50} values for AS against the tumor cell lines in the NCI panel. As tumor cells contain much less iron than erythrocytes, but more than other normal tissues (Shterman et al., 1991), the question arises as to whether iron may be critical for ART's activity against tumor cells (Payne, 2003). The growth of tumors in rats was significantly retarded by daily oral administration of ferrous sulfate followed by dihydroartemisinin, while treatment with each drug applied alone had no effect (Moore et al., 1995). Cellular iron uptake and internalization are mediated by binding of transferrin-iron complexes to the transferrin receptor (CD71) expressed on the cell surface membrane which leads to subsequent iron endocytosis. CD71 is normally expressed in the basal epidermis, endocrine pancreas, hepatocytes, Kupfer cells, testis, and pituitary, while most other tissues are CD71-negative. In contrast, CD71 is highly expressed in proliferating and malignant cells (Sutherland et al., 1981) and it is widely distributed among clinical tumors (Gatter et al., 1983).

Interestingly, exposure of ART and its derivatives produces no or only marginal cytotoxicity to non-tumor cells. Human breast cells do not respond to treatment with transferrin plus DHA, while the growth of breast cancer cells is significantly inhibited (Singh and Lai, 2001). Similarly, ART tagged to transferrin has been shown to be more cytotoxic to MOLT-4 leukemia cells than to normal lymphocytes (Lai et al., 2005).

2.4.6. Oncogenes and tumor suppressor genes

Oncogenes and tumor suppressor genes frequently affect downstream processes in tumor cells. The expression of several oncogenes and tumor suppressor genes has been shown to correlate with response to artesunate, including the epidermal growth factor receptor (*EGFR*), the tumor growth factor ß (*TGFB*), FBJ murine osteosarcoma viral oncogene homologue B (*FOSB*), *FOS*-like antigen-2 (*FOSL2*), the multiple endocrine neoplasia 1 gene (*MEN1*), *v-myb* avian myeloblastosis viral oncogene homolog (*MYB*), *v-myc* avian myelocytomatosis viral oncogene homolog

(*MYC*), *c-src* tyrosine kinase (*CSK*), *v-raf* murine sarcoma viral oncogene homolog B1 (*BRAF*), the *RAS* oncogene family members *ARHC, ARHE, RAB2 and RAN*, the breast cancer susceptibility gene 2 (*BRCA2*), and others (Efferth et al., 2003).

The epidermal growth factor receptor (*EGFR*) represents an exquisite target for therapeutic interventions, and molecular approaches to study the expression of the EGFR gene have yielded some very interesting findings. Glioblastoma cells transfected with a deletion-activated *EGFR* cDNA were more resistant to AS than the control cells which agrees well with microarray gene expression data (Efferth et al., 2003). In addition to playing a role in drug resistance, the activation of *EGFR*-coupled signaling routes drives mitogenic and other cancer-promoting processes, e.g. proliferation, angiogenesis, and inhibition of apoptosis (Efferth 2006). In addition, combination treatment of the EGFR tyrosine kinase inhibitor, OSI-774, plus AS was investigated and synergistic effects were found in glioblastoma cells transfected with a deletion-activated *EGFR* cDNA, and additive effects were shown to occur in cells transfected with wild-type *EGFR* (Efferth et al., 2004a). A profile of chromosomal gains and losses was determined by comparative genomic hybridization in nine non-transfected glioblastoma cell lines, and this profile correlated well with the IC_{50} values determined after treatment of the same glioblastoma cell lines with the combination treatment of AS and OSI-774. Genes located at genomic loci correlating to cellular response to AS and OSI-774 may serve as candidate genes to determine drug sensitivity and resistance (Efferth 2007).

By screening a panel of isogenic *Saccaromyces cerevisiae* strains with defined genetic mutations in DNA repair, DNA checkpoint, and cell proliferation genes, one yeast strain with a defective mitosis-regulating *BUB3* gene showed increased sensitivity to AS treatment. Another strain with a defective proliferation-regulating *CLN2* gene showed increased AS resistance over the wild-type strain. None of the other DNA repair or DNA check-point deficient isogenic strains were different from wild-type yeast (Efferth et al., 2001). The conditional expression of the *CDC25A* gene by a tetracycline repressor expression vector (tet-off system) has been shown to increase cellular sensitivity to AS treatment (Efferth et al., 2003). CDC25A is a key regulator of the cell cycle, which drives cells from the G1 phase into S phase. AS has been shown to down-regulate the expression of the CDC25A protein which supports the hypothesis that AS interferes with cell cycle regulation (Efferth et al., 2003).

The IC_{50} values for artesunate were correlated with the constitutive mRNA expression levels measured by microarray hybridization. Scientists selected expression data of 559 genes deposited in the NCI's database (http://dtp.nci.nih.gov). The mRNA expression has been determined as reported. These genes belong to different categories of biological functions (63 apoptosis-regulating genes, 113 proliferation associated genes, 140 anti-oxidative stress response genes, 90 angiogenesis-regulating genes, 123 oncogenes and tumor suppressor genes). For example, p53, the "guardian of the genome", is a transcription factor that can bind to promoter regions of hundreds of genes where it either activates or suppresses gene expression. Thereby, p53 serves as a tumor suppressor by inducing cell cycle arrest, apoptosis, senescence and DNA repair. In normal cells, p53 is frequently undetectable due to fast ubiquitination by mdm-2 and subsequent proteasomal degradation. However, upon DNA damage and several other stresses, including drug stress, the amount of p53 is increased due to disruption of its degradation. Artesunate could inhibit HSCs proliferation in vitro through increase the expression of p53 (Efferth et al., 2006; Hou et al., 2008; Lu et al., 2008).

2.4.7. Multidrug resistance

A prominent feature of ART and its derivatives in malaria treatment shows early signs of cross-resistance to other antimalarial drugs. ARTs are therefore very valuable for the treatment of otherwise unresponsive, multidrug-resistant malaria parasites (Li and Weina 2011). Therefore, it is reasonable to ask whether ARTs are involved in the multidrug-resistance phenotypes observed in tumor cells. A comparison of the microarray-based mRNA expression of the multidrug resistance-conferring *ABCB1* gene (*MDR1*; P-glycoprotein) was conducted with the IC_{50} values determined for tumor cells treated with AS and dihydroartemisinyl ester stereoisomer 1, but no significant relationships were observed.

Similarly, the flow cytometric measurement of the fluorescent probe rhodamine 123, which represents a functional assay for P-glycoprotein, did not reveal significant correlations, and similar results were obtained with other ARTs. As a control, we used the established antitumor drug docetaxel (taxotere), which is a known substrate of *MDR1* (Shirakawa et al., 1999). The IC_{50} values determined for cells treated with docetaxel correlated both with rhodamine 123 efflux and *MDR1* mRNA expression. To validate these results obtained by correlation analyses, cell lines over-expressing *MDR1*/P-glycoprotein as well as other drug resistance-conferring genes were used. AS was shown similarly active towards drug-sensitive and multidrug resistant cell lines (Efferth et al., 2002; 2003). Likewise, methotrexate-resistant CEM/MTX1500LV cells with an amplification of the dihydrofolate reductase (*DHFR*) gene and hydroxyurea-resistant CEM/HUR90 cells with over-expression of ribonucleotide reductase (RRPM2) were not cross-resistant to AS. In addition, other research has shown that ART increased the tissue permeability for standard cytostatic drugs. i.e. doxorubicin in mouse embryonic stem cell-derived embryoid bodies (Wartenberg et al., 2003).

3. Anti-cancer effect of ARTs *via* an anti-angiogenic activity

In the process of angiogenesis, the formation of new blood vessels from pre-existing ones is essential for the supply of tumors with oxygen and nutrients and for the spread of metastatic cells throughout the body. Normal angiogenesis is strictly controlled by some transient, typical physiological processes such as reproduction, development, wound healing; continued angiogenesis is also a characteristic of pathological alteration such as neoplasia. Neoplasia is an angiogenesis-dependent disease, and the growth of tumors, intravasation and metastases require angiogenesis. In human and experimental cancers, new vessels are required for increased delivery of nutrients and are a target for invading tumor cells, and there is a large body of evidence to support a key role for angiogenesis in disease progression. The growth, invasion and metastasis of tumors have been shown to be dependent on angiogenesis. A summary of the anti-angiogenic effects of ARTs is shown in Table 1.

Artemisinins	Effects/Mechanism	References
Artesunate (AS)	1) Induction of apoptosis in KS-IMM cells	Dell'Eva et al., 2004
	2) Reduced F1t-1 and KDR/flk-1 expressions	Huan-huan et al., 2004
	3) Lowered VEGF and KDR/flk-1 expression	Chen et al., 2004a
	4) inhibited the proliferation of HUVEC	Chen et al., 2004b
	5) Inhibited HUVEC and VEGF expression	Chen et al., 2004c
	6) Suppress angiogenic ability & Decreased VEGF	Zhou et al., 2007
	7) Decreased HIF-1α levels	Zhou et al., 2007
	8) Decreased VEGF and Ang-1 secretion	Chen et al., 2010a
	9) Decreased the secretion of VEGF and IL-8	He et al., 2011
	10) Either increased cytotoxicity or cytostasis	Liu et al., 2011
Dihydro-artemisinin (DHA)	1) DHA was more effective than AS	Chen et al., 2003
	2) Reduced VEGF binding to its receptors	Chen et al., 2004a
	3) Induced K562 cells apoptosis, inhibited VEGF	Lee et al., 2006
	4) Reduced VEGF secretion by RPMI8226 cells	Wu et al., 2006
	5) Attenuated the levels of VEGFR-3/Flt-4.	Wang et al., 2007
	6) Decreased KDR levels and NF-kB DNA binding	Chen et al., 2010b
	7) Inhibition of PKCalpha/Raf/MAPKs	Hwang et al., 2010
	8) Decreased VEGF receptor KDR/flk-1	Zhou et al., 2010
	9) Inhibited the expression of several MMPs	Rasheed et al., 2010
	10) DHA inactivates NF-kappaB and potentiates	Wang et al., 2010
	11) Down-regulated VEGF	Aung et al., 2011
	12) Inducted iron-dependent endoplasmic reticulum stress	Lu et al., 2011
	13) DHA inhibits formation of HUVECs, MMP9	Wang et al., 2011
Artemisinin (ART)	1) Decreased VEGF-A transcription	Anfosso et al., 2006
	2) Decreased MMP2, MMP9 and BMP1 levels	Anfosso et al., 2006
	3) Decreased VEGF-C, IL-1 β-induced p38	Wang et al., 2008
	4) Decreased αvβ3 transcription	Buommino et al., 2009
2nd Artemisinin artemisone	less anti-angiogenic effect than DHA in all the experimental models	D'Alessandro et al., 2007
Artemisinin-like compounds (ART-like)	1) Active against solid tumor-derived cell lines and good correlation with other ARTs 2) More active in vitro and in vivo than the commonly used AS	Galal et al., 2009 Soomro et al., 2011
Thioacetal ARTs	inhibitiory activity upon HUVEC	Oh et al., 2003
ART-glycolipid hybrids	Showed potent in vivo anti-angiogenic activity on CAM	Ricci et al., 2010

VEGF = vascular endothelial growth factor; HIF = hypoxia-inducible factor; NF-kB = nuclear factor of kappa light polypeptide gene enhancer in B cells 1; KDR = kinase insert domain protein recepto; MMP = matrix metalloproteinase; BMP = bone morphogenic protein; αvβ3 = Transmembrane heterodimeric protein expressed on sprouting endothelial cells; HUVEC = human umbilical vein endothelial cells. CAM = chorioallantoic membrane

Table 1. Anti-angiogenic effects of ART and its derivatives

3.1. Anti-angiogenic effects of ARTs

3.1.1. In vitro anti-angiogenic effects of ART and its derivatives

While most of the research on the anti-cancer activities of ARTs has been performed with cell lines *in vitro*, there are a few reports in the literature showing activity *in vivo* against xenograft tumors, e.g., breast tumors, ovarian cancer, Kaposi sarcoma, fibrosarcoma, or liver cancer. The *in vitro* data in the literature supports the hypothesis that ART and its derivatives kill or inhibit the growth of many types of cancer cell lines, including drug-resistant cell lines, suggesting that ART could become the basis of a new class of anti-cancer drugs. In addition, the co-administration of holotransferrin and other iron sources with ARTs has been shown to increase the potency of ARTs in killing cancer cells.

Artemisinin (ART)

ARTs are antimalarial agents, but also reveal profound antitumor activity *in vitro* and *in vivo*. Ina microarray study of cancer cells treated at the 50% inhibition concentration with eight ARTs, (ART, AS, arteether, artemisetene, arteanuine B, dihydroartemisinylester stereoisomers 1 and 2) the mRNA expression data of 89 known angiogenesis-related genes was obtained and correlated against the sensitivity of these tumor cells to ARTs treatment. The constitutive expression of 30 genes correlated significantly with the cellular response to ARTs. The finding cell sensitivity and resistance of tumor cells could be predicted by the mRNA expression of angiogenesis related genes supports the hypothesis that ARTs reveal their antitumor effects at least, in part, by inhibition of tumor angiogenesis. As many chemopreventive drugs exert anti-angiogenic features, ARTs might also be chemo-preventive in addition to their cytotoxic effects (Anfosso et al., 2006).

A recent study demonstrated that ART-induced cell growth arrest in A375M malignant melanoma tumor cells also affected the viability of A375P cutaneous melanoma tumor cells with both cytotoxic and growth inhibitory effects, while ART was not effective in inhibiting the growth of other tumor cell lines (MCF7 and MKN). In addition, ART treatment affected the migratory ability of A375M cells by reducing metalloproteinase 2 (MMP-2) productions and down-regulating $\alpha v\beta 3$ integrin expression. These findings support the hypothesis that ART may serve as a chemotherapeutic agent for melanoma treatment (Buommino et al., 2009). Furthermore, IL-1beta-induced p38 mitogen-activated protein kinase (MAPK) activation and upregulation of VEGF-C mRNA, and VEGF-C receptor protein levels in LLC cells were also suppressed by ART or by the p38 MAPK inhibitor SB-203580, suggesting that p38 MAPK could serve as a mediator of pro-inflammatory cytokine-induced VEGF-C expression. These data support the hypothesis that ART may be useful for the prevention of lymph node metastasis by downregulating VEGF-C and reducing tumor lymphangiogenesis (Wang et al., 2008).

Dihydroartemisinin (DHA)

DHA and AS have been shown to be remarkable inhibitors of tumor cell growth and suppression of angiogenesis *in vitro*. The anti-cancer activity of ARTs has been demonstrated by an MTT (3-(4,5-dimethylthiazol-2-yl)-2,5-diphenyltetrazolium bromide) growth inhibition assay of four human cancer cell lines, cervical cancer HeLa, uterus chorion cancer JAR, embryo transversal cancer RD and ovarian cancer HO-8910 treated with DHA and AS. IC_{50} values obtained through this MTT growth inhibition assay demonstrated that DHA was more effective at inhibiting cancer cell lines than AS. The anti-angiogenic activities of DHA and AS were tested on *in vitro* models of angiogenesis by assessing the proliferation, migration and tube formation of human umbilical vein endothelial (HUVE) cells. The results showed that DHA and AS significantly inhibited angiogenesis in a dose-dependent manner. These results also showed that DHA was more effective than ART in inhibiting angiogenesis (Chen et al., 2003).

The effect of DHA on human multiple myeloma-induced angiogenesis under hypoxia and elucidated its mechanism of action has been performed. An *in vivo* chicken chorioallantoic membrane model was used to examine the effect of DHA on multiple myeloma-induced angiogenesis. Compared with conditioned medium of control, conditioned medium from human multiple myeloma RPMI8226 cells pretreated with 3 μM DHA in hypoxia was observed to reduce microvessel growth on chicken chorioallantoic membranes by approximately 28.6% ($P < 0.05$). The level of VEGF in conditioned medium was determined by enzyme-linked immunosorbent assay. The results confirmed that 3 μM DHA could significantly decrease VEGF secretion by RPMI8226 cells ($P < 0.05$), which correlated well with the reduction of multiple myeloma-induced angiogenesis on chicken chorioallantoic membranes. Western blot and reverse transcription-PCR results revealed that DHA downregulated the expression of VEGF in RPMI8226 cells in hypoxia. Therefore, DHA possesses potential as an antiangiogenic drug in multiple myeloma therapy and thereby may improve patient outcome (Wu et al., 2006).

The effect of DHA on VEGF expression and apoptosis in chronic myeloid leukemia (CML) K562 cells was assessed. The results demonstrated that in addition to its anti-proliferation effect on CML cells, DHA was also found to induce K562 cells apoptosis. The percentage of apoptotic cells was increased to 6.9 and 15.8% after being treated with 5 and 10 μM DHA for 48 h, respectively ($P < 0.001$). All these experiments suggested that DHA could inhibit the VEGF expression and secretion effectively in K562 cells, even at a lower concentration (2 μM, $P < 0.05$). Moreover, we further assessed the stimulating angiogenic activity of CM from K562 cells on CAM model. Also, the angiogenic activity was decreased in response to the CM from K562 cells pretreated with DHA in a dose-dependent manner. Taken together, these results from our study together with its known low toxicity make it possible that DHA might present potential anti-leukemia effect as a treatment for CML therapy, or as an adjunct to standard chemotherapeutic regimens (Lee et al., 2006)

DHA was found to have a potent ability in influencing lymphatic endothelial cells (LECs) behavior. DHA also exerted a significant inhibitory effect on migration and tube-like formation of LECs in a dose-dependent manner. Quantitative RT-PCR further showed that DHA remarkably downregulated the expression of antiapoptotic bcl-2 mRNA, but upregulated that of the proapoptotic gene bax mRNA. In addition, DHA could strongly attenuate the mRNA and protein levels of VEGFR-3/Flt-4. In summary, these findings indicate that DHA may be useful as a potential lymphangiogenesis inhibitor under induction of cell apoptosis, inhibition of the migration, and formation of tube-like structures in LECs (Wang et al., 2007). In addition, to investigate the effects of DHA on cell cycle progression and NF-kappaB activity in pancreatic cancer cells, the cell cycle progression was determined. The translocation and DNA-binding activity of NF-kappaB were inhibited in DHA-treated cells in a dose-dependent manner, indicated the inactivation effects of DHA in pancreatic cancer cells. Study shows that DHA induces cell cycle arrest and apoptosis in pancreatic cancer cells, and this effect might be due to inhibition of NF-kappaB signaling (Chen et al., 2010b).

One study showed that DHA is an effective anti-metastatic agent that functions by down-regulating the MMP-9 gene which is associated with metastasis. 1) DHA was shown to reduce phorbol myristate acetate (PMA)-induced activation of MMP-9 and MMP-2 and further inhibited cell invasion and migration. 2) DHA was also shown to suppress the PMA-enhanced expression of the levels of MMP-9 protein and mRNA, and enhanced transcriptional activity of the MM-9 gene through suppression of NF-kappaB and activation of AP-1 without changing the level of tissue inhibition of metalloproteinase (TIMP)-1. 3) DHA has been shown to reduce PMA-enhanced MMP-2 expression by suppressing membrane-type 1 MMP (MT1-MMP), but was not shown to t alter TIMP-2 levels. 4) DHA was shown to inhibit PMA-induced NF-kappaB and c-Jun nuclear translocation, which are upstream of PMA-induced MMP-9 expression which enhances metastasis. 5) DHA strongly repressed the PMA-induced phosphorylation of Raf/ERK and JNK, which are dependent on the PKC alpha pathway. In summary, this study demonstrated that the anti-invasive effects of DHA may occur through inhibition of PKC alpha/Raf/ERK and JNK phosphorylation and reduction of NF-kappaB and AP-1 activation, leading to down-regulation of MMP-9 expression. (Hwang et al., 2010)

Wang et al. demonstrated that DHA enhances gemcitabine-induced growth inhibition and apoptosis in both BxPC-3 and PANC-1 cell lines *in vitro*. The effect is at least partially due to the DHA-driven deactivation of gemcitabine-induced NF-kappaB activation, which in turn leads to a tremendous decrease in the expression of NF-kappaB target gene products, such as c-myc, cyclin D1, Bcl-2, Bcl-xL (Wang et al., 2010). DHA was also shown to exhibit significant anti-cancer activity against the renal epithelial LLC cell line. In addition, DHA was shown to induce apoptosis of LLC cells and influenced the expression of the vascular endothelial growth factor (VEGF) receptor KDR/flk-1. Furthermore, in both tumor xenografts, a greater degree of growth inhibition was achieved when DHA and chemotherapeutic drugs were used in combination. The combined effect of DHA administered with chemotherapy drugs on LLC tumor metastasis was shown to be significant (Zhou et al., 2010).

The effect of DHA was investigated using *in vitro/in vivo* optical imaging combined with cell/tumor growth assays of the pancreatic cancer cell line BxPc3-RFP which stably expresses red fluorescence protein. DHA inhibited the proliferation and viability of pancreatic cancer cells in a dose-dependent manner and induced apoptosis. The results of this experiment demonstrated DHA-induced down-regulation of PCNA and Bcl-2, and up-regulation of Bax. VEGF expression was down-regulated by DHA in cells under normoxic, but not hypoxic, conditions. The anti-angiogenic effect of DHA appears to be a complicated process (Aung et al., 2011). DHA was shown to significantly inhibit NF-κB DNA-binding activity, which in turn results in a tremendous decrease in the expression of NF-κB-targeted pro-angiogenic gene products such as VEGF, IL-8, COX-2, and MMP-9 in *vitro*: These findings suggest that DHA could be developed as a novel agent against pancreatic cancer (Wang et al., 2011). Additional supporting evidence of the potential of DHA to be used as an anti-pancreatic cancer agent were shown through a DHA driven up-regulation of glucose-regulated protein 78 (GRP78), which is known to be involved in endoplasmic reticulum stress (ER stress),. Further study demonstrated that DHA could enhance expression of GRP78 as well as the growth arrest and DNA-damage-inducible gene 153 at both the mRNA and protein levels. These studies suggest that redox imbalance may result in DHA-induced ER stress, which may contribute, at least in part, to its anti-cancer activity (Lu et al., 2011).

Artesunate (AS)

AS has been shown to inhibit the growth of Kaposi's sarcoma cells, a highly angiogenic multifocal tumor, and the degree of cell growth inhibition correlated with the induction of apoptosis. AS was also shown to inhibit the growth of normal human umbilical endothelial cells and of KS-IMM cells that were established from a Kaposi's sarcoma lesion obtained from a renal transplant patient. The inhibition of cell growth correlated with the induction of apoptosis in KS-IMM cells. Apoptosis was not observed in normal endothelial cells, which showed drastically increased cell doubling times upon AS treatment (Dell'Eva et al., 2004).

AS has been shown to greatly inhibit cell proliferation and differentiation of endothelial cells in a dose-dependent manner in the range of 12.5-100 μM. AS was also shown to reduce Flt-1 and KDR/flk-1 expression of endothelial cells when dosed *in vitro* in a range of 0.1-0.5 μM. In subsequent studies by the same author, the AS-driven apoptosis of a human microvascular dermal endothelial cell line was studied. The apoptosis was detected utilizing a morphological dual staining assay composed of ethidium bromide and acridine orange as well as a DNA fragmentation TUNEL assay quantified by a flow cytometric propidium iodide (PI) assay. The results suggest that the anti-angiogenic effect induced by AS treatment might occur by the induction of cellular apoptosis (Huan-huan et al., 2004). In addition, the inhibitory effect of AS on *in vitro* angiogenesis was tested using aortic cells cultured in a fibrin gel. AS was shown to effectively suppress the stimulating angiogenic ability of chronic myeloid leukemia cells (line K562) when the K562 cells were pretreated for 48 h with AS in a time-dependent manner (days 3-14). AS treatment was also found to decrease the VEGF level in chronic myeloma K562 cells, even at a lower concentration (2 μmol/l, $P < 0.01$). (Zhou et al., 2007).

The addition of Fe(II)-glycine sulfate and transferrin has been shown to enhance the cytotoxicity (10.3-fold) of free AS *in vitro*. AS microencapsulated in maltosyl-ß- cyclodextrin, and ARTs were tested against CCRF-CEM leukemia and U373 astrocytoma cells *in vitro* (Efferth et al., 2004). Treatment with AS at more than 2.5 μM for 48 h inhibited the proliferation of human vein endothelial cells (HUVEC) in a concentration dependent manner using an MTT (3-(4,5-dimethylthiazol-2-yl)-2,5-diphenyltetrazolium bromide) based growth proliferation assay ($p < 0.05$). The IC_{50} value of this growth inhibition assay was 20.7 μM, and HUVEC cells were also shown to be growth inhibited by 88.7% after treatment with 80 μM AS (Chen et al., 2004b).

AS at low concentration was shown to significantly decrease VEGF and Ang-1 secretion by human multiple myeloma cells (line RPMI8226, $P < 0.05$), which correlated well with the reduction of angiogenesis induced by the myeloma RPMI8226 cells. This study also showed that AS down-regulated the expression of VEGF and Ang-1 in RPMI8226 cells and reduced the activation of extracellular signal regulated kinase 1 (ERK1) as well. Therefore, AS has been shown to block ERK1/2 activation, downregulate VEGF and Ang-1 expression and inhibit angiogenesis induced by human multiple myeloma RPMI8226 cells. Combined with previous published data, the results from this study supports the hypothesis that AS possesses potential anti-myeloma activity (Chen et al., 2010a).

AS has also been shown to decrease the secretion of VEGF and IL-8 from TNFα- or hypoxia-stimulated rheumatoid arthritis fibroblast-like synoviocyte (line RA FLS) in a dose-dependent manner. In addition, AS treatment resulted in the inhibition of TNFα- or hypoxia-induced nuclear expression and translocation of HIF-1α. AS treatment was shown to prevent Akt phosphorylation, but there was no evidence that phosphorylation of p38 and ERK was averted. TNFα- or hypoxia-induced secretion of VEGF and IL-8 and expression of HIF-1α were hampered by treatment with the PI3 kinase inhibitor LY294002, suggesting that inhibition of PI3 kinase/Akt activation might inhibit VEGF, IL-8 secretion, and HIF-1α expression induced by TNFα or hypoxia. Therefore, AS has been shown to inhibit angiogenic factor expression in the RA FLS cell line, and this latest study provides new evidence that, as a low-cost agent, AS may have therapeutic potential for rheumatoid arthritis (He et al., 2011).

Using a polyploid cell line, research on the role of AS in impacting cell cycle arrest was assessed. The results of this study show that AS treatment of polyploid cells resulted in a dose-dependent decreases in cell number, which was associated with either increased cytotoxicity or cytostasis. Of the two possibilities, cytostasis, a simultaneous arrest at all phases of the cell cycle, appeared to be a more likely possibility. This deduction was supported by molecular profiling, which showed reductions in cell cycle transit proteins. AS appeared to maintain cells in this arrested state, however, reculturing these treated cells in drug-free medium resulted in significant reductions in cell viability. Taken together, these observations indicate AS and its related compounds may be effective for the treatment of polyploid tumors, and that activity is related to the cell cycle schedule. Therefore, it is important to carefully select the most appropriate schedule to maximize AS efficacy when using AS as a primary or adjuvant anti-tumor therapy (Liu et al., 2011)

3.1.2. In vivo anti-angiogenic effects of ART and its derivatives

There are many reports discussing the *in vivo* anti-cancer activity of ARTs which may provide insight into the potential activity of ARTs as anti-cancer agents.

Artemisinin (ART)

The effect of ART on tumor growth, lymphangiogenesis, metastasis and survival in mouse Lewis lung carcinoma (LLC) models was examined. The results of this study showed that orally administered artemisinin inhibited lymph node and lung metastasis and prolonged survival without retarding tumor growth. ART-treated mice showed significant decreases in lymph node metastasis, tumor lymphangiogenesis and expression of VEGF-C as compared to control mice. (Wang et al., 2008).

Dihydroartemisinin (DHA)

The anti-angiogenic activity of DHA *in vitro* and *in vivo*, and investigated DHA-induced apoptosis in human umbilical vein endothelial cells (HUVEC). DHA markedly reduced VEGF binding to its receptors on the surface of HUVEC. The expression levels of two major VEGF receptors, Flt-1 and KDR/flk-1, on HUVEC were lower following DHA treatment as shown by an immunocytochemical staining assay. The *in vivo* anti-angiogenic activity was evaluated in the chicken chorioallantoic membrane (CAM) neovascularization model. DHA significantly inhibited CAM angiogenesis at low concentrations (5-30 nmol/100 microl per egg). This group also investigated both qualitatively and quantitatively the induction of HUVEC apoptosis by DHA. A dose-related (5-80 μM) and time-dependent (6-36 h) increase in DHA-induced HUVEC apoptosis was observed by flow cytometry. These results suggest that the anti-angiogenic effect induced by DHA might occur by induction of cellular apoptosis and inhibition of expression of VEGF receptors. These findings and the known low toxicity of DHA indicate that it might be a promising candidate angiogenesis inhibitor (Chen et al., 2004a).

The anti-angiogenic effect of DHA on pancreatic cancer was assessed using BxPC-3 xenografts subcutaneously established in BALB/c nude mice. DHA demonstrated remarkable activity against pancreatic cancer studies concuted *in vivo*. DHA treatment resulted in reduced tumor volume and decreased microvessel density, and there were additional transcriptional effects demonstrated in these studies as well regarding the expression of NF-κB-related pro-angiogenic gene products which were down-regulated. This finding of relating to the inhibition of NF-κB activation is likely one of the mechanisms involved in DHA anti-angiogenic activity against human pancreatic cancer. This suggests that DHA could be developed as a novel agent against pancreatic cancer (Wang et al., 2011). In a further study, the co-administration of the chemotherapeutic agent gemcitabine with DHA was shown to result in remarkably enhanced anti-tumor effects, as demonstrated by significantly increased apoptosis, as well as a decreased Ki-67 index, reduced NF-kappaB activity, reduced downstream angiogenic gene products, and predictably, significantly reduced tumor volume. The authors conclude that inhibition of gemcitabine-induced NF-kappaB activation is one of the mechanisms by which DHA could promote its anti-tumor effect on pancreatic cancer (Wang et al., 2010).

Artesunate (AS)

The anti-angiogenic effect *in vivo* of artesunate was evaluated in nude mice f implanted with human ovarian cancer cells (HO-8910). The effects of artesunate on angiogenesis in this *in vivo* study were evaluated by immune-histochemical staining for microvessel associated antigens (CD31), VEGF and the VEGF receptor KDR/flk-1. AS significantly inhibited angiogenesis in a concentration-dependent form in the range of 0.5-50 μM. The IC_{50} of AS for HUVE cells was 21 μM. Growth of the xenograft tumor was decreased and microvessel density was reduced following drug-treatment with no apparent toxic effects on the nude mice. AS administration was shown to dramatically reduce VEGF expression on tumor cells and KDR/flk-1 expression on endothelial cells as well as tumor cells. Accordingly, these results support the hypothesis that AS is capable of inhibiting angiogenesis in *vitro* and *in vivo*. These findings together with the known low toxicity of AS are clues that AS may be a promising angiogenesis inhibitor (Chen et al., 2004c).

Further studies on the anti-angiogenic effects of AS have been conducted *in vivo* and *in vitro*. The anti-angiogenic effect of AS *in vivo* was evaluated utilizing the chicken chorioallantoic membrane (CAM) neovascularization model. At low concentrations of 10 nM/100 µl/egg, AS was shown to significantly inhibit CAM angiogenesis, and completely inhibited angiogenesis at concentrations of 80 nM/100 µl/egg. The results of this study suggest that the anti-angiogenic effect induced by AS might occur by the induction of cellular apoptosis. These findings and the known low toxicity of AS support the hypothesis that AS might be a promising candidate as an angiogenesis inhibitor (Huan-huan et al., 2004). Similarly, AS was shown to significantly impair primary tumor growth and metastasis in the chicken embryo metastasis (CAM) model where AS was shown to suppress invasion and metastasis of non-small cell lung cancer (NSCLC) cells. The transcriptional findings of these experiments showed AS treatment reduced transcription of u-PA, MMP-2 and MMP-7, supporting the hypothesis that AS has promise as a novel therapeutic for NSCLC (Rasheed et al., 2010).

Also, AS has been studied in a variety of tumor models as a potential antitumor drug. In one study of vascularization, a critical element of tumor metastasis, AS was shown to strongly reduce angiogenesis of Kaposi's sarcoma cells *in vivo* by inhibiting vascularization in Matrigel plugs injected subcutaneously into syngenic mice. This data suggests that AS represents a promising candidate drug for the treatment of the highly angiogenic Kaposi's sarcoma. As a low-cost drug, it might be of particular interest for use in areas of the world where Kaposi's sarcoma is highly prevalent. (Dell'Eva et al., 2004).

The efficacy of AS, as an anti-cancer agent, to reduce tumor growth was studied in rats given AS subcutaneously at a dose of 50 mg/kg/day and at a dose of 100 mg/kg/day for 15 days. The results of this experiment showed animals with AS treated tumors showed a reduction in tumor growth by 41%, in the 50 mg/kg treatment group and 62% in the 100 mg/kg treatment group. The density of micro-vessels which was used as a measure of angiogenic activity in the tumors of animals treated with 100 mg/kg of AS daily was at least four times lower than in the control group (Chen et al., 2004b). The anti-angiogenic activity of AS *in vivo* was also evaluated in nude mice implanted with a human ovarian cancer cell line (HO-8910). Evaluation of angiogenesis in the AS treated and control animals with an ovarian cancer xenograft were determined through immunohistochemical staining for microvessel formation (CD31), VEGF and the VEGF receptor KDR/flk-1. Tumor growth was noted to be decreased, and the density of the tumor microvessels was reduced following AS treatment with no apparent toxicity to the animals (Chen et al., 2004a, 2004b).

The anti-angiogenic effect of AS was further evaluated *in vivo* in the chicken chorioallantoic membrane (CAM) neovascularization model. The results showed that stimulating angiogenic activity was decreased in response to the treatment of myeloblastic K562 cells with ART, and tumor growth was inhibited when K562 cells were pretreated with ART in a dose-dependent manner (3-12 μmol/l). Further analyses of the level of VEGF expression by Western blot and also assays of VEGF mRNA by RT-PCR in K562 cells showed that ART could inhibit VEGF expression, and the inhibition correlated well with the level of VEGF secreted in the culture medium. These findings suggest that AS may have potential as a treatment for chronic myelogenous leukemia (CML) or as an adjunct to standard chemotherapeutic regimens (Zhou et al., 2007).

3.1.3. Anti-angiogenic effects of novel ARTs and ART-like compounds

Artesunate has been shown to exhibit anti-angiogenic, anti-tumorigenic and anti-viral properties in addition to its known antimalarial properties. The array of activities of the ARTs, and the recent emergence of malaria resistance to AS, prompted one group to synthesize and evaluate several novel ART-like derivatives. Sixteen distinct derivatives were therefore synthesized, and the *in vitro* cytotoxic effects of each were tested with different cell lines. The *in vivo* anti-angiogenic properties were evaluated using a zebrafish embryo model. This groupreported the identification of several novel ART-like compounds that are easily synthesized, stable at room temperature, may overcome drug-resistance pathways and are more active *in vitro* and *in vivo* than the commonly used AS. These promising findings raise the hopes of identifying safer and more effective strategies to treat a range of infections and cancer (Soomro et al., 2011).

Twelve ART acetal dimers were synthesized and tested for antitumor activity against 60 *in vitro* tumor cell lines compiled by the National Cancer Institute (NCI), producing a mean GI_{50} concentration between 8.7 (least active) and 0.019 μM (most active). The significant activity of the compounds in this preliminary screen led to additional *in vitro* antitumor and anti-angiogenesis studies. Several active dimers were also evaluated in the *in vivo* NCI hollow fiber assay followed by a preliminary xenograft study. The title compounds were found to be active against solid tumor-derived cell lines and showed good correlation with other artemisinin-based molecules in the NCI database (Galal et al., 2009).

In addition, various thioacetal ART derivatives can inhibit the angiogenesis and might be angiogenesis inhibitors. In particular, 10 alpha-phenylthiodihydroartemisinins, 10 beta-benzenesulfonyl-9-epi-dihydroartemisinin and 10 alpha-mercaptodihydroartemisinin exhibit strong growth inhibition activity against HUVEC proliferation. Compound 11 have a good inhibitory activity upon HUVEC tube formation, and 5 and 11 show a strong inhibitory effect on angiogenesis using CAM assay at 5 μg/egg by 90% (Oh et al., 2004).

Artemisone is a novel 10-alkylamino derivative which is not metabolized to DHA. It was selected as a clinical drug candidate on the basis of its potency *in vitro* against *Plasmodium falciparum* and its lack of detectable neurotoxicity in both *in vitro* and *in vivo* screens. Artemisone was tested *in vitro* and *in vivo* for anti-angiogenic effects which may support its use as an anti-angiogenic agent as an adjunct to standard tumor chemotherapy. The various studies of artemisone's anti-angiogenic activity include proliferation of human endothelial cells and their migration on a fibronectin matrix, the sprouting of new vessels from rat aorta sections grown in collagen, and the production of pro-angiogenic cytokines such as vascular endothelial growth factor (VEGF) and interleukin-8 (CXCL-8). The data showed that artemisone is significantly less anti-angiogenic than DHA in all the experimental models tested, suggesting that artemisone will be safer to use than the current clinical artemisinins during pregnancy for an antimalarial indication but perhaps less efficacious for an anti-angiogenic indication as part of a anti-cancer regimen (D'Alessandro et al., 2007).

3.2. Mechanistic perspectives for the anti-angiogenic activities of ARTs

Angiogenesis and vasculogenesis refer to the growth of blood vessels. Angiogenesis is the growth most often associated with repair of damaged vessels or the growth of smaller blood vessels, while vasculogenesis is the process by which the primary blood system is being created or changed. Vasculogenesis occurs during the very early developmental stages of an organism when the blood vessel pathways are created. Angiogenesis, while a similar process, does not depend on the same set of genes as vasculogenesis, and this process is activated instead in the presence of an injury to a blood vessel. In the last three decades, considerable research has been reported that supports the hypothesis that tumor growth and metastasis require angiogenesis. Angiogenesis, the proliferation and migration of endothelial cells resulting in the formation of new blood vessels, is an important process for the progression of tumors (Figure 3). ARTs have been shown in a number of published reports to have anti-angiogenic effects.

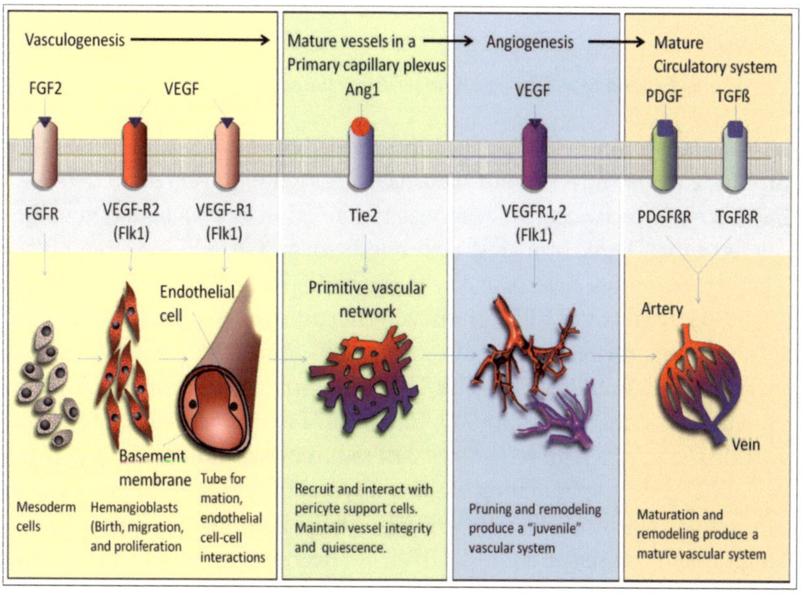

Figure 3. The modes of vasculogenesis and angiogenesis. Vasculogenesis occurs during the very early developmental stages of an organism when the blood vessel pathways are created. Angiogenesis, while a similar process, does not depend on the same set of genes as vasculogenesis, and this process is activated instead in the presence of an injury to a blood vessel. Angiogenesis finishes the circulatory connections begun by vasculogenesis and builds arteries and veins from the capillaries (Modified from Hanahan, 1997

As malignant tissues grow, metastases and solid tumors require extra blood supply for thriving and survival. Thus, cancer cells induce neovascularization by regulating proteins and pathways involved in the generation and restructure of new vasculature. Angiogenesis process leads to enhanced proliferation of endothelial cells through induction of VEGF, fibroblast growth factor (FGF), its receptors, and cytokines. This event occurs via multiple effects including hypoxia-driven activation of expression of HIF-1α and the aryl hydrocarbon receptor nuclear translocator (ARNT). Angiogenesis control is mediated by angiostatin, endostatin, thrombospondin, TIMPs, PAI-1, and others. Due to their role in tumor survival, the pro-angiogenic factors and the molecules involved in their regulatory networks are relevant drug targets (Crespo-Ortiz and Wei, 2012)

Cancers are capable of spreading through the body by two mechanisms: invasion and metastasis. Invasion is the direct migration and penetration by cancer cells into neighboring tissues. Metastasis is the ability of cancer cells to penetrate into lymphatic and blood vessels, circulate through the bloodstream, and then grow in a new focus (metastasize) in normal tissues elsewhere in the body. Without a connection to a network of blood vessels, a tumor can only grow to about the size of a pinhead (1-2 mm), that is to say a tumor is in a vascular, quiescent status. When a subgroup of cells within the tumor switches to an angiogenic phenotype by changing the local equilibrium between positive and negative regulators of angiogenesis, tumor starts to grow rapidly and becomes clinically detectable. Anti-angiogenesis therapy is a novel approach in cancer treatment and prevention of tumor metastasis. It is therefore expected that angiogenesis inhibitors may be clinically useful for the treatment of tumors.

3.2.1. Anti-cancer mechanism of ARTs on angiogenesis-related genes

Angiogenesis involves tissue restructuring, and genes that regulate angiogenesis, such as chemokine receptors, can also affect tumor metastasis. A vital requirement of neovasculogenesis is endothelial mitosis, which occurs in response to activation by pro-angiogenic signaling from VEGF and its receptors. Three human genes encode for VEGF (VEGFA, VEGFB and VEGFC) and splice variants add more heterogeneity to the biological actions of the VEGF gene family (Tischer et al., 1991). Analysis of VEGF transcripts in cultured vascular smooth muscle cells by PCR and cDNA cloning revealed three different forms of the VEGF coding region, which has also been previously reported in HL60 cells. The three forms of the human VEGF protein chain predicted from these coding regions are 189, 165, and 121 amino acids in length. Comparison of cDNA nucleotide sequences with sequences derived from human VEGF genomic clones indicates that the VEGF gene is split among eight exons and that the various VEGF coding region forms arise from this gene by alternative splicing. Analysis of the VEGF gene promoter region revealed a single major transcription start, which lies near a cluster of potential Sp1 factor binding sites. Northern blot analysis demonstrated that the level of VEGF transcripts is elevated in cultured vascular smooth muscle cells after treatment with the phorbol ester 12-O-tetradecanoyl-phorbol-13-acetate (Tischer et al., 1991).

In a study using an US National Cancer Institute (NCI) panel of 60 tumor cell lines, ART and related compounds displayed anti-angiogenic activities based on the altered expression of genes implicated in angiogenesis. The mRNA expression data of angiogenesis-related genes correlated well with the 50% growth inhibition concentration values for eight ARTs (ART, AS, arteether, artemisetene, arteanuine B, dihydroartemisinylester stereoisomers 1 and 2). The constitutive expression of 30 different genes correlated significantly with the cellular response to ARTs. The finding that drug sensitivity and resistance of tumor cells could be predicted by the mRNA expression of angiogenesis related genes supports the hypothesis that the antitumor activity of ARTs may be due, at least in part, by inhibition of tumor angiogenesis. As many chemo-preventive drugs exert anti-angiogenic features, ARTs might also have a chemo-preventive effect in addition to their cytotoxic effects (Anfosso et al., 2006).

These findings are consistent with previous published work (Wartenberg et al., 2003) showing an artemisinin-dependent decrease in expression levels of hypoxia-inducible factor 1a (HIF-1a; H1F1A), which is known to be a transcriptional activator of VEGFA and is critical in neovasculogenesis in hypoxic tissues. The inhibition of angiogenesis by ART (at a concentration of 12 mM) involving VEGF and HIF-1a was also demonstrated in leukemic and glioma cells (Huang et al., 2008; Zhou et al., 2007). Loss of HIF-1α and VEGF expression by artemisinin appears to depend on ROS as co-treatment with free-radical scavengers such as vitamin E and mannitol reversed the effects of artemisinin (Wartenberg et al., 2003). The sensitivity and resistance of these tumor cells has been shown to correlate with mRNA expression of angiogenesis-related genes. This suggests that the anti-tumor effects of ARTs are potentially due to their role in inhibiting tumor angiogenesis (Anfosso et al., 2006). The finding that tumor cell drug sensitivity and resistance could be predicted by mRNA expression of angiogenesis-related genes supports the hypothesis that artemisinins their anti-tumor effects at least in part by inhibition of tumor angiogenesis.

In addition, an investigation to determine the sensitivity and resistance of cancer cells towards AS was conducted. The gene-hunting approach applied by us delivered several novel candidate genes that may regulate the response of cancer cells to AS. These results merit further investigations to prove the contribution of these genes for AS resistance. Study demonstrated that AS was no inhibitor of ABC transporters ABCB1 and ABCG2. Although AS may exhibit specific inhibitory functions towards particular ABC transporters, but not towards a wide spectrum of several different ABC transporters. This approach showed that response of tumor cells towards AS is multi-factorial in nature and is determined by gene expression associated with AS sensitivity on the one hand and with gene expression associated with AS resistance on the other hand (Sertel et al., 2010).

3.2.2. Anti-proliferative mechanisms of ARTs

The anti-cancer mechanism of ARTs is likely to be related to the cleavage of the iron- or heme-mediated peroxide bridge, followed by the generation of ROS (Mercer et al., 2011; Zhang et al., 2010). The anti-cancer potential of ARTs is possibly connected to the expression of TfR. The synergism of AS and iron (II)-glycine sulfate co-treatment is unsuitable for all types of tumor cells. Endoplasmic reticulum stress is partially involved in some cases of ARTs-mediated anti-proliferation (Lu et al., 2010; Stockwin et al., 2009).

In normal cells, cyclin-dependent kinases (CDK) are the proteins translating signals in order to guide cells through the cell-division cycle. Normal growth relies on the ability to translate signals in order to replicate and divide in an effective manner (McDonald and El-Deiry, 2000). Uncontrolled proliferation in cancer cells is known to result from mutations inducing amplification of growth signals, deregulation of checkpoints, and loss of sensitivity to growth inhibitors. Abnormal cell growth is also triggered by deregulation of programmed cell death or apoptosis (Vogelstein and Kinzler, 2004). ARTs have been shown to effectively induce cell growth arrest in cancer lines either by disrupting the cell cycle kinetics or by interfering with proliferation-interacting pathways.

DHA and AS are very potent growth inhibitors, and multiple studies have demonstrated that DHA is the most potent anti-cancer artemisinin-like compound (DHA > AS > AM) (Efferth et al., 2003; Woerdenbag et al., 1993). Recently, artemisone has shown impressive anti-tumor efficacy in 7 cells lines including melanoma and breast cancer cells (Gravett et al., 2010). ART compounds have been shown to exert cytostatic and cytotoxic action on cancer cells (Efferth et al., 2003; Hou et al., 2008). ART-induced growth arrest has been reported at all cell cycle phases; however, arrest at the G0/G1 to S transition seems to be more commonly affected (Efferth et al., 2003). Arrest at all cell cycle phases at the same time has been interpreted as a cytostatic effect. Disruption of the cell cycle at G2/M was observed after DHA treatment in osteosarcoma, pancreas, leukemia (Yao et al., 2008) and ovarian cancer cells (Jiao et al., 2007). Similarly, AS interferes with G2 in osteosarcoma, ovarian, and other different cancer lines (Ji et al., 2011).

Several ART derivatives displayed higher cytotoxicity to murine bone marrow cells than to murine Ehrlich ascites tumor cells in a clonogenic assay (Beekman et al., 1998). The IC_{50} values for HeLa cervical cancer cells, uterine chorion cancer JAR cells, embryo transversal cancer RD and ovarian cancer HO-8910 cell lines after 48-h treatment with ART and DHA ranged from 15 to 50 μM and from 8 to 33 μM, respectively (Chen et al., 2003). ART potentiated the differentiation of 1α, 25-dihydroxyvitamin-D3-induced HL-60 leukemia cell predominantly into monocytes and all-*trans* RA-induced cell differentiation into granulocytes, respectively (Kim et al., 2003). Signal transducers involved in the differentiation process, such as extracellular-signal regulated kinase (ERK) and protein kinase C ß1 (PKCB1) were affected by ART.

Inhibition of proliferation may also be attributed to down-regulation of interacting proteins targeting multiple pathways (Firestone and Sundar, 2009). It has been shown that DHA treatment of pancreatic cells (BxPC3, AsPC-1) inhibited cell viability by decreasing the levels of proliferating cell nuclear antigen (PCNA) and cyclin D with parallel increase in p21 (Chen et al., 2009). Another study in the same system showed that DHA counters NF-κB factor activation leading to inhibition of its targets in the proliferation (c-myc, cyclin D) and apoptotic pathways (Bcl2, Bcl-xl) (Wang et al., 2010). In prostate cancer, DHA has been shown to induce cell cycle arrest by disrupting the interaction of Sp1 (specificity protein 1) and the CDK4 promoter (Willoughby et al., 2009). Dissociation of the Sp1-CDK4 complex promotes caspase activation and cell death. In addition, another study has identified AS as a topoisomerase II inhibitor which inhibits growth by interaction with multiple pathways (Youns et al., 2009).Overall, a wide body of research supports the hypothesis that ARTs are capable of interfering with several pathways known to be involved in neoplasia.

3.2.3. *Anti-VEGF mechanisms of ARTs*

Angiogenesis is promoted by numerous factors including cytokines such as VEGF, bFGF, PDGF and others. It is negatively regulated by angiostatin, endostatin, thrombospondin, TIMPs and other factors. The factors that are produced in tumor cells as well as in surrounding stromal cells act in a balance to promote either pro-angiogenic or anti-angiogenic processes. Among the cytokines for regulating angiogenesis, VEGF and angiopoietin-1 (Ang-1) have specific modulating effects on the growth of vascular endothelial cells, and they play a key role in the process of angiogenesis (Thurston 2002). VEGF is a homodimeric 34-42 kDa, a heparin-binding glycoprotein with potent angiogenic, mitogenic and vascular permeability-enhancing activities specific for endothelial cells. Two receptor tyrosine kinases have been described as putative VEGF receptors, Flt-1 and KDR. Flt-1 (fms-like tyrosine kinase), and KDR (kinase-insert-domain-containing receptor) proteins have been shown to bind VEGF with high affinity.

ART and DHA have been shown to significantly inhibit angiogenesis in a dose-dependent manner as demonstrated by measurement of the proliferation, migration and tube formation of human umbilical vein endothelial (HUVE) cells (Chen et al., 2003). DHA was shown to markedly reduce VEGF binding to its receptors on the surface of HUVE cells and reduced the expression levels of two major VEGF receptors, Flt-1 and KDR/flk-1, on HUVE cells. ART derivatives also inhibited HUVE cell tube formation and exhibited anti-angiogenic effects (Oh et al., 2004). By utilizing the chicken chorioallantoic membrane (CAM) culture technique, it is possible to detect the microangium-like structures formed by *in vitro* cultivated arterial rings associated with angiogenesis. By using this method, AS has been shown to also have anti-angiogenic effects. Treatment with AS significantly inhibited chicken chorioallantoic membrane (CAM) angiogenesis, proliferation, and differentiation of human microvascular dermal endothelial cells in a dose-dependent manner and reduced Flt-1 and KDR/flk-1 expression (Huan-Huan et al., 2004).

Tumor hypoxia activates the transcription factor hypoxia inducible factor-1α (HIF-1α). This adaptation increases tumor angiogenesis to support the survival of poorly nourished cancer cells. Hypoxic tumors are resistant to radiation and many anti-cancer agents. HIF-1α is activated during angiostatic therapy, and HIF-1α has also been shown to up-regulate the expression of transferrin receptors. Since ART is selectively toxic to iron-loaded cells, radio and drug-resistant tumors might be selectively susceptible to attack by a treatment strategy consisting of iron-loading and ART treatment (Li et al., 2008; Zhou et al., 2007).

These findings are consistent with previous findings (Wartenberg et al., 2003) that noted ART-dependent decreases in expression levels of HIF-1α. HIF-1α is known to be a transcriptional activator of VEGF, and it plays a crucial role in neo-vasculogenesis in hypoxic tissues. ART treatment of leukemic and glioma cells in vitro at a concentration of 12 mM was shown in another study to inhibit angiogenesis. This ART driven angiogenesis inhibition was shown to involve suppression of VEGF and HIF-1α expression at the transcriptional level. (Huang et al.,

2008; Zhou et al., 2007). Loss of HIF-1α and VEGF expression after ART treatment appears to be dependent on production of ROS because co-treatment with free-radical scavengers such as vitamin E and mannitol reversed the effects of ART (Wartenberg et al., 2003).

In vitro, VEGF is a potent endothelial cell mitogen. In cultured endothelial cells, VEGF has been shown to activate phospholipase C and induce rapid increases of free cytosolic Ca^{2+}. VEGF has also been shown to stimulate the release of von Willebrand factor from endothelial cells and induce expression of tissue factor activity in endothelial cells as well as in monocytes, and. VEGF has been shown to be involved in the chemotaxis of monocytes and osteoblasts. *In vivo,* VEGF can induce angiogenesis as well as increase microvascular permeability. As a vascular permeability factor, VEGF acts directly on the endothelium and does not degranulate mast cells. It promotes extravasation of plasma fibrinogen, leading to fibrin deposition which alters the tumor extracellular matrix. The modified extracellular matrix subsequently promotes the migration of macrophages, fibroblasts and endothelial cells. Based on its *in vitro* and *in vivo* properties, VEGF is believed to play important roles in inflammation and also in normal and pathological aspects of angiogenesis, a process that is associated with wound healing, embryonic development, growth, and metastasis of solid tumors. Elevated levels of VEGF have been reported in synovial fluids of rheumatoid arthritis patients and in sera from cancer patients.

In the last three decades, there is a growing body of evidence on the role of angiogenesis in tumor growth and metastases of tumors (Firestone and Sundar, 2009). Angiogenesis can be divided into a series of temporally regulated responses, including induction of proteases, migration of endothelial cells, cell proliferation and differentiation. This is a highly complex process, in which a number of cytokines and growth factors released by endothelial cells, tumor cells and matrix cells are involved. The expression of VEGF has been suggested to be related to some fundamental features of solid tumors, such as the growth rate, the density of tumor microvessels, and the development of tumor metastases.

It is interesting to note that torilin, another sesquiterpene (derived from the fruits of *Torilis japonica),* has also been shown to be a potent anti-angiogenic factor which also inhibits blood vessel formation by disrupting VEGFA expression. A similar finding was also shown by using DHA (Kim et al., 2007). Hence, the ability of ART to inhibit angiogenesis may be due to its chemical nature as a sesquiterpene. Another compelling finding is that other phytosesquiterpene lactones, such as costunolide from *Saussurea lappa,* can inhibit KDR signaling (Jeong et al., 2002). Comparisons with other sesquiterpenes may shed more light on the unique features of the anti-cancer actions of ART, and potentially lead to better angiostatic drug design. Taken together, ART and its derivatives, and other sesquiterpene lactones, have been shown to have potent anti-angiogenic effects in tumor cells. These observations have many implications in terms of cancer therapy as well as cancer prevention since angiogenesis is a promotional event.

3.2.4. Other anti-angiogenic mechanisms of ARTs

Anti-cancer activity of ARTs has been reported both *in vitro* and *in vivo*. The inhibitory effects of ART on the migratory ability of melanoma cell lines (A375P and A375M) were analyzed, and the results demonstrated that ART induces cell growth arrest in the A375M cell line, and affects the viability of A375P melanoma cells through both cytotoxic and growth inhibitory effects. In addition, ART was shown to affect the migratory ability of A375M melanoma cells by reducing metalloproteinase 2 (MMP-2) production and down-regulating alpha v beta 3 integrin expression (Buommino et al., 2009). Other studies, however, showed ART was not effective in inhibiting proliferation of other tumor cell lines such as MCF7, a breast adenocarcinoma cell line, and MKN, a gastric carcinoma line.

Similarly, ARTs have been shown to inhibit Matrigel invasion of 6 non-small cell cancer (NSCLC) cell lines and inhibited urokinase-type plasminogen activator (u-PA) activity, -protein and -mRNA expression. Furthermore, in a PCR-metastasis array, ARTs were shown to inhibit the expression of several matrix metalloproteinases (MMPs), especially MMP-2 and MMP-7 mRNA/protein. In luciferase reporter assays, ARTs were shown to down-regulate MMP-2-, MMP-7- and u-PA-promoter/-enhancer activity, in parallel to AP-1- and NF-kB-transactivation. Si-RNA knockdown of u-PA, MMP-2 and MMP-7 abolished ART's ability to inhibit invasion, further supporting hypotheses of the anti-cancer activity of ARTs In conclusion, this study showed that ART treatment suppresses invasion and metastasis in NSCLC, specifically targeting transcription of u-PA, MMP-2 and MMP-7. These studies all support the utility of ART compounds as novel therapeutic agents or adjunct therapies for NSCLC (Rasheed et al., 2010).

DHA displayed significant anti-proliferative activity in human colorectal carcinoma HCT116 cells, which may be attributed to its induction of G1 phase arrest and apoptosis. To further elucidate the mechanism of action of DHA, a proteomic study employed two-dimensional gel electrophoresis (2-DE) and matrix-assisted laser desorption/ionization time-of-flight mass spectrometry (MALDI-TOF MS) was performed. Glucose-regulated protein 78 (GRP78), which is related with endoplasmic reticulum stress (ER stress), was identified to be significantly up-regulated after DHA treatment. Further study demonstrated that DHA enhanced expression of GRP78 as well as growth arrest and DNA-damage-inducible gene 153 (GADD153, another ER stress-associated molecule) at both mRNA and protein levels. DHA treatment also led to accumulation of GADD153 in cell nucleus. Moreover, pretreatment of HCT116 cells with the iron chelator deferoxamine mesylate salt (DFO) abrogated induction of GRP78 and GADD153 upon DHA treatment, indicating iron is required for DHA-induced ER stress. This result is consistent with the fact that the anti-proliferative activity of DHA is also mediated by iron. Accordingly, it is possible that a redox imbalance may be the mechanism behind DHA-induced ER stress, which may contribute, at least in part, to its anti-cancer activity (Lu et al., 2011).

DHA has been shown to enhance gemcitabine-induced growth inhibition and apoptosis in both BxPC-3 and PANC-1 cell lines. The mechanism is at least partially due to DHA's role in deactivating gemcitabine-induced NF-kappaB activation, which, in turn, so as to dramatically decreases the expression of its target gene products, such as c-myc, cyclin D1, Bcl-2, Bcl-xL. *In vivo* studies have shown that, gemcitabine also manifested remarkably enhanced anti-tumor effects when combined with DHA, as demonstrated by significantly increased apoptosis, as well as decreased Ki-67 index, NF-kappaB activity and its related gene products, and predictably, significantly reduced tumor volume. The inhibition of gemcitabine-induced NF-kappaB activation is one of the mechanisms that is known by which DHA dramatically promotes its anti-tumor effect on pancreatic cancer (Wang et al., 2010).

Embryotoxicity appears to be connected with defective angiogenesis and vasculogenesis in certain stages of embryo development. This may prevent the use of ART derivatives in malaria during pregnancy, when both mother and fetus are at high risk of death. Artemisone is a novel 10-alkylamino derivative which is not metabolized to DHA. It was selected as a clinical drug candidate on the basis of its high efficacy against *Plasmodium falciparum in vitro* and its lack of detectable neurotoxicity in both *in vitro* and *in vivo* screens. A comparative study of the anti-angiogenic properties of both artemisone and dihydroartemisinin in different model systems was conducted. In this study, the effects of both artemisone and DHA were evaluated by measuring the proliferation of human endothelial cells and their migration on a fibronectin matrix, the sprouting of new vessels from rat aorta sections grown in collagen, and the production of pro-angiogenic cytokines such as VEGF and interleukin-8 (CXCL-8). The data show that artemisone is significantly less anti-angiogenic than DHA in all the experimental models, suggesting that it will be safer to use than the current clinical ARTs during pregnancy (D'Alessandro et al., 2007).

3.3. Anti-cancer clinical trials and case treatments of ARTs

Antitumor activity of ARTs has also been documented in human trials and individual clinical cases. ART, AM and AS have been used in cancer therapy, and they have been shown to be well tolerated without significant side effects (Table 3).

3.3.1. Clinical trials of ARTs as anti-cancer agents

Clinical evidence has accumulated showing that ART-derived drugs have promise for treatment of laryngeal carcinomas, uveal melanomas and pituitary macroadenomas. AS is also in phase I-II trials for treatment of breast, colorectal and non-small cell lung cancers. Similarly, a clinical trial in 120 patients with advanced non-small cell lung cancer has shown that artesunate in combination with a chemotherapy regimen of vinorelbine and cisplatin elevated 1-year survival rate by 13% with a significant improvement in disease control and time to progression. No additional AS-related side effects were reported (Zhang et al., 2008).

1. Phase I study of oral AS to treat colorectal cancer (Completed)

The primary objective of this study was to determine the effects of oral AS in inducing apoptosis in patients awaiting surgical treatment of colorectal adenocarcinoma. The secondary objective of this study was to establish the tolerability of oral AS for the treatment of colorectal cancer. Subjects were randomized to receive either 200 mg AS or placebo orally once daily for 14 days while awaiting surgery for definitive surgical treatment of colorectal adenocarcinoma. A significant difference in the proportion of colorectal adenocarcinoma cells exhibiting apoptosis was noted between the two treatment groups (placebo and AS), assessed at the time of surgery after two weeks of drug treatment. No result was publicly issued (Protocol Number: ISRCTN05203252, 2008. http://www.controlled-trials.com/ISRCTN05203252/).

2. Phase II study of AS treatment as an adjunct to treat non-small cell lung cancer (Completed)

This study was designed to compare the efficacy and toxicity of AS treatment combined with NP (a chemotherapy regimen of vinorelbine and cisplatin) and NP alone in the treatment of advanced non-small cell lung cancer (NSCLC). One hundred and twenty cases of advanced NSCLC were randomly divided into an NP chemotherapy group and a combined AS with NP therapy group. Patients in the control group were treated with the NP regimen of vinorelbine and cisplatin. Patients in the trial group were treated with the NP regimen supplemented with intravenous AS injections (120 mg, once-a-day intravenous injection, from the 1st day to 8th day, for 8 days). At least two 21-day-cycles of treatment were performed. There were no significant differences in the short-term survival rates, mean survival times and the 1-year survival rates between the trial group and the control group, which were 44 weeks and 45 weeks, respectively. The disease controlled rate of the trial group (88.2%) was significantly higher than that of the control group (72.7%) ($P < 0.05$), and the trial group's time to disease progression (24 weeks) was significantly longer than that of the control group (20 weeks). No significant difference was found in toxicity between the two treatment groups. Therefore. AS combined with NP can increase the disease controlled rate and prolong the time to progression of patients with advanced NSCLC without significant side effects (Zhang et al., 2008).

3. Phase I study with metastatic breast cancer (Completed)

The purpose of this study was to evaluate the tolerability of an adjunctive therapy with AS for a period of 4 weeks in patients over the age of 18 years with advanced metastatic breast cancer, which was defined as a histologically or cytologically confirmed. Women of child-bearing potential were tested to rule out pregnancy prior to their treatment. Relevant neurological symptoms, adverse events, and the relation between adverse events and the use of AS, as an adjunct, saliva cortisol profile, overall response rate, clinical benefit, and assessment of patients' expectations will be monitored as study endpoints. No result of this study has yet been publicly issued (Protocol Number: NCT00764036, 2011, http://www.cancer.gov/clinicaltrials/search/view/print?cdrid=616937&version=HealthProfessional).

3.3.2. *Treatment reports of ARTs used to treat cancers*

AS was successfully used in the treatment of laryngeal squamous cell carcinoma where treated patients showed a substantial reduction in tumor size (by 70%) after two months of treatment (Singh and Verma, 2002). Furthermore, AS used in combination with standard chemotherapy increased survival and substantially reduced metastasis in patients with malignant skin cancer (Berger et al., 2005). Another report describes a beneficial improvement in a patient with pituitary macroadenoma who was treated with artemether for 12 months (Singh and Panwar, 2006). Other cases describing the use of ARTs for treatment of cancer have been reported in the Cancer Smart Bomb Part I and II study (White, 2002)

1. Metastatic uveal melanomas treated with AS

Berger et al. reported on the first long-term treatment of two cancer patients with AS in combination with standard chemotherapy. These patients with metastatic uveal melanoma were treated on a compassionate-use basis, after standard chemotherapy alone was ineffective in stopping tumor growth. The therapy regimen was well tolerated with no additional side effects other than those caused by standard chemotherapy alone. One patient experienced a temporary response after the addition of AS to Fotemustine while the disease was progressing under therapy with Fotemustine alone. The second patient first experienced a stabilization of the disease after the addition of AS to Dacarbazine, followed by objective regressions of splenic and lung metastases. This patient is still alive 47 months after first diagnosis with stage IV uveal melanoma, a diagnosis with a median survival of 2-5 months, without additional side effects. One patient experienced a temporary response after the addition of AS while the disease was progressing under standard therapy with Fotemustine alone. This patient died after 24 months.

Despite the small number of treated patients, AS may be a promising adjuvant drug for the treatment of melanoma and possibly other tumors in combination with standard chemotherapy. AS is well tolerated, and the lack of serious side effects will facilitate prospective randomized trials in the near future. From *in vitro* studies already conducted (Efferth et al., 2004b), it is further conceivable that loading tumor cells with bivalent iron, by simply providing Fe^{2+} in tablet form, might increase the susceptibility of cancer cells to AS treatment. It is tempting to speculate that, in the case of the second patient previously discussed, the addition of Fe^{2+} had an actual clinical impact and resulted in an improved response to therapy (Berger et al., 2005).

2. Laryngeal carcinoma treated with AS

AS injections and tablets were used in one study to treat a laryngeal squamous cell carcinoma patient over a period of nine months. The tumor was significantly reduced in size by 70% after two months of treatment. Overall, AS treatment of the patient was beneficial in prolonging and improving quality of life. Without treatment, laryngeal cancer patients die within an average of 12 months. The patient lived for nearly one year and eight months until his death due to pneumonia.

The observations that the patient regained his voice, appetite, and weight after a short term treatment with AS, and the fact that the tumor was significantly reduced in size without any apparent adverse side effects suggests that AS treatment could be an effective and economical alternative treatment for cancer, especially in cases of late cancer detection where available treatments are limited. Since this case report was published, several patients with different types of cancers have begun treatment with ART and its analogs with promising results. AS therapy has potential to prevent and treat a wide range of cancers given its efficacy, low cost, and due to the common mechanisms of action demonstrated against various cancer cells (Singh and Verma, 2002).

3. Pituitary macroadenoma treated with AM

AM, an ART analogue, was used to treat a 75-year old male patient with pituitary macroadenoma. This patient presented with vision, hearing, and locomotion-related problems as a consequence of his disease. AM was administered orally to the patient over a period of 12 months. Although the tumor remained consistent in size, CT scans showed a reduction in tumor density, and clinically, the related symptoms and signs improved significantly as therapy progressed. Overall, the AM treatment was beneficial in improving the patient's quality of life. AM and other ART analogs appear to have promise for treatment of this type of cancer (Singh and Panwar, 2006).

3.4. Why are not there more trials or more wide-spread use of ARTs?

ARTs are largely non-toxic, with related compounds having been administered to over 2 million patients; both children and adult, world-wide without reports of significant serious side effects, and ARTs are very inexpensive when compared to conventional cancer drugs. The final results of current clinical trials utilizing ARTs as therapy or adjunct against a wide variety of cancers have not yet been published although initial findings released suggest positive results. How positive or efficacious these results are remains to be seen until full and final results are published. One question, however, remains - why are there not more trials or more wide-spread use of ARTs as an off-label cancer treatment?

3.4.1. PK mismatch of ARTs in cancer therapy

ARTs as angiogenesis inhibitors are unique cancer-fighting agents because they tend to inhibit the growth of blood vessels rather than tumor cells. Therefore, the angiogenesis inhibitor therapy does not necessarily kill tumors but instead may prevent tumors from growing. This type of therapy may therefore need to be administered over a long period.

Following oral administration, however, AS and DHA have short mean residence times (MRT) of 1.95 and 2.71 hr, respectively, and ART has a longer MRT of 7.4 hr. Intramuscular AM and arteether have longer MRTs ranging from 13.9 - 42.9 hrs in humans s due to prolonged absorption and accumulation at the injection sites. The shortest MRT (0.90 hr) was found in humans following intravenous injection of AS (Table 2). It is obvious that the different ARTs administered in different regimens have significant differences in pharmacokinetic (PK) characteristics in humans, and only intramuscular ARTs can provide a long period of therapy. Therefore, injectable AM has been recommended as a longer acting compound that may be suitable for cancer treatment (White, 2002).

Pharmacokinetics (PK) studies of ARTs show three phases (absorption, distribution, and elimination) of ART drugs in blood following oral, intravenous, or intramuscular administration. After multiple daily administrations, four ARTs showed declining daily drug concentrations (ART, DHA, AS, and AM) which has been shown is believed to be due to an auto-induced metabolism pathway during multiple oral treatments in patients and health subjects (van Agtmael et al., 1999; Ashton et al., 1996; 1998; Khanh et al., 1999; Park et al., 1998). The C_{max} and AUC values of ARTs are markedly reduced from one-third to one-seventh on the last dose day compared with the first day. The decrease in drug exposure levels during treatment is not disease-related, since the PK profile of ART drugs on the last day shows a similar decrease to that reported in healthy subjects. Similar time-dependent de-

PK Parameters	AS	AS	DHA	ART	AM	AE
Route of administration	Intravenous	Oral	Oral	Oral	Intramuscular	Intramuscular
First loading dosage	120 mg	100 mg	200 mg	500 mg	3.2 mg/kg	4.8 mg/kg
Maintaining dosage	Oral 100 mg at 8 hr	50 mg b.i.d. x 4	100 mg x 4	250 x 2 x 5	1.6mg/kg x 4	1.6mg/kg x 5
Total dose	220 mg and mefloquine**	500 mg	600 mg	3000 mg	9.6 mg/kg	12.8 mg/kg
C_{max} (ng/ml)	2646 (DHA); 11343(AS)	1052 (DHA); 198 (AS)	437.5	588.0	74.9	110.1
T_{max} (hr)	0.13	0.75	1.4	2.4	6.0	8.2
T_{lag} (hr)			0.2	0.45		
$AUC_{0\text{-}24\,hr}$ (ng·h/ml)	2378 (DHA); 1146 (AS)	1334 (DHA); 210 (AS)	1329	2601	1230	4702
$t_{1/2}$ (absorption, hr)		0.36 (DHA)	0.67	1.21	1.88	3.2
$t_{1/2}$ (elimination, hr)	0.67 (DHA); 0.05 (AS)	0.70 (DHA)	0.85	2.3	7.83	22.7
MRT (hr)	0.90 (DHA)	1.95 (DHA)	2.71	7.41	13.94	42.9

*The data was fitted with WinNonlin (V5.0) by author. **Oral 750 mg mefloquine at 24 hr after IV injection. PK = pharmacokinetics; PD = pharmacodynamics; MRT = Mean residence time; PC_{50} = Mean time for parasitemia to fall by half; AUIC = area under inhibitory curve; QHS = Artemisinin; DHA = Dihydroartemisinin; AM = Artemether; AE = Arteether; AS = Artesunic acid; MPC = minimum parasiticidal concentration; IM = intramuscular.

Table 2. Pharmacokinetics (PK) parameters of intravenous artesunate (AS), oral AS, oral dihydroartemisinin (DHA), oral artemisinin (ART), intramuscular artemether (AM) and arteether (AE) in human treatments with uncomplicated and severe/complicated malaria on day 1*.

clines have been reported in animals dosed with oral AM (Classen et al., 1999). One possible explanation for the decrease in plasma concentration-time during treatment is an increase in metabolic capacity due to auto-induction of hepatic drug-metabolizing enzymes.

Similar observations have shown that decreasing absorption of ART derivatives may be a problem for the longer-term use required for treatment of cancer. In treating malaria, the ART derivatives are given for a short four or five day course. In these short treatments, no absorption resistance has been observed to occur. Recent information has come to light that indicates that the intestine builds up resistance to absorbing oral ART compounds very quickly, within several days. Resistance is demonstrated by a >30% drop of the original rate of absorption. Research indicates that this resistance can be overcome very quickly by discontinuing use of the ART compounds for several days to a week; when resumed, their absorption will be at the previous higher level. One study author, Dr. Lai, pointed out that this intestinal resistance and subsequent lowered absorption rate may be the basis of the plateau that many patients reach after treatment with these compounds. After an initial quick response, many patients seem to stabilize without a complete remission (White, 2002).

Artemisinins	Cancer targets	Clinical studies	Protocols & References
Artesunate	Colorectal cancer	Clinical trial, Phase I	ISRCTN05203252, 2011 UK
Artesunate	Non-small cell lung cancer Metastatic uveal melanoma Laryngeal carcinoma Metastatic breast cancer	Clinical trial Phase I-II Case report Case report Clinical Trial, Phase I-II	Zhang et al., 2008 CHINA Berger et al., 2005 GERMANY Singh & Verma, 2002 INDIA NCT00764036 2008 GERMANY Verified Feb. 2009
Artemether	Pituitary macroadenoma	Case report	Singh& Panwar 2006 INDIA
All clinical trials listed here are completed			

Table 3. Anti-cancer effects of artemisinin (ART), artesunate (AS), and artemether (AM) in case reports of treatments and clinical trials (Ghantous et al., 2010)

3.4.2. Possible optimization of clinical trials with ARTs

ARTs are anti-angiogenic agents with a variety of targets that inhibit tumor angiogenesis in two ways: 1) blockade of angiogenic pathways and 2) inhibition of endogenous angiogenesis (Efferth, 2006; 2007; Crespo-Ortiz and Wei, 2012). Cancers produce a variety of angiogenic factors or cytokines to stimulate angiogenesis, which is essential for tumor growth and metastasis (Cao and Liu, 2007). These cancer-derived angiogenic factors include VEGF, fibroblast growth factor-2 (FGF-2), platelet-derived growth factor (PDGFs), angiopoietins (Angs), hepatocyte growth factor (HGF), and insulin-like growth factors (IGFs). The angiogenic signals triggered by these angiogenic factors are mediated by their specific tyrosine kinase receptors (TKRs) expressed in endothelial cells (Nissen *et al.*, 2007; Xue *et al.*, 2008).

ARTs responses seem to be mediated by those angiogenic factors with strong multi-targeted anti-angiogenic potency. However, ART targets cancer cells is cleavage of the endoperoxide bridge by the relatively high concentrations of iron in cancer cells, resulting in generation of free radicals such as reactive oxygen species (ROS) and subsequent oxidative damage as well as iron depletion in the cells. Studies demonstrated that co-administration of holotransferrin and other iron sources with ARTs have been shown to increase the potency of ARTs in killing cancer cells (Lai et al., 2009; Mercer et al., 2011; Zhang et al., 2010). Also, DHA in combination with butyric acid acts synergistically at low dose (Singh and Lai, 2005).

Current combinations with chemotherapy for the treatment of patients with cancer have produced only modest beneficial effects (Cao *et al.*, 2009). Optimization of anti-angiogenic therapy is urgently needed in order to maximize therapeutic efficacy of these drugs. Obviously, defining novel therapeutic targets other than VEGF would be an important approach to increase clinical responses as a majority of cancer patients have been shown to demonstrate intrinsic resistance to anti-VEGF therapy. Given the fact that most tumors produce a broad spectrum of angiogenic factors to stimulate angiogenesis and to sustain the established vasculature, it is not surprising that blockade of a single angiogenic pathway would be insufficient to suppress tumor growth and multitargeted "dirty drugs" would be more effective. In support of this view, anti-angiogenic monotherapy with tyrosine kinase inhibitors such as sunitinib and sorafenib targeting multiple signaling pathways has been shown to result in increased survival in patients treated for metastatic renal cell carcinoma (Escudier *et al.*, 2007; Motzer *et al.*, 2006)

ARTs are delivered to cancer patients by systemic administration, which may lead to a universal impact on healthy vasculatures distributed in multiple tissues and organs (Cao, 2010). In the conventional view of anti-cancer drugs, off-tumor targets would be associated with unwanted adverse effects of drugs. Interestingly, clinical benefits of ARTs have been positively associated with neurotoxicity and embryotoxicity, which have been shown to result from the systemic effects of these drugs (Li et al., 2009). In preclinical tumor models, it has been demonstrated that anti-angiogenic agents administered at a low dose normalize vasculatures in healthy tissues including those fenestrated vasculatures in endocrine organs such as bone marrow, liver and adrenal gland without affecting the tumor vasculature (Xue *et al.*, 2008). Normalization of tumor VEGF-induced vascular tortuosity in non-tumor tissues has been shown to significantly prolong the survival of tumor-bearing mice by improving the cancer associated systemic syndrome. These findings suggest that the off-tumor targets of anti-angiogenic agents such as ARTs may provide clinical benefits to cancer patients. Unfortunately, clinical trials based on improvement of paraneoplastic syndrome and cancer cachexia by ARTs have neither been designed nor reported (Cao, 2011).

3.4.3. Animal model results differ from human cancer patients

Preclinical models for assessment of anti-angiogenic and antitumor activities are xenograft tumor models in mice that carry implanted mouse or human tumors. Although this is a commonly used animal tumor model for studying anti-angiogenic and antitumor effects of different molecules, the relevance of this xenograft model to the clinical setting is far from reality. The subcutaneous implantation site does not usually represent physiologically orthotropic sites where human tumors arise. The tissue site is probably one of the most important issues related to response of tumors to drugs because angiogenic vessels in various tissues may express different receptors that are activated by specific ligands. Selective expression of different subsets of the same ligand receptors exists in different tissues. Differential expression of angiogenic factor receptors in various tissues and organs may lead to distinctive ARTs specific responses.

It is known that angiogenesis occurs at different rates in various aged populations (Rivard *et al.*, 1999). Thus, a difference between human cancers and mouse tumor models is the speed of cancer development. In human patients, spontaneous development of a clinical detectable cancer may take years whereas development of a similar sized mouse tumor may only take weeks (O'Reilly *et al.*, 1994). The differential growth rates between human and mouse tumors may create completely different environments, leading to dissimilar angiogenic profiles and drug responses. Young human or animal subjects are susceptible to angiogenic stimuli by triggering relatively robust angiogenic responses under physiological and pathological settings. In contrast, older human or animal subjects often show delayed or impaired angiogenic responses under the same conditions.

In animal tumor models, the endpoint of any drug study is the effect of the drug on tumor size, whereas in human patients, survival improvements by ARTs are often the clinical endpoints measure. Therapeutic efficacy of anti-angiogenic agents is often assessed as monotherapy in animals whereas the same agents are delivered to cancer patients as combinatorial therapy with chemotoxic drugs. In animal tumor models, delivery of chemotherapeutic drugs alone at the conventional dose levels often produces overwhelming anti-tumor effects and addition of anti-angiogenic agents as an extra component would be difficult to enhance the chemotherapeutic effect. Thus, the anti-angiogenic monotherapy with most available drugs has not demonstrated clinical benefits in cancer patients (Cao, 2009; 2011; Hurwitz et al., 2004).

Unlike humans, inbred experimental homogenous mice represent the same genetic background and tumors are artificially manipulated to grow at the same or at least a similar pace. Unsurprisingly, these genetically identical animals would produce a similar response to the same drug. Indeed, anti-angiogenic monotherapy in mice regardless of whether the tumor implanted is a xenograft or derived from a genetically prone mouse tumor model shows the predicted power of drug tumor suppression. Thus, this type of animal model would not be appropriate for assessment of the therapeutic efficacy of ARTs in human cancer patients. Therefore, the difference in anti-angiogenic profiles between human and mouse cancers in relation to the therapeutic efficacy of drug treatment may well explain the variation in human cancer patient responses to ARTs therapy.

3.4.4. Potential toxicities of ARTs in the cancer therapy

There have been a variety of reasons to believe that anti-angiogenic drugs for clinical use as a cancer treatment may have a number of side effects. First, the generation of new blood vessels is a very complicated, multi-step biological process, and VEGF plays an important role in a variety of biological processes such as hematopoiesis, myelopoiesis and endothelial cell survival. Therefore, anti-angiogenic therapy could cause several toxicities due to these pleiotropic biologic effects. Furthermore, many of the angiogenic inhibitors tested target multiple tyrosine kinases in several different pathways, and thus toxicities may not only arise from the inhibition of one pathway but also possibly from the concomitant inhibition of several pathways. Moreover, many of these biological agents are used or will be used in combination with other cytotoxic agents as a treatment strategy. It is not surprising that there is more toxicity in some studies using combination therapies involving angiogenesis inhibitors than those using single agents. The toxicities associated with administration of angiogenesis inhibitors have been shown to include bleeding, disturbed wound healing, thrombosis, hypertension, hypothyroidism and fatigue, proteinuria and edema, skin toxicity, leukopenia, lymphopenia, and immunomodulation (Wu et al., 2008).

In addition, there are published studies showing potential toxicities associated with the use of ARTs as anti-angiogenic agents. Various animal studies have documented neurotoxicity and embryotoxicity associated with ARTs administration, which has raised the question of whether those toxicities might occur in humans, particularly, in anti-cancer therapy and prevention of metastasis.

Neurotoxicity of ARTs

Studies with laboratory animals have demonstrated neurotoxicity associated with a number of adverse effects including movement disturbances, spasticity, balance deficits, brainstem tissue damage, and even death following administration of some intramuscular doses of oil-soluble AM and arteether, or intragastric water-soluble artelinate. There are significant differences in neurotoxicity observed between rats, dogs and rhesus monkeys after treatment with different ARTs suggesting that the exposure time required to induce neurotoxicity after dosing with ARTs is likely to be longer in humans. Since toxicity is dependent on chemical/drug exposure levels and time (Rangan et al., 1997; Rozman and Doull 2000), the neurotoxicity of ARTs has been demonstrated to occur through continued drug exposure over a longer period of time rather than through an elevated drug exposure level over a shorter period of time (Jorgensen 1980; Li et al., 2002 and 2006; Rozman 1998). Accordingly, the 3-5 days dosing duration currently used in ART antimalarial therapy should be quite safe. Neurotoxicity may be caused in humans, however, with inappropriate dose regimens, and therefore, sustained drug exposure times appear to be the critical factor to assess and prevent neurotoxicity (Li and Hickman, 2011).

The current clinical dose regimens of three-day ART combined therapies (ACTs) for uncomplicated cases of malaria, and the dose regimens recommended for intravenous AS treatments for severe malaria which include a few days of a loading doses may be too short of a drug exposure time to induce neurotoxicity in humans. Also, with regard to acute toxicity, humans appear to be less sensitive than animals (Geyer et al., 1990; Kimbrough 1990), and humans appear to have much better repair capabilities than animals to respond to such toxicity (Culotta and Koshland 1994). TK/TD analysis of neurotoxicity after ART treatment has provided a wealth of data to provide a means of predicting the neurotoxic exposure time of ARTs in humans (Li and Hickman, 2011). Based on this data, we predict the safe dosing duration of ARTs in the neurotoxic exposure time should be longer than 7 days (168 hr). Advances in our knowledge of ART-induced neurotoxicity can help refine the treatment regimens used to treat malaria with ACTs as well as injectable AS products to avoid the risk of neurotoxicity. If the drug exposure time of ARTs administered for anti-cancer therapy occurs over 14 days or even longer anti-cancer, ARTs-induced neurotoxicity may well occur (Li and Hickman, 2011).

Embryotoxicity of ARTs

In animal work, there is clear evidence of ARTs-induced embryo death and some evidence of morphological abnormalities in mice, rats, hamsters, guinea pig, rabbits and monkeys in early pregnancy especially after administration of injectable AS (Li and Weina, 2010b). The mechanisms and the pharmacokinetic profiles that affect reproductive toxicity in animal species are currently understood. These animal studies have shown that only injectable AS (intramuscular, intravenous, or subcutaneous) induces reprotoxicity at a lower dose (0.6-1.0 mg/kg) than the therapeutic dose (2-4 mg/kg) in humans. Other doses in different regimens (oral artemisinins or intramuscular AM) are safe at higher levels (6.1-51.0 mg/kg) than the therapeutic doses used. Orally dosing, the most commonly used route of administration in pregnant women with Artemisinin-based combination therapies (ACTs), has been shown to result in lower peak drug concentrations and shorter exposure times, which is less likely to induce embryotoxicity.

Toxicokinetic and tissue distribution data has shown that the severe embryotoxicity induced by injectable AS is associated with six risk factors: 1) Injectable AS can provide much higher peak concentrations (3–25 fold) than oral ARTs or intramuscular AM when administered to animals. *In vitro* results have shown that the drug exposure level and time are important factors required for induction of embryotoxicity (Longo et al., 2006a; 2006b; 2008). *In vivo* studies have shown that the drug exposure level, however, is more important than the drug exposure time as AS and DHA both have been shown to have very short half–lives (< 1 h) when administered to various animal species. 2) AS is completely converted to DHA, and therefore, AS serves as a prodrug of DHA. DHA has been shown to be more effective than AS in inhibition of angiogenesis and vasculogenesis *in vitro* (Chen et al., 2004a; White et al., 2006). 3) Among the ARTs, AS has been shown to have the highest conversion rate to DHA. The conversion rate of AS to DHA was shown to range from 38.2–72.7% while of the conversion rate of AM and AE to DHA ranges from 12.4–14.2%. 4) The conversion rate of AS to DHA was significantly increased in pregnant animals than in non–pregnant rats following multiple injections. 5) The buildup of high peak concentrations of AS and DHA in the plasma of pregnant rats was significantly higher than those of non–pregnant animals after repeated dosing. 6) Injectable AS administration results in a higher distribution of AS and DHA in the tissues of feto–placental units in pregnant animals after multiple administrations (Li et al., 2008).

It is not clear how these findings from animals translate to human patients treated for malaria in with a 3-5 day treatment regimen (WHO, 2006b; Wang, 1989). Data from limited clinical trials in pregnant women (1837 cases) exposed to ART compounds and ACTs, including a small number (176 cases) in the first trimester, have not shown an increase in the rates of abortion or stillbirth; they have also not shown evidence of abnormalities. Since more than 99% of pregnant patients have been treated with oral ARTs or intramuscular AM in the previously referenced trials, the lack of sensitivity and enhanced repair capabilities of humans to respond to ARTs induced embryotoxicity may explain the lack of embryotoxicity observed.

The possible embryotoxicity associated with ARTs therapy should be avoided by limiting exposure of pregnant women in the first trimester which is the critical period for induction of embryo damage and resorption. In addition, to protect pregnant women from embryotoxicity associated with ARTs treatment, injectable AS should be used very cautiously. There is agreement that ART derivatives should not be withheld at any stage of pregnancy, in cases of severe and complicated malaria, if the life of the mother is at risk. It is believed that oral ARTs regimens are much safer than parenteral administrations in pregnant patients. When relating the animal and human toxicity associated with ARTs administration, there are differences in sensitivity, the timing of the most vulnerable period of the embryo to ARTs administration, and the different pharmacokinetic profiles between animals and humans which may possibly provide a greater margin of safety for the use of ARTs by pregnant women.

In accordance with WHO recommendations and the new research described above, the two major issues for considering ART drug use in a program for prevention or management of malaria in pregnant women are safety and efficacy (WHO, 2006a). First, the exposure to injectable AS should be very limited, during the early sensitive period (GD 15 to week 6 in humans), which is the likely critical phase for induction of embryo damage. This is essentially the same recommendation that the WHO has provided where ARTs should not be used in the first trimester of pregnancy in women. Secondly, in uncomplicated malaria WHO recommends that the oral ARTs, including ACTs, should only be used in the second and third trimester when other treatments are considered unsuitable? We feel that oral regimens could be used to treat pregnant women in all trimesters, however, when other treatments are considered unavailable, because the common oral ARTs regimens utilized provide a lower peak concentration and short exposure time, and that can make these ARTs combination drugs safer for use in pregnant women than intravenous or intramuscular injection of AS. Therefore, this policy should also suitable in anticancer therapy and prevention (Li and Weina, 2011).

4. Therapeutic implications of new and alternative mechanisms of anti-angiogenesis

Until recently, normal and abnormal processes of angiogenesis were considered to be based on a limited number of known mechanisms. Recent advances have been made in identifying a number of novel alternate processes involved in angiogenesis. If these new findings of alternate mechanisms are confirmed, cancer therapy strategies may also be affected

4.1. New signaling molecules and pathways that influence the angiogenic response

The first generation of clinically useful anti-angiogenic agents including ARTs focused on VEGF and targets in the VEGF pathway. VEGF and its receptors represent one of the best-validated signaling pathways in angiogenesis (Ferrara et al., 2003), and the current FDA approved anti-angiogenic agents inhibit the VEGF pathway (Ferrara, 2010). The strengths and limitations of this therapeutics are now clear. Some tumors do not respond to VEGF-directed therapies *de novo*, and others become non-responsive or resistant over time by switching to other angiogenic pathways. The next generation of angiogenesis-directed therapeutics will expand the field beyond the VEGF pathway and become more disease selective. New signaling molecules and pathways, including new VEGF-independent cancer angiogenesis pathways, have been recently reported (Teicher, 2011):

http://dx.doi.org/10.5772/54109

1. Over-expression of VEGF results in increased angiogenesis in normal and pathological conditions. The existence of an alternative splicing site at the 3'untranslated region of VEGF mRNA results in the expression of isoforms with a C-terminal region which are down-regulated in tumors and may have differential inhibitory effects. This suggests that control of splicing can be an important regulatory mechanism of angiogenesis in cancer cells (Biselli-Chicote et al., 2012).

2. The VEGF family includes VEGF-A, -B, -C, -D, -E factors and the placenta growth factor (PIGF). The most studied and best characterized member of the VEGF family is VEGF-A or VEGF, which is secreted by tumors- and plays an important role in both normal and tumor-associated angiogenesis. The biologic effect of VEGF-A is exerted through interaction with cell surface receptors that include VEGF receptor-1 (VEGFR-1, flt-1) and VEGF receptor-2 (VEGFR-2, KDR/flk-1), which are selectively located on vascular endothelium and are up-regulated during angiogenesis, and VEGFR-3, a lymphatic growth factor. The role of VEGFR-1 seems to be complex, and studies indicate that VEGFR-1 may negatively regulate angiogenesis, although it has also been shown that it contributes to vascular sprouting and metastasis. The VEGF-A–VEGFR-2 interaction also plays a crucial role in angiogenesis, through the coordinated signaling of endothelial cell proliferation, migration and recruitment of endothelial cell progenitor cells. VEGF-B has recently been found to be largely necessary for vascular survival rather than angiogenesis (Ferrara, 2009; 2010; Zhang et al., 2009).

3. Placental growth factor (PlGF), a member of the VEGF family of growth factors, is induced as tumors lose responsiveness to VEGF-directed therapies (Van de Veire et al., 2010). PlGF was first described, crystallized and identified as a ligand for VEGFR1 in the early 1990s (Ribatti, 2008). The functional biology of PlGF is still being explored. PlGF appears to have direct effects on some malignant cells and has been shown to increase cell proliferation and migration (Chen et al., 2009d).

4. Angiopoietins (Angs) are another family of endothelial cell-specific molecules that bind Tie receptors, and they play an important role in vessel maintenance, growth and stabilization. There are four types of angiopoietins known: Ang-1, -2, -3 and -4. Tie1 mRNA is highly expressed in embryonic vascular endothelium, angioblasts, endocardium, and lung capillaries while it is weekly expressed in the endocardium of adults The Tie2 receptor takes part in vessel maturation by transducing survival signals for endothelial cells. Ang-1 acts as an agonist promoting vessel stabilization in a paracrinal manner, whileAng-2 is an autocrine antagonist inducing vascular destabilization at high concentrations. Ang-2 has been found to be dramatically increased during vascular remodeling, and it has been implicated in tumor-associated angiogenesis and tumor progression. It has been found that VEGF also activates the Tie2 receptor (Makrilia et al., 2009).

5. The Notch signaling pathway is critical for many developmental processes including physiologic angiogenesis. The Notch pathway has also been shown to have a key role in tumor angiogenesis. Preclinical and clinical studies of various anti-angiogenic combinations suggests that the mechanism associated with poor efficacy may involve tumor re-

sistance and recurrence, which has led to the search for alternative angiogenic treatment strategies. Significant progress has been made in shedding light on the complex mechanisms by which Notch signaling can influence tumor growth by disrupting vasculature in an array of tumor models (Ridgway et al., 2006). The Notch pathway is being investigated as a target for anti-angiogenesis treatment. The VEGF and Notch pathways interact and intersect such that the VEGF pathway stimulates angiogenesis while the Notch pathway helps to guide cell fate decisions that appropriately shape activation (Li and Harris, 2009; Garcia and Kandel, 2012).

Delta-like ligand 4 (Dll4) is a key endothelial Notch ligand. The Notch pathway and the VEFG pathway interrelate via the interaction between Dll4 and VEGF. This cross-talk occurs through VEGF-induced upregulation of Dll4 and Dll4 downregulation of the VEGFR signaling. Both pathways are essential for normal angiogenesis, and blockade of one may produce compensatory changes in the other. Dll4–Notch signaling has sparked high interest in exploring molecular targets in these interconnected pathways for cancer therapy (Oon and Harris, 2011)

6. Fibroblast growth factors (FGFs) in signaling pathways are a family of heparin-binding proteins required for the development and differentiation of various organs from the early stages of embryogenesis. Acidic and basic fibroblast growth factors (aFGF or FGF1 and bFGF or FGF2 respectively) are described as inducers of angiogenesis. FGFs stimulate endothelial cell proliferation and migration, as well as production of collagenase and plasminogen activator. FGFs induce sprouting of blood vessels *in vivo* in the chick chorioallantoic membrane and cornea, thus supporting their role in angiogenesis (Makrilia et al., 2009). In addition, the HGF/c-Met pathway is upregulated in some tumors as an alternate angiogenic pathway. The HGF/c-Met tyrosine kinase signaling pathway is upregulated in many cancers resulting in invasive growth consisting of physiological processes including proliferation, invasion and angiogenesis (Eder et al., 2009).

7. The CXCL12 (SDF-1)/CXCR4 pathway represents a stromal chemokine axis involved in tumor angiogenesis. CXCR2 is a G-protein coupled receptor with several ligands including interleukin-8 and other angiogenic cytokines and may represent a useful target for anti-angiogenic agents. The CXCL12/CXCR4 axis is involved in tumor progression, angiogenesis, metastasis and survival (Teicher and Fricker, 2010).

8. Sphingosine-1-phosphate (S-1-P) is a bioactive lipid that regulates many cellular and physiological processes including cell proliferation, survival, motility, angiogenesis, vascular maturation, immunity and lymphocyte trafficking. Sphingosine-1-phosphate can be neutralized with a monoclonal antibody. Anti-S-1-P antibodies are under investigation as an anti-angiogenic agent. (Hait et al., 2009).

9. Several small molecules and antibodies targeting additional pro-angiogenic cell surface molecules are under investigation as anti-angiogenic agents. Tumor necrosis factor-a (TNF-α), transforming growth factor-α (TGF-α), epidermal growth factor (EGF), colony-stimulating factors (CSFs) and others have been implicated in the process of angiogenesis. Several multi-targeted kinase inhibitors each with a unique pattern of

inhibitory potency are in clinical trials with a focus on anti-angiogenic activity. Matrix metalloproteinases (MMPs) are a family of enzymes that cleave the extracellular matrix, a process which is considered important for the formation of new blood vessels. Inhibition of MMPs activity seems to be a crucial step in the process of vessel stabilization during the resolution phase of angiogenesis, since uncontrolled proteolysis results in regression of newly formed vessels (Makrilia et al., 2009).

4.2. Potential targets in angiogenesis and angioprevention

Angiogenesis is an essential process in tumor growth, and new basic science research findings in angiogenesis have had considerable impact on cancer therapy research, as the survival and proliferation of cancer is fundamentally dependent on angiogenesis,. In past years, numerous anti-angiogenic agents were developed, and some of them have been applied clinically. Angiogenesis is a complex and multistep process, however, and the intertwining of interrelated angiogenesis pathways is still not completely understood. Discoveries of new and alternative angiogenesis signaling molecules and pathways, combined with studies on the major signaling proteins and pathways related to tumor angiogenesis, have led to new drug development research to target tumor angiogenesis.

Similarly, angiopreventive strategies may involve various targets including angiogenic molecules from tumors cells, inflammatory system and their respective receptors on endothelial cells such as VEGF, PDGF, FGF and their receptors, angiopoietin (Ang) family, endothelial cells, matrix metalloproteinases (MMPs), cyclooxygenases (COXs), lipoxygenases (LOXs) etc. Inflammation, for example, has been shown to be one of the most important processes in mediating angiogenesis, and may be a valid target for mediating anti-angiogenic therapies. Accordingly, long-term angiostasis treatments will likely be an important element in preventing metastasis of tumors that have been treated and are in remission. Emphasis should be placed on screening and identification of non-toxic anti-angiogenic molecules or compounds and their further evaluation in clinical trials to discover the most efficacious anti-angiogenic treatments for cancer therapy.

VEGF-A (VEGF)

VEGF has a number of different gene family members including VEGF-A, -B, -C, -D, and -E and placental growth factor (PlGF). Among them, VEGF-A (or VEGF) has been the most well-characterized and is considered a key angiogenic factor with various splicing variants such as VEGF-A_{125}, -A_{145}, -A_{165}, -A_{183}, -A_{189}, and -A_{206}. VEGF-A is indispensable during embryonic vascular development, and even the loss of a single VEGF-A allele in mice has been shown to result in embryonic lethality due to defective vasculature. Hypoxia, often seen in the center of tumors, strongly up-regulates VEGF-A expression via increased production of hypoxia inducible factor (HIF). Under normal conditions, HIF is ubiquitinated and degenerated by binding to von Hippel-Lindau (VHL) proteins, but, in under hypoxic conditions, HIF cannot bind to VHL, resulting in increased active HIF. HIF acts as a transcriptional activator by mediating transcription at the HIF-1 binding site, the hypoxia response element (HRE), and by enhancing transcription of many pro-angiogenic genes including VEGF-A gene (Ichihara et al., 2011).

VEGF Receptors (VEGFR)

VEGF family members bind to VEGFR (VEGFR-1, VEGFR-2, and VEGFR-3), and VEGF-A binds to VEGFR-1 and VEGFR-2. Although the affinity of VEGF-A to VEGFR-1 is 10-fold higher than it's binding to VEGFR-2, VEGF-A signaling is mainly mediated by VEGFR-2 because of its intense kinase activity (Olsson et al., 2006). VEGFR-2 signaling in endothelial cells is mediated through downstream cascades such as PI3K/AKT, p38/MAPK, and PLCγ/MAPK, triggering proliferation and migration of endothelial cells, production of proteases, and hyperpermeability of vessels. Currently, researchers agree that VEGF-A/VEGFR-2 signaling is the key pathway for tumor angiogenesis.

VEGF-B and PlGF bind only to VEGFR-1, in contrast to VEGF-A, which binds to both VEGFR-1 and -2. VEGFR-1 signaling has more complex roles in angiogenesis compared with that of VEGFR-2. VEGFR-1 exists as a decoy receptor with high affinity for VEGF-A, and its low kinase activity prevents VEGF-A from binding to VEGFR-2, so VEGFR-1 actually functions as a negative regulator of angiogenesis. In fact, VEGFR-1 tyrosine kinase-deficient mice, with normal ligand binding ability and deficient signal transduction, have been shown to develop normally, which means VEGFR-1 tyrosine kinase activity is not indispensable, at least during development. On the other hand, there is growing evidence that VEGFR-1 can mediate signaling to downstream cascades. VEGFR-1 signaling in bone marrow cells such as macrophage lineage cells has been shown in a subcutaneous injected tumor model to mobilize them to tumor tissues, contributing to angiogenesis and tumor progression (Muramatsu et al., 2010). It has also been reported that VEGFR-1 signaling might be associated with metastasis. Lymphangiogenesis plays an important role in the tumor microenvironment and the formation of new lymphatic blood vessels is considered the first step of tumor metastasis. VEGFR-3 has been shown to induce lymphangiogenesis after binding VEGF-C or –D (Ichihara et al., 2011).

Angiopoietin/Tie2

Ang/Tie2 signaling is an endothelial cell-specific pathway, like VEGF/VEGFR signaling, but it is difficult to target for cancer therapy because of the complex nature of this signaling pathway which will be reviewed in depth later in this chapter. Angiopoietins play an important role in vessel stabilization and maturation, although they cannot directly induce tumor angiogenesis. There are four types of angiopoietins that are known: Ang-1, -2, -3 and -4. Tie1 mRNA is highly expressed in embryonic vascular endothelium, angioblasts and in the endocardium; however, in adult tissues it is expressed strongly in lung capillaries but weakly in the endocardium. The Tie2 receptor takes part in vessel maturation by mediating survival signals for endothelial cells. Ang-1 acts as an agonist promoting vessel stabilization in a paracrinal manner, whereas Ang-2 is an autocrine antagonist inducing vascular destabilization at high concentrations. Ang-2 has been found to be dramatically increased during vascular remodeling and is implicated in tumor-associated angiogenesis and tumor progression. As a further demonstration of the interrelated nature of angiogenic pathways, it has been shown that VEGF also activates the Tie2 receptor (Singh and Milner, 2009; Thomas and Augustin, 2009).

http://dx.doi.org/10.5772/54109

PDGF

The role of platelet-derived growth factor (PDGF) in angiogenesis is not yet fully understood. More recently, PDGF has been found to stimulate angiogenesis *in vivo,* and experiments with knockout mice have suggested a role for PDGF in the recruitment of pericytes that are needed for the development of capillaries in tumors. PDGF has also been implicated in the vascular aging process. It has been shown that some tumors overcome inhibition of VEGF-mediated angiogenesis by upregulating members of the PDGF family. Epithelial cancers are characterized by paracrine PDGF signaling, whereas autocrine PDGF signaling is implicated in neoplasms such as leukemias, gliomas and sarcomas (Yang et al., 2009). Thus far, four PDGF family members have been identified, PDGF-A, -B, -C, and -D. They form 5 different forms of homodimers and heterodimers, PDGF-AA, -AB, -BB, -CC, and -DD. PDGFs generally act in a paracrine manner in epithelial cancers, while they have been shown to act in an autocrine manner in gliomas, sarcomas, and leukemia. PDGFs are secreted from various cells, and PDGF-A and -C are mainly secreted from epithelial cells, muscle, and neuronal progenitors while PDGF-B is secreted from vascular endothelial cells. PDGF-D secretion is, unfortunately, not well understood (Andrae et al., 2008).

PDGF Receptors (PDGFR)

PDGFs transmit their signal via PDGFRs. When PDGFRs bind PDGFs, PDGFRs dimerize, are autophosphorylated at tyrosine residues in the PDGFR intracellular domain, and the phosphoyrlated PDFGR dimer has been shown to activate downstream pathways, including PI3K, Ras-MAPK, and PLCγ. There are 2 types of PDGFRs, PDGFR-α and PDGFR-β. PDGFRs can form 3 kinds of homodimers and heterodimers, PDGFR-$\alpha\alpha$, -$\beta\beta$, and $\alpha\beta$. Considering the five PDGF dimers described above, there could be multiple and complex PDGF/PDGFR pairings. To date, however, there are only three PDGF/PDGFR pairs proven to be functional *in vivo*, PDGF-AA/PDGFR-$\alpha\alpha$, PDGF-CC/PDGFR-$\alpha\alpha$, and PDGF-BB/PDGFR-$\beta\beta$. PDGFR-α has been shown to be involved in embryonic development, while PDGFR-β has been shown to be involved in angiogenesis (Cao et al., 2008).

The PDGFR-α-induced pathway is involved in organogenesis such as in alveogenesis, villus morphogenesis, hair morphogenesis, and oligodendrogenesis. In addition, PDGFR-α may indirectly promote angiogenesis by recruiting stromal fibroblast-producing VEGF-A and other pro-angiogenic factors. PDGFR-β is expressed in pericytes but not in endothelial cells, and PCGFR-β signaling is believed to play a role in angiogenesis. Due to PDGFR-β's expression in pericytes as opposed to endothelial cells, the PDGFR-β signaling pathway does not increase the number of tumor vessels but acts to form mature tumor vessels by recruiting PDGFR-β-expressing pericytes, and, in turn, acting to accelerate tumor growth. Blocking the PDGFR-β pathway inhibits the maturation of blood vessels, eliciting detachment of pericytes and disruption of tumor vessels, while blocking the VEGFR pathway impairs formation of early-stage immature vessels lacking pericyte coverage but does not affect existing mature, large blood vessels well-covered with pericytes (Ichihara et al., 2011).

Delta-like ligand 4 (DLL4)

Delta-like ligand 4 (DLL4) belongs to the Delta/Jagged family of transmembrane ligands that binds to Notch receptors. Delta–Notch signaling has been shown to mediate cell–cell communication and regulates cell fate determination. Delta/Notch signaling is also critically important for proper vascular development. One particular endothelial cell Notch ligand, DLL4, has been shown to be required for regulation of tip cell formation during angiogenesis. Activation of the Delta/Notch signaling pathway has been shown to decrease endothelial tip cell numbers. Conversely, decreased DLL4 signaling increases tip cell formation. Upregulation of DLL4 was also found in tumor vessels. Two groups have demonstrated independently that inhibiting DLL4 leads to tumor growth suppression by deregulating angiogenesis, resulting in increased, but non-functional vessels. Importantly, this strategy is also effective in slowing the growth of tumors that are relatively resistant to anti-VEGF therapy, and DLL4 inhibition also exhibits an additive effect when combined with anti-VEGF therapy to slow the growth of anti-VEGF resistant tumors (Dufraine et al., 2008, Ferrara, 2010).

In fact, not all of the endothelial cells are stimulated, due to a mechanism deciding which endothelial cells should react to angiogenic stimulus and which should not. The DLL4/Notch pathway plays a key role in this mechanism. DLL1, DLL3, DLL4, Jagged1, and Jagged2 bind to the Notch receptor as ligands. Among these ligands related to tumor angiogenesis, DLL4 has been the most intensely investigated, because DLL4 is strongly expressed in tumor vascular endothelial cells but more weakly in normal vascular endothelial cells. DLL4 is a transmembrane ligand, and its expression in tumor vessels is regulated by VEGF-A. VEGF-A up-regulates DLL4 in sprouting endothelial cells (tip cells), and up-regulated DLL4 interacts with Notch in the adjacent endothelial cells (stalk cells). In reverse, the DLL4/Notch pathway down-regulates VEGFR-2 expression in Notch-expressing endothelial cells, resulting in the reduction of VEGF-A-induced sprouting and branching (Lobov et al., 2007). Thus the DLL4/Notch pathway can be considered a negative feedback VEGFR pathway (Ichihara et al., 2011).

Notch

Notch receptors are single-pass transmembrane proteins in a family consisting of Notch1, Notch2, Notch3, and Notch4. The Notch receptor signaling pathway has a characteristic mechanism for signal transduction. After ligand binding, the Notch receptor is cleaved at an extracellular domain by proteases such as ADAM10 or TACE, followed by cleavage at a transmembrane domain by γ-secretase. As a consequence, the Notch intracellular domain translocates to the nucleus and activates the transcription of target genes. Blocking the DLL4/Notch signaling pathway leads to increased angiogenesis, such as the enhancement of tip-cell formation, branching, and vessel density. Paradoxically, blockade of the DLL4/Notch signaling also leads to the inhibition of tumor growth in a variety of tumor models. This is possibly due to an increase in the number of non-functional tumor vessels induced by the DLL4/Notch blockade which in turn results in tumor hypoxia (Scehnet et al., 2007).

FGF1 and FGF2

The fibroblast growth factor (FGF) family has been implicated in neurogenesis, organ development, branching morphogenesis, angiogenesis and various pathologic processes including cancer. Acidic and basic fibroblast growth factors (aFGF or FGF1 and bFGF or

FGF2 respectively) have been shown to be inducers of angiogenesis. FGFs stimulate endothelial cell proliferation and migration, as well as production of collagenase and plasminogen activator. FGFs have also been shown to induce sprouting of blood vessels *in vivo* in the chick chorioallantoic membrane and cornea, thus supporting their role in angiogenesis (Makrilia et al., 2009).

The FGF signaling pathway plays an important role in embryonic organogenesis, and disturbance of this pathway leads to various kinds of developmental defects. In the adult organism, FGF/FGFR signaling is involved in important physiological processes such as the regulation of wound healing and angiogenesis. FGFs are heparin-binding growth factors that are part of a family that includes 23 members, FGF1-23 (Turner and Grose, 2010). Only 18 FGF members work as FGF ligands, because FGF11, 12, 13, and 14 are not functional ligands for FGFR, and the FGF15 gene does not exist in humans. Among these family members, FGF1 and FGF2 have been shown to possess a potent pro-angiogenic effect and they play a role in inducing proliferation and migration of endothelial cells (Daniele et al., 2012).

FGF Receptors (FGFR)

FGFRs belong to a receptor family consisting of FGFR-1, -2, -3, and -4 (Turner and Grose, 2010). FGFRs are expressed in most cells and have various functions, including normal cell growth, differentiation, and angiogenesis., FGFR over expression or mutation has been shown to be associated with a variety of different neoplasms FGFR activation has been shown to induce angiogenesis in both cell cultures and in animal models (Cao et al., 2008; Korc and Friesel, 2009).

TGF-β

The transforming growth factor-β (TGF-β) is thought to have both pro- and anti-angiogenic properties. Low TGF-β levels contribute to a switch in angiogenesis, by up-regulating angiogenic factors and proteinases. On the other hand, high TGF-β levels have been shown to inhibit endothelial cell growth, stimulate smooth muscle cells differentiation and recruitment and promote basement membrane reformation. In cancer cells, multiple mutations in the TGF-β signaling pathway have been described. Elevated TGF-β levels have been shown to induce proliferation of cancer cells, the surrounding stromal cells, immune cells, endothelial cells and smooth muscle cells. High levels of endoglin, which is part of the TGF-β receptor complex, have been detected in cancer patients and are directly correlated with tumor metastasis. More specifically, during the initial stages of tumorigenesis, TGF-β inhibits tumor growth and development by inhibiting cell proliferation and by inducing apoptosis. In later stages, tumor stages become resistant to the tumor suppressioni activity of TGF-β, TGF-β takes on a pro-oncogenic role (Pardali and Dijke, 2009).

Other important tumor angiogenesis targets include:

1. The role of integrin αvβ3 in mediating angiogenesis has been shown through its binding of extracellular matrix components and matrix metalloproteinase-2, thus helping to connect new vessels with pre-existing ones, to produce the intra-tumoral vascular network. Ephrin ligands and ephrin receptors play a critical role in blood vessel assembly.

2. The role of VE-cadherin in neovascularization has been shown in a number of studies.

3. Cadherins have been shown to establish endothelial cell junctional stability in the vessel wall and enhance endothelial cell survival by promoting the transmission of the anti-apoptotic signal of VEGFs.

4. Cyclooxygenase-2, an enzyme known to regulate cellular processes such as apoptosis, also has been shown to have an angiogenic effect via thromboxane-A2.

5. The fibrinolytic system is another angiogenesis target, and the activation of this system depends on the conversion of plasminogen to plasmin by the tissue-type plasminogen activator (tPA) and the urokinase-type plasminogen activator (uPA).

6. Matrix metalloproteinases (MMPs) are a family of enzymes that cleave the extracellular matrix, a process which is considered important for the formation of new blood vessels. Inhibition of the activity of MMPs seems to be a crucial step in the process of vessel stabilization during the resolution phase of angiogenesis, as uncontrolled proteolysis results in regression of newly formed vessels.

7. The hypoxia-inducible factors (HIFs) mediate transcriptional responses to localized hypoxia in normal tissues and in cancers, and HIFs have been shown to promote tumor progression by altering cellular metabolism and stimulating angiogenesis. Under conditions of abundant oxygen (N8–10%), HIF-α proteins are translated, but the proteins are rapidly degraded. Stabilization of HIF proteins in hypoxic cancer cells is thought to promote tumor progression, largely by inducing the localized expression of specific target genes encoding VEGF, glycolytic enzymes (PGK, ALDA), glucose transporters (GLUT1) and proteins regulating motility (lysl oxidase) and metastasis (CXCR4, E-cadherin). (Makrilia et al., 2009)

4.3. Vascular normalization in anti-angiogenic cancer therapy

Normal vasculature comprises organized layers of endothelial cells (ECs) and pericytes. There is evidence for paracrine signaling between ECs and specialized organ-specific cells; hence, there is some variation in the structure and function of blood vessels depending on their anatomic location. Pericyte-EC crosstalk facilitates vascular growth and homeostasis, and once vessels mature, these cells become dormant. Blood vessel proliferation is an essential physiological process, and vessel sprouting is one of the major mechanisms of expansion in the network of vessels in growing tumors through filopodia and endothelial stalk cells.

Unlike blood vessels in normal tissue, the tumor-associated vasculature is irregular and unstable, probably due to the over-production of pro-angiogenic proteins such as VEGF. Tumor vessels are distinct in several respects relative to normal vasculature as they are disorganized and tortuous and their spatial distribution is significantly heterogeneous, resulting in uneven drug distribution in tumors. Tumor vessels do not follow the hierarchy of arterioles, capillaries and venules, and tumor vessels are leakier than normal vessels since tumor-associated endothelial cells are widened and loosely connected. Recent studies suggest that tumor ECs have cytogenetic abnormalities including aneuploidy, multiple chromosomes, and multiple centrosomes, raising the possibility that such instability may contribute to resistance to anti-angiogenic therapies. Tumor-associated blood vessels are excessively branched and hemorrhagic, and blood flow through these malformed vessels is often chaotic and may impede delivery of chemotherapy to the tumor itself (Ferrara, 2010; Gordon et al., 2010).

A new therapeutic strategy targeting tumor vasculature has gained increased attention in the scientific community. This method involves targeting abnormal tumor vessel function by inducing vessel normalization. It is well known that tumor blood vessels are highly abnormal in structure and function, characterized by a tortuous, chaotic, and irregular branching network. In the tumor vasculature, ECs are highly activated, lose their polarity and alignment, and detach from the basement membrane, all resulting in a leaky, fenestrated network that facilitates bleeding and increases interstitial fluid pressure. Apart from the ECs, the entire vessel wall, including the basement membrane and the covering pericytes, becomes abnormal in most tumors. Tumor ECs are typically covered with fewer and more abnormal pericytes, and their associated basement membrane is only loosely associated and inhomogeneous in structure. It is suspected that this abnormal vasculature impedes the distribution of chemotherapy and oxygen. Traditional anti-angiogenic therapy aims to maximally inhibit angiogenesis and to prune existing tumor vessels, however, this strategy can also increase the risk of aggravating hypoxia and enhancing tumor cell invasiveness (Carmeliet and Jain, 2011).

Recent genetic and pharmacological studies have revealed that targeting abnormal tumor vessel function by the induction of vessel normalization can offer alternative options for anti-angiogenic therapy. Vessel normalization can be achieved by several different approaches, including blockade of VEGF, genetic modulation of the oxygen sensors prolyl hydroxylase domain containing protein 2 (PHD2), targeting of mechanisms that affect pericyte coverage and vessel maturation, and targeting myeloid cells via blockade or genetic loss of PlGF. Vessel normalization could provide a means to increase the responsiveness to chemotherapy, immunotherapy, or radiation, and may contribute to restricting tumor dissemination (Rolny et al., 2011; Schmidt and Carmeliet, 2011).

One recent study demonstrated that boron targeting of the largest possible proportion of tumor cells contributes to the success of boron neutron capture therapy (BNCT), and tumor blood vessel normalization improves the delivery of boron to the tumor. In this study, blood vessel normalization was induced by administering two doses of thalidomide (Th) in tumor-bearing hamsters on two consecutive days. The effect of blood vessel normalization to enhance the efficacy of boronophenylalanine (BPA) administration was assessed through *in vivo* BNCT studies at the RA-3 Nuclear Reactor utilizing tumor-bearing hamsters. Overall tumor control at 28 days post-treatment was significantly higher for Th+ BPA-BNCT than for Th- BPA-BNCT with a tumor volume reduction of 84 ± 3% in the Th+ BPA-BNCT group compared to 67 ± 5% in the Th- BPA-BNCT group. Pretreatment with thalidomide enhanced the therapeutic efficacy of BNCT and reduced precancerous tissue toxicity (Molinari et al., 2012). Some studies confirmed, however, that antibodies to VEGF in combination with chemotherapeutic agents produce synergistic cytotoxicity in a range of cancers. Research data shows that the process of normalization of tumor blood vessel structure is not always beneficial. In the case of cerebral tumors, for example, the process of tumor vessel normalization may induce a re-establishment of the low permeability characteristics of normal brain microvasculature, preventing the delivery of chemotherapeutics (Ribatti, 2011).

Despite having an abundant number of vessels, tumors are usually hypoxic and nutrient-deprived because their vessels malfunction. Such abnormal milieu can fuel disease progression and resistance to treatment. Traditional anti-angiogenesis strategies attempt to reduce the tumor vascular supply, but their success is restricted by insufficient efficacy or development of resistance. Preclinical and initial clinical evidence have shown that normalization of tumor vascular abnormalities is emerging as a complementary therapeutic paradigm for cancer therapy and other vascular disorders, which affect more than half a billion people worldwide. Clearly, additional randomized prospective multi-centered trials should be conducted in larger patient populations to confirm these initial clinical data. In addition, critical questions regarding whether vessel normalizing agents can improve tumor oxygenation and drug delivery in human cancers remain to be answered (Carmeliet and Jain, 2011).

4.4. New vascularization/angiogenesis mechanisms in cancer therapy

Before discussing the different ways a tumor is vascularized, we should emphasize that these mechanisms are not mutually exclusive. In fact, in most cases, angiogenesis and neovascularization mechanisms are interlinked, being involved concurrently in physiological as well as in pathological angiogenesis. Although the molecular regulation of endothelial sprouting has been extensively studied and reviewed in the literature, the morphogenic and molecular events associated with alternative cancer vascularization mechanisms are not nearly as well understood. Cancer cells are not generally controlled by normal regulatory mechanisms, but tumor growth is highly dependent on the supply of oxygen, nutrients, and host-derived regulators. It is now established that tumor vasculature is not necessarily derived from endothelial cell sprouting. Cancer tissue can acquire vasculature by a variety of mechanisms to include co-opting pre-existing vessels, intussusceptive microvascular growth, postnatal vasculogenesis, glomeruloid angiogenesis, or vasculogenic mimicry. The best-known molecular pathway driving tumor vascularization is the hypoxia-adaptation mechanism. Other pathways involving a broad and diverse spectrum of genetic aberrations, however, are associated with the development of the "angiogenic phenotype." Based on this knowledge, novel forms of antivascular modalities have been developed in the past decade.

When applying these targeted therapies, the stage of tumor progression, the type of vascularization of the given cancer tissue, and the molecular machinery behind the vascularization process all need to be considered. A further challenge is finding the most appropriate combinations of antivascular therapies and standard radio- and chemotherapies. The most promising therapeutic plan of action will involve the integration of recent discoveries in this field into a rational strategy to for developing effective clinical modalities using antivascular therapy for cancer (Döme et al., 2007).

Neovascularization is essential for tumor growth and metastasis. An adequate vasculature feeds tumor growth and enhances the potential of metastasis. For many years, tumor vessels were thought to be lined exclusively by endothelial cells (ECs). Therapeutic benefits from promising anti-angiogenic strategies targeting genetically stable ECs, however, are frequently limited by the development of resistance, implying an oversimplified view of tumor vasculature. Recently, great advances in our understanding of cancer vascularization have emerged with several novel mechanisms proposed. In fact, the latest studies of the most lethal ovarian cancers characterized by widespread metastases within the peritoneal cavity have revealed that in addition to ECs, other cells, including bone marrow-derived and plastic tumor cells, contribute to tumor vascularization There are two proposed mechanisms by which tumor-infiltrating bone marrow-derived cells might participate in tumor angiogenesis: (1) direct incorporation in the tumor vasculature and (2) as a source of angiogenic factors such as VEGF-A and MMP-9, which may in turn increase the bioavailability of angiogenic factors.

Current anti-angiogenic therapies have been designed on the assumption that endothelial cells forming the tumor vasculature exhibit genetic stability. Recent studies demonstrate that this is not the case. Tumor endothelial cells possess a distinct phenotype, differing from normal endothelial cells at both the molecular and functional levels. This finding challenges the concept that tumor angiogenesis exclusively depends on normal endothelial cell recruitment from the surrounding vascular network. Indeed, recent data suggest alternative strategies for tumor vascularization, and it has been reported that tumor vessels may be derived from an intratumor embryonic-like vasculogenesis. This condition might be due to differentiation of normal stem and progenitor cells of either hematopoietic origin or cells resident in tissues. Cancer stem cells may also participate in tumor vasculogenesis by virtue of their stem and progenitor cell properties (Bussolati et al., 2011).

During cancer progression, tumors require a blood supply for growth and use the blood supply for metastatic dissemination. It is logical that a stronger ability to form *de novo* networks and channels providing a stable blood supply may confer a survival advantage for tumors. Ovarian cancers, as discussed previously, can generate tumor vasculature from diverse origins, including EC, EPC, and tumor cells, reflecting a vast capacity for neovascularization, which may help to explain its high malignancy. Thus, anti-angiogenic and vascular targeting strategies against alternative tumor vascularization mechanisms are clearly promising as improved, more efficacious cancer therapies.

The existence of multiple signal pathways and complex regulatory systems in vascular formation means that inhibition of just a single pathway will presumably trigger alternative vascularization mechanisms and additional signal pathways. Therefore, exploring other novel signals in neovascularization is essential for further studies to efficiently target blood vessels in cancer therapy. On the other hand, with the emergence of the concept of normalization of tumor vasculature as a novel form of anti-angiogenic therapy, new vascular signals involved in vascular remodeling are becoming appealing therapeutic strategies to researchers, as a better understanding of these normalization mechanisms may ultimately lead to more effective therapies. Indeed, several novel ligand/receptor pathways are emerging to include: Slit/Robo, semaphoring/plexins, Netrin-1/UNC5B, Delta-like 4/Notch, and others. Interestingly, the first three ligand/receptor pairs are all formerly known to be involved with neuronal axon guidance, implying a possibility that other neural guidance cues may also function as vascular signals. Agents developed from these pathways that control the morphology of the vascular system can induce tumor vascular normalization and, thus, alleviate hypoxia and increase the efficacy of conventional therapies if both are carefully scheduled. Alternatively, blockade of these pathways may result in increased amounts of immature, nonfunctioning vessels, which results in reduced tumor growth, as is the case with blockade of Delta-like 4 (Tang et al., 2009)

In addition, newly published findings suggest that vessels in many non-malignant diseases are also abnormal. Pharmacological approaches used to normalize vessels in cancer can also induce vessel normalization in other angiogenic disorders in animal models and in patients. Moreover, vascular normalization with bevacizumab has provided the first medical treatment to improve hearing in patients with type II neurofibromatosis. Despite treatment advances for coronary and peripheral arterial disease, the burden of these illnesses remains high. To this end, normalization of abnormal vessels has been proposed as a novel strategy to stabilize vulnerable atherosclerotic plaques. One of the challenges for this therapeutic approach is that these strategies stimulate the formation of immature, leaky and disorganized vessels that are poorly perfused, exhibit signs of vessel disorganization and are prone to regression once therapy is halted. Therapeutic normalization of such neovessels would offer the advantage of creating more mature vessels that could deliver oxygen and nutrients more rapidly and efficiently to the ischemic tissue and thereby restore tissue performance (Carmeliet and Jain, 2011).

In contrast with the anti-angiogenic therapy, vascular targeting therapy aims at destroying the existing vasculature of a tumor. Three different classes of vascular targeting therapeutics have been proposed, cytoskeletal disruption, targeted gene delivery, and drug targeting of tumor endothelial cells. The first class, cytoskeletal disruptors, utilizes a combination of combretastatin derivatives which stops blood flow and inhibits tumor growth through the disruption of the tubulin cytoskeleton of endothelial cells which, in turn, leads to vasculature thrombosis. The second class of vascular targeted therapeutics is targeted gene delivery to the neovasculature. This is achieved by using cationic nanoparticles bound to an integrin $\alpha v\beta 3$ directed ligand that delivers a mutant gene to tumor vessels. The third class of vascular targeting therapeutics is cationic liposome-based vascular targeting therapy, which relies on a selective propensity for drug delivery to activated tumor endothelial cells. The mechanism on which this targeted drug delivery is based relies on the negative charge associated with angiogenic endothelial cells which in turn attracts cationic liposomes which can actively bind negatively charged angiogenic endothelial cells and deliver cytotoxic drugs (Makrilia et al., 2009).

4.5. Anti-angiogenic gene therapy for cancer

Tumor growth and progression depends on angiogenesis, a process of new blood vessel formation from preexisting vascular endothelial cells. Tumors promote angiogenesis by secreting or activating angiogenic factors that stimulate endothelial proliferation and migration and capillary morphogenesis. The newly formed blood vessels provide nutrients and oxygen to the tumor, increasing its growth. Thus, angiogenesis plays a key role in cancer progression and development of metastases. Anti-angiogenic therapies have demonstrated significant efficacy in some patients, however, several side effects of anti-angiogenic therapy have been noted in the literature. In addition, the cost of several of these therapies is very high and may not affordable for many patients worldwide

VEGF is an important growth factor that promotes angiogenesis and participates in a variety of physiological and pathological processes. Over-expression of VEGF results in increased angiogenesis in normal and pathological conditions. There is significant evidence that alternative splicing of VEGF gene and other genes involved in angiogenesis can regulate the angiogenic process in tumors. Alternative therapies might replace or improve existing ones. In particular, there is a place for pharmaceutical modulation of angiogenic factors affecting pre-mRNA splicing. This can be brought about not only by alteration in the splicing of heparin-binding isoforms of VEGF but also by the relative balance of pro- and anti-angiogenic isoforms. The concept of an angiogenic splicing phenotype, which controls a number of different proteins that can be activated or deactivated by over-expression or activation of key splicing control factors, is an opportunity for intervention that should be explored in greater detail in the near future (Biselli-Chicote et al., 2012).

In eukaryotes genes consist of coding sequences (exons) interspersed with non-coding sequences (introns). The regulation of alternative inclusion/exclusion of exons, or parts of exons, during RNA processing of pre-mRNA into mRNA (alternative splicing) allows a dramatic increase of the protein repertoire versus the gene repertoire. In a number of cases, alternative splicing of mRNA has been shown to generate proteins with distinct, sometimes opposite, functions from a given gene. Angiogenesis is the process of vascularization in physiological conditions, and there are a number of pathologies, including cancer, where angiogenesis favors tumor progression and dissemination of metastasis. In this chapter, we discuss some key examples showing how alternative splicing may induce a switch from anti-angiogenic to pro-angiogenic functions reciprocally. For some of these splicing events, the molecular mechanisms that trigger alternative splicing toward one or the other direction are now becoming known. The emergence of strategies enabling the regulation of alternative splicing opens new routes for anti-angiogenic therapies (Munaut et al., 2010).

In tumors of the nervous system, tumor derived endothelial cells (TECs) may present the same genetic amplification or chromosomal aberrations of the tumor of origin. In human xenografts of renal carcinoma, melanoma, and liposarcoma, murine TECs are aneuploid, bearing alterations similar to those observed in human TECs. This observation remains unexplained. It cannot be ascribed to cell fusion among tumor and endothelial cells, as no human DNA was present in murine TECs. The researchers who conducted this research speculated that the tumor microenvironment may produce factors capable of inducing genetic instability, or loss of tumor suppressors and/or check point activity, resulting in aneuploidy. Altogether, these data suggest two different explanations for the origin of TECs. The first is that they originate from a common progenitor of tumor and endothelial cells targeted by neoplastic transformation; the second is that the effect of the tumor microenvironment leads to genetic instability (Gardlik et al., 2011a).

In addition, the differentiation of cancer stem cells into endothelial cells and the consequent involvement of these cells in tumor vascularization have been recently described in different tumors. The definitive proof that tumor stem cells are bipotent relies on the ability of clones of tumor stem cells to differentiate *in vitro* and *in vivo* into both tumor epithelial and endothelial cells (Bussolati et al., 2008; 2009). More recently, the ability of tumor cells to differentiate into endothelial cells has also been reported for cancer stem cells present in neuroblastomas (Alvero et al., 2009). In particular, only a fraction of stem cells, characterized by CD133 and CD144 co-expression (Wang et al., 2010), or in a recent report, by co-expression of Oct4 and tenascin C, shows vasculogenic potential and is selectively localized in the proximity of tumor vessels (Pezzolo et al., 2011). An alternative mechanism of tumor blood perfusion implies the possibility that tumor cells form channels connected to the tumor vasculature, a process defined as "vasculogenic mimicry". Alternatively, the process of tumor vasculogenic mimicry could be interpreted as being dependent on tumor stem cells (El Hallanti et al., 2010; Yao et al., 2011), as a transitional step in stem cell differentiation toward endothelial cells (Bussolati et al., 2011).

In cancer therapy, recent investigations have focused on using genetically modified bacteria to actually block tumor angiogenesis. Despite recent progress, only a few studies on bacterial tumor therapy have focused on anti-angiogenesis. Bacteria-mediated anti-angiogenic therapy for cancer, however, is an attractive approach given that solid tumors are often characterized by increased vascularization.

The first modern attempts at using bacteria for therapeutic purposes were made more than 40 years ago by showing that bacteria could predominantly replicate in solid tumors. The first indications of this phenomenon, however, date back to the 19th century. These findings remained largely unexplored until the turn of the 20th century, when oncolytic bacteria capable of lysing host cells were first studied by various research groups. The utilization of bacterial systems for therapeutic anti-cancer purposes is further enhanced by genetic modifications, which make them a very promising tool for targeted delivery of genes and their products. Specific advantages of using bacteria for anti-cancer gene therapy include the natural oncolytic potential of some strains/species, direct targeting of tumor tissues and the ease of positive regulation/eradication. The anti-cancer effect of tumor-targeting bacteria can also be achieved after oral administration, which may circumvent the use of intravenous routes of delivery and associated adverse events of intravenous therapy (Chen et al., 2009; Gardlik et al., 2011b).

5. Further development of ARTs as anti-angiogenic cancer agents

Cancer angiogenesis has been confirmed by measurement of high proliferation indices for endothelial cells, not only in rapidly growing animal tumors, but also in human tumors. The rationale for developing anti-angiogenic strategies for cancer therapy was based on the fact that physiological angiogenesis only occurs in a limited number of situations, such as in wound healing and during menstrual cycle. This suggests there is an opportunity for developing highly tumor-specific anti-angiogenic applications which utilize drugs such as the ARTs which have demonstrated anti-angiogenic efficacy with little toxicity.

5.1. Further targeting anti-angiogenesis of ART and its derivatives

Our current knowledge of the anti-cancer mechanism of ARTs is derived from our knowledge of the antimalarial activity of ARTs. The potent anti-cancer activity of ARTs can be attributed to the endoperoxide bond of the ARTs compounds which is shared with the antiparasitic activity of ARTs. In most of the cancers studied, preloading of cancer cells with iron or iron-saturated holotransferrin triggers ART cytotoxicity with an increase in the activity of ARTs. It has been hypothesized that iron-activated ARTs induce damage by release of highly alkylating carbon-centered radicals and radical oxygen species (ROS). Generation of free radicals may play a role in the cell alterations reported in ARTs-treated cancer cells such as enhanced apoptosis, arrest of growth, inhibition of angiogenesis, and DNA damage. In addition, ARTs-sensitive cancer cells have been shown to have down-regulated expression of oxidation enzymes while cancer cells with over-expression of these molecules are more resistant to ARTs therapy. The antineoplastic toxicity of ARTs appears to be also modulated by calcium metabolism, endoplasmic reticulum (ER) stress, and the expression of the translationally controlled tumor protein, TCTP, a binding calcium protein which has been also postulated as a parasite target. Although the expression of the TCTP gen, *tctp,* was initially correlated with cancer cell responses to ARTs, a functional role for TCTP in the anti-cancer activity of ARTs has yet to be found. As for malaria parasites, the role of sarcoendoplasmic $Ca^{2}+$ ATPase (SERCA) as a target of ARTs in cancer cells has also been explored (Crespo-Ortiz and Wei, 2012).

ART and its bioactive derivatives elicit their anti-cancer effects by concurrently activating, inhibiting and/or attenuating multiple complementary cell signaling pathways, especially those associated with the VEGF family, based on published data. The precise mechanism of new and alternative actions and other primary targets of ARTs, however, will require further study. In anti-cancer therapy, it has been postulated that ARTs may target organelles such as pathways involving PlGF growth factors (a VEGF subfamily),, angiopoietins, such as the Angs proteins, the Notch signaling pathway, signaling pathways involving fibroblast growth factors (FGFs), and the matrix metalloproteinase (MMPs) family of enzymes (Crespo-Ortiz and Wei, 2012). In a recent study, investigators discovered a panel of genes containing many fundamental regulators of angiogenic regulators, such as VEGF, was found that correlate with the cellular response to AS. These genes govern the stimulation, proliferation and migration of endothelial cells, a fundamental step in vessel formation. The investigators decided to further limit their cluster analysis by including in the cluster analysis only those genes whose mRNA expression correlated with GI_{50} values of at least four ARTs (Anfosso et al., 2006). Three human genes coding for VEGF (VEGFA, VEGFB, and VEGFC) were discovered in this cluster of ARTs-affected angiogenic regulating genes.. Despite the continuous investigations on new targets, the ART compounds exert common as well as distinct cellular effects depending on the phenotype and tissue origin of the human cancer cells examined. (Firestone and Sundar, 2009).

In addition, most of these studies were based on the consideration that an ideal ARTs as an anti-angiogenic drugs may target different types of tumor, assuming endothelial cells to be similar in different tumor types and genetically stable. The therapeutic efficacy of ARTs, however, was not as successful as expected and endothelial cells acquired drug resistance. This setback is possibly due to the fact that most anti-angiogenic drugs were tested on normal endothelial cells. In light of the involvement of angiogenesis and vasculogenesis in tumor vascularization, it can be speculated that tumor cytotoxic therapies, radiotherapy, and anti-angiogenic drugs, may stimulate vasculogenesis by inducing tumor hypoxia and/or an epithelial mesenchymal transition. Therefore, targeting both angiogenesis and vasculogenesis in tumors may be required to inhibit tumor vascularization, growth, and invasion. In particular, an improved knowledge of the relative contribution of vasculogenesis to tumor vascularization is likely to be critical for development of specific therapeutic strategies (Li et al., 2011).

5.2. Prevention and therapy strategies of ARTs for cancer treatments

Angiogenesis inhibition therapy does not necessarily kill tumors but instead may prevent tumors from growing. Therefore, this type of therapy may need to be administered over a long period of time. Some common components of human diets also act as mild angiogenesis inhibitors and have therefore been proposed for angioprevention, the prevention of metastasis through the inhibition of angiogenesis. Phytochemicals and ART-mediated anti-angiogenic intervention is a growing area of research that may provide an effective cancer prevention strategy. Suppression of pathological angiogenesis by phytochemicals and ARTs could have potential applications in cancer prevention and therapy as well as in other diseases with similar etiology. Chemopreventive phytochemicals are generally non-toxic and hence will produce minimal side effects. In addition, endothelial cells lack induced drug resistance and, therefore, angioprevention could be a preferred strategy for cancer control in comparison to other therapies such as radiotherapy and chemotherapy.

Several anti-angiogenic strategies have been developed to inhibit tumor growth by targeting different components of tumor angiogenesis. Non-toxic natural chemopreventive agents that could be part of the daily human diet have been shown to safely target and inhibit different aspects and components of the process of angiogenesis. ART and its derivatives, and other sesquiterpene lactones, have been shown to have potent anti-angiogenic effects in tumor cells as well as in healthy rat embryos in culture. These observations have many implications in terms of cancer therapy as well as cancer prevention since angiogenesis is a promotional event (Firestone and Sundar, 2009).

Studies have shown that, the upper limit of a tumor mass in the absence of angiogenesis is 1-2 mm, and this size limit is related to the maximum size possible for simple diffusion of nutrients and gases like CO_2 and O_2. This 1-2 mm tumor size can be maintained by the balance of cell proliferation and apoptosis leading to dormancy of small tumors for many years. Therefore, for tumor growth and the development of vasculature is critical to proceed towards tumor progression and metastasis., Endothelial cells are a preferential target for therapy because they are common to all solid tumors, and endothelial cell proliferation normally occurs only in pathological conditions such as injury or endometrial development. Large number of angiogenic factors, such as VEGF and bFGF. etc., is secreted by tumor cells are required to cause endothelial cell recruitment and proliferation (Ferrara et al., 2003).

These stimuli are constantly present so the differentiation of the tumor endothelium into a mature vessel network is rarely complete, and tumor vessels show an abnormal morphology. The immature vessel network of tumors is a promising anti-angiogenic target for ARTs compounds. The body of knowledge of endothelial cell physiology and tumor angiogenesis obtained through recent research has been crucial to actually understand some of the mechanisms of how ARTs actually exert their anti-angiogenic effects (Efferth, 2005; 2007).Endothelial cells are non-transformed cells, and they should be quite accessible to treat with physiologically achievable concentrations of ARTs (Efferth, 2006; Crespo-Ortiz and Wei, 2012). This therapeutic strategy may involve various targets including angiogenic molecules from tumors cells and inflammatory system (such as neutrophils and macrophages) such as VEGF, bFGF, TNFa, IL-8, etc. and their respective receptors on endothelial cells, endothelial cells itself, matrix metalloproteinases (MMPs), cyclooxygenases (COXs), lipoxygenases (LOXs) etc (see Section 3). Therefore, long-term angiostasis treatment will likely be necessary for cancer prevention and control. This multitargeted anti-angiogenic strategy suggests drug discovery and development should be focused on finding small, non-toxic anti-angiogenic molecules or compounds to be used in a multifaceted cancer control regimen (Firestone and Sundar, 2009).

Large numbers of chemopreventive agents, such as ARTs, have been shown to possess anticancer activities in many studies. These agents achieve anti-cancer activities through various mechanisms by targeting different aspects of cancer progression and development. Since angiogenesis is a pre-requisite for the growth of solid tumors, vascular targeting has been explored as a potential strategy to suppress tumor growth and metastasis. In this regard, many phytochemicals or ARTs have been shown to target tumor angiogenesis using *in vitro* and *in vivo* model systems (Chen and Cleck, 2009a; Cao et al., 2009; 2011).

Since, angiogenesis is critically important for physiological process such as wound-healing, acute injury healing, and healing of chronic ulceration of the gastrointestinal mucosa, administration of ARTs compounds that inhibit tumor angiogenesis might also suppress physiological angiogenesis and produce critical side effects when dosed over a long period of time. Therefore, anti-angiogenic chemopreventive ARTs and phytochemicals should be studied and analyzed first for their selective targeting of tumor specific angiogenesis to find the most effective anti-tumor combinations (Bhat and Singh, 2008; Crespo-Ortiz and Wei, 2012).

5.3. Combination strategies to enhance efficacy and to prevent resistance of ARTs

Anti-angiogenesis is a cytostatic therapy that is likely to have greatest effect when combined with cytotoxic therapy. It has recently been suggested that anti-angiogenic drugs represent the universal chemosensitizing agents for cancer treatment. There are a number of mechanisms for the observed synergism between anti-angiogenic agents and anti-cancer chemotherapeutic agents that have been proposed 1) the normalization of tumor microvessels by anti-angiogenic therapy which enhances chemotherapeutic drug delivery, 2) prevention of tumor cell repopulation by anti-angiogenic drugs during the break periods after maximum tolerated dose chemotherapy and 3) augmentation of the antivascular effects of chemotherapeutics by anti-angiogenic drugs (Makrilia et al., 2009). There is growing evidence supporting the use of ART and its derivatives in cancer therapy given their potent antiproliferative, antimetastatic and anti-angiogenic activity, which makes them potential anti-cancer drugs. In a combination therapy for cancer, the antineoplastic action of ART may contribute to an independent antitumor activity with no additional side effects. The benefits of combining ARTs with other anti-cancer agents have been investigated showing that the multifactorial activity of ARTs in different pathways may provide synergism and improve overall activity (Liu et al., 2011).

Drug combinations that involve ARTs have been reported *in vitro*, which show value in this approach, both as a sensitizing agent to chemotherapy in solid tumors (Sieber et al., 2009), and as a synergistic partner with doxorubicin in leukemia (Efferth et al., 2007). Incubation of cancer cells with DHA alone was found to be less effective than in combination with holo-transferrin, indicating that intracellular iron plays a role in the cytotoxic effects of DHA (Lai and Singh, 1995). In addition to conventional chemotherapies, ART was also shown to be effective when combined with the immune modulatory drug LEN (Galustian and Dalgleish, 2009). These *in vitro* studies demonstrated the effects of ARTs on the cell cycle, and these studiesalso demonstrated restoration of cytotoxicity in an ART-resistant cell by adopting a pulsed-schedule of combination treatment.

Many anti-angiogenic and antivascular agents are now in clinical trials for the treatment of cancer. It is conceivable that loading tumor cells with bivalent iron by simply providing Fe^{2+} in tablet form might increase the susceptibility of cancer cells to the action of AS. In a clinical study of humans with uveal melanoma, one of the patients enrolled was treated with bivalent iron and artesunate, and it is tempting to speculate the addition of Fe^{2+} had an actual clinical impact and resulted in an improved response to therapy (Berger et al., 2005). Continued research in this area is encouraged by the recent success of a Phase II clinical trial of AS combined with NP chemotherapy in treatment of advanced non-small cell lung cancer. The disease controlled rate of the trial group of AS plus NP chemotherapy (88.2%) was significantly higher than that of the NP chemotherapy alone group (72.7%), and the trial group's time to progression (24 weeks) was significantly longer than that of the NP chemotherapy alone group (20 weeks). AS combined with NP chemotherapy can increase the short-term survival rate of patients with advanced non-small cell lung cancer and prolong the time to progression without extra side effects (Zhang et al., 2008). The diversity in the targets of ART supports the possibility that it could be used in combination with other agents.

In addition, it has been reported that resistant cancer cell lines become sensitive by adding ART to the conventional treatment (chemosensitization). Interestingly, DHA and AS have exhibited the strongest chemosensitizing/synergistic effects, while other ARTs shows only additive and antagonistic interactions (Singh and Lai, 2005). DHA was shown to synergistically enhance tumor growth inhibition by 45% when administered in combination with gemcitabine, while other ARTs showed only additive effects (Wang et al., 2010). Consistent with this observation, a greater antitumor activity was observed when DHA was used in a combination with cyclosphosphamide in murine Lewis lung carcinoma cell line or in combination

http://dx.doi.org/10.5772/54109

with cisplatin in non-small cell lung cancer A549 in mice (Zhou et al., 2010). In rat C6 glioma cells, addition of 1 μM DHA increased the cytotoxic effect of temozolomide, a DNA alkylating agent used in the treatment of brain cancer, by 177%,. Further investigation showed that DHA promotes apoptotic and necrotic activity of temozolomide through ROS generation (Huang et al., 2008).

Recently, an enhancement of the anti-cancer activity of AS was shown in different combination regimens. A striking synergy was achieved in combinations of AS and the immunomodulator drug, lenalidomide (Liu et al., 2011). Overall, this evidence suggests that DHA and AS have remarkable ability to potentiate antitumor agents and to counter tumor resistance. ARTs also have been shown to improve ionizing-based therapies. In the glioma cell line U373MG, DHA treatment was shown to inhibit the radiation- induced expression of GST with concomitant ROS generation. A combination treatment with DHA has been shown to be more effective than radiation or DHA alone (Kim et al., 2006). The adjuvant effect of ARTs in other cancer treatments including hyperbaric oxygen has also been reported (Ohgami et al., 2010).

Current available ARTs in combination with chemotherapy for the treatment of cancer patients have produced only modest beneficial effects (Cao *et al.*, 2009). Optimization of anti-angiogenic therapy is urgently needed in order to maximize therapeutic efficacy of these drugs. Thus, development of a new generation of drugs targeting diverse angiogenic pathways is expected to improve the anticancer benefits of ARTs therapy. In preclinical tumor models, it has been shown that a combination of anti-angiogenic agents with different mechanistic principles yielded a synergistic effect on tumor suppression. Translation of this preclinical finding to patient therapy would suggest acombination of different of anti-angiogenic agents combined with a chemotherapeutic agent will enhance cancer therapy, and such a combination should be considered in future clinical trials (Cao, 2011).

The mechanism(s) underlying the interaction of combinations of anti-angiogenic agents such as the ARTs plus chemotherapeutic treatment, and, indeed, the mechanism of ART action against cancer is still not fully understood, however, many studies in this field of research are ongoing and will guide the basis of further studies and clinical trials (Liu et al., 2011). Scientists investigating the cancer-fighting properties of ARTs have found early evidence that combining it with an existing cancer drug has the potential to make each drug more effective in combination versus when these drugs are used alone. There is currently limited published data exploring the value of ARTs as a combination partner in treatment regimens. These studies have used simple approaches to studying drug–drug interactions, and as a consequence, their conclusions are still open to debate (Liu, 2008).

5.4. Strategies to avoid potential drug toxicities of ARTs

At high concentrations, ARTs appear to be active against cancer *in vivo.* The use of ARTs at high concentrations or for long drug exposure times, however, has substantial risk of severe toxicities, including embryotoxicity and neurotoxicity. Animal studies have shown that high peak concentrations of AS and DHA can induce embryotoxicity, and the longer exposure times associated with therapy using oil-soluble ARTs, such as AM, will produce fatal neurotoxicity (Li et al., 2007a). To prevent embryotoxicity in pregnant women with malaria, current WHO policy recommendations on the use of ARTs in uncomplicated malaria state that ARTs should be used only in the second and third trimester, limiting the use of ARTS in the first trimester to cases where it is the only effective treatment available (WHO 2006b).

Studies with laboratory animals have demonstrated fatal neurotoxicity associated with intramuscular administration of AM and AE or oral administration of artelinic acid. These effects suggest that the exposure time of ARTs was extended in these studies due to the accumulation of drug in the bloodstream, and this accumulation, in turn, resulted in neurotoxicity. In one study, the drug exposure time with a neurotoxic outcome (neurotoxic exposure time) was evaluated as a predictor of neurotoxicity *in vivo* (Li and Hickman, 2011). The neurotoxic exposure time represents a total time spent above the lowest observed neurotoxic effect levels (LONEL) in plasma. The dose of AE required to induce minimal neurotoxicity required a 2-3 fold longer exposure time in rhesus monkeys (179.5 hr) than in rats (67.1 hr) and dogs (113.2 hr) when using a daily dose of 6-12.5 mg/kg for 7-28 days, indicating that the safe dosing duration in monkeys should be longer than 7 days under this exposure. Oral artelinic acid treatment required much longer LONEL levels (8-fold longer) than intramuscular AE to induce neurotoxicity, suggesting that water-soluble ARTs appear to be much safer than oil-soluble ARTs. Due to the lower doses (2-4 mg/kg) used with current ARTs and the more rare use of AE in treating humans, the exposure time is much shorter in humans. Therefore, the current regimen of 3-5 days dosing duration should be quite safe. Advances in our knowledge of ART-induced neurotoxicity can help refine the treatment regimens used to treat malaria with oral ARTs as well as injectable AS products to avoid the risk of neurotoxicity. Although the water-soluble ARTs, like AS, appear to be much safer, further study is needed in when employing ARTs as anti-cancer agents (Li and Hickman, 2011).

Thus, rapid elimination of ARTs in oral formulations is safer than slow-release or oil-based intramuscular formulations (Efferth and Kaina, 2010). Remarkably, although ARTs derivatives have been widely used as antimalarials, their toxicity in humans have been shown to be negligible. In cancer therapy, ARTs may have multiple benefits as it can be used in combination with no additional side effects, but also it enhances potency and reduces doses of more toxic anti-cancer partners. Clinical doses used in malaria treatment after ART administration of 2 mg/kg in patients raise plasma concentrations to 2640 ± 1800 μg/L (approximately 6.88 ± 4.69 mM) which can be considered up to 3 orders of magnitude higher than those ART concentrations with antitumor activity (Efferth et al., 2003). It becomes relevant to closely monitor the safety of long-term ARTs-based therapies as severe side effects may be highly unusual but significant. So far, ARTs treatments for as long as 12 months have been reported with no relevant side effects (Berger et al., 2005; Singh and Verma, 2002; Singh and Panwar 2006).

5.5. Strategies to utiliize current and novel ARTs as anti-cancer agents

A number of first generation derivatives of ART have been created (DHA, AS, AM and AE), and other novel compounds have been synthesized as second generation derivatives designed to improve the anti-cancer activities of ART. This second generation ART derivatives have shown remarkable anti-angiogenic effects and cytotoxicity towards tumor cells (D'Alessandro et al., 2007; Krishna et al., 2008). Ether-linked dimers of DHA, for example, have been shown to cause accumulation of tumor cells in the G1 phase of the cell cycle (Morrissey et al., 2010). New growth-inhibitory ART derivatives containing cyan and aryl groups have been shown to cause accumulation of P388 and A549 cells in the G1 phase (Li et al., 2001). Finally, deoxoartemisinyl cyanoarylmethyl ART derivatives with cytotoxic activity have been shown to induce a significant accumulation of L1210 and P388 cells in the G1 phase (Wu et al., 2001)., ART-like endoperoxides have also been synthesized chemically which show greater cytotoxicity towards tumor cells than native ART, which aids in preserving the natural resources of the *A. annua* plants (Soomro et al., 2011).

As mentioned above, AS is completely converted to DHA and is best described as a prodrug of DHA. DHA has been shown to be more effective than AS in inhibition of angiogenesis and vasculogenesis *in vitro* (Longo et al., 2006a; 2006b; Chen et al., 2004b; White et al., 2006). In addition, the embryotoxicity and neurotoxicity of ARTs can be reduced by using artemisone, which is a novel derivative of ART that is not metabolized to DHA (D'Alessandro et al., 2007; Schmuck et al., 2009).

Artemisone is a novel amino alkyl ART that has recently entered Phase II clinical trials (D'Alessandro et al., 2007). The compound was rationally designed to have reduced lipophilicity in order to impede transport to the brain and embryo. In addition, the inclusion of a thiomorpholine 1,1-dioxide group at the C10 position blocks the conversion of artemisone to the more lipophilic DHA. This structural modification does not affect anti-parasitic activity but reduces neurotoxicity and embryotoxicity, as assessed *in vitro* against primary neuronal brain stem cell cultures from fetal rats and *in vivo* in female rats (Schmuck et al., 2009). The retention of artemisone antimalarial activity infers that chemical activation of the peroxide bridge to a toxic parasiticidal chemical species remains unchanged, but recent literature also suggests that artemisone has a direct cytotoxic activity without activation of the endoperoxide bridge. In fact, two subsequent studies have provided conflicting results concerning the dependence of the pharmacological activity of artemisone on iron-activation of the endoperoxide group.

Interestingly, an *in vitro* study by D'Alessandro et al, showed that the anti-angiogenic effects of artemisone were reduced compared with DHA, and it was suggested that this reduction may limit the potential of artemisone to cause embryotoxicity mediated by defective angiogenesis and vasculogenesis during embryo development (D'Alessandro et al., 2007). Together these studies suggest that, while artemisone was designed to optimize safety by physicochemical means, the structural changes induced to create artemisone may also affect the intracellular chemical and molecular pathways which underlie toxicity, perhaps via reduced or alternative mechanisms of bio-activation and/or reduced cellular accumulation, when compared with the traditional ARTs. Therefore, artemisone represents an exciting novel compound in which increased anti-parasitic activity is combined with a reduced potential to cause both embryotoxicity and neurotoxicity.

Increased knowledge of the molecular mechanisms of ART-derived drugs and recent synthesis of novel ART derivatives demonstrates that further pharmacokinetic and pharmacodynamic analyses of novel ART derivatives are needed to understand why these compounds differ in efficacy and toxicity. This information will prove useful for the rationale design of more-effective ART-based molecules for use as anti-cancer agents. New derivatives of ARTs may act not only as treatment drugs, but also may have potential as potent cancer preventative agents due to their inhibition of tumor promotion and progression.

Recently, a series of DHA derivatives were synthesized via an aza-Michael addition reaction, and these novel compounds showed a high selectivity index and an IC_{50} in the nanomolar range against HeLa cells (0.37 μM) (Feng et al., 2000). In another study, a series of deoxoartemisinins and carboxypropyldeoxoartemisinin compounds were synthesized, and the antitumor effects of these compounds were not associated with lipophilicity, as has commonly been assumed, but instead was associated with distinctive boat/chair molecular conformations which facilitated the interaction of these novel compounds with receptors (Lee et al., 2000). In many studies, there has been an emphasis on the nature and stereochemistry of the dimer linker which may influence anti-cancer activity. It has also been shown, however, that the linker by its own is inactive. Morrisey et al. have described that an ARTs dimer exhibits up to 30-fold more activity than ARTs against prostate cancer lines (Morrissey et al., 2010). This dimer selectively exerted both higher cytostatic activity and apoptosis in C4-2 (a cell line derived from LNCaP) and LNCaP cells compared to ARTs (Morrissey et al., 2010). The stereoisomery of the linker may be associated with enhanced anti-cancer activity (Alagbala et al., 2006). In another study, C12 non-acetal dimers and one trimer of deoxoartemisinin showed similar potency to that of the conventional anti-cancer drugs against many cell lines. The linker with one amide or one sulfur-centered 2 ethylene group was essential for potent anti-cancer activity (Jung et al., 2003). The mechanism underlying the antiproliferative action of the ARTs-derived dimers is not clear and requires further study.

Recently, a series of easily synthesized, potent ARTs-like derivatives with anti-cancer activity were created. These endoperoxides exhibit high chemical stability and greater cytotoxicity than AS against cancer cell lines. These compounds also exhibit relevant anti-angiogenic properties as judged by studies in a zebrafish model (Soomro et al., 2011). To overcome the short half-lives of ARTs, novel, longer lasting derivatives will be required. One such example is synthetic trioxolanes, endoperoxide drugs which were created to provide long lasting efficacy against *Schistosoma* species. ARTs compounds share the endoperoxide bridge structural feature of the trioxolanes, and they have been shown to have prophylactic activity towards the younger developmental stages of *Schistosoma* but are ineffective as curative agents. The synthetic trioxalane compounds incorporate the endoperoxide "warhead" with enhanced pharmacokinetic properties and exhibit greater efficacy as curative agents against established Schistosoma infections (Xiao et al., 2007). Given that ARTs may be potentially used as anti-cancer drugs and possibly in other parasitic and viral infections, the development of novel endoperoxide compounds with enhanced pharmacokinetic properties and targeted anti-cancer activity is essential. These promising research findings suggest it is possible to identify safer and more effective strategies to treat a range of infections and cancer (Crespo-Ortiz and Wei, 2012).

http://dx.doi.org/10.5772/54109

6. Perspectives and conclusion

ART and its bioactive derivatives are potent anti-cancer phytochemicals that pose minimal risks to human patients. ART has been shown to arrest cancer cell growth, induce apoptosis, disrupt angiogenic pathways and has other anti-cancer properties through pleiotropic effects as shown against a variety of human cancer cell lines. In addition, ART-related compounds have been shown to inhibit tumor promotion and progression, suggesting these molecules is not only effective as treatment therapeutics, but also as potential anti-cancer preventive agents. ARTs have been recommended and widely used as antimalarials for six years, and they have saved the lives of many patients infected with malaria (WHO, 2006a). Supporting evidence indicates that ART-like compounds may be a therapeutic alternative or adjunct for use in treating highly metastatic and aggressive cancers that have no other long term effective therapy (Morrissey et al., 2010) particularly against cancer cells that have developed drug resistance (Wang et al., 2010). Furthermore, antimalarial endoperoxides may act synergistically with other anti-cancer drugs with no additional side effects. The many antitumor activities, both direct and indirect, of ARTs compounds, however are not entirely explained. So far, the precise molecular events involved in how, when, and where radical oxygen species (ROS) production is initially triggered in cancer cells remain to be defined. In addition, the relevance of any ROS-independent mechanism should be also addressed; these might not be obvious but possibly important for ART-mediated cytotoxicity in some cancer cells. Some other aspects such as the direct DNA damage induced by ART-like compounds and the role of p53 status in genotoxicity need to be further analyzed.

Characterizing the anti-cancer effects of existing and novel ARTs derivatives remains an important research goal, and research also needs to be focused on unveiling the mechanisms of cancer cell cytotoxicity by identifying their relation to particular cancer biomarkers and molecules. ARTs seem to regulate key players participating in multiple pathways such as VEGF, NF-κB, survivin, NOXA, HIF-1α, and BMI-1. These molecules and others are to be revealed, which in turn may be involved in drug response, drug interactions, mechanisms of resistance, and collateral effects in normal cells. A better understanding of common mechanisms under similar conditions in different cell systems will greatly aid the development of targeted ART derivatives. This will improve ARTs cytotoxicity by lowering IC_{50}, emerging of resistance, drug associated toxicity, and potentiating drug interactions. Furthermore, novel endoperoxide compounds and combinational therapies can be addressed to target or co-target markers of carcinoma progression and prevent invasiveness and metastatic properties in highly recurrent and aggressive tumors or advanced stage cancers.

Even though the utility of ARTs in the clinical setting have already been assessed, specific interactions with established chemotherapy regimens need to be further dissected in different cancer cell lines and their associated phenotypes. This will be crucial to implement clinical trials and treatment of individual cases. Due to the toxicity of ARTs, long-term therapy also requires close monitoring. It is important to note that the prototype drug, ART, seems to modulate responses leading to antagonistic interactions with other anti-cancer drugs. While it may be useful to have the prototype drug as a control *in vitro*, however, its pharmacokinetic properties may differ from the semisynthetic ARTs. Therefore, ART antagonistic reactions and resistance must be cautiously validated using different semisynthetic derivatives. DHA,

AS, and AM are the only endoperoxides currently licensed for therapeutic use. So far, AM has been shown to share similar anti-cancer properties as DHA and AS (Wu et al., 2009).

Cancer research is a permanent discovery of new genes and pleiotropic interactions. The study of the antitumor activity of ARTs compounds may become even more complex as immunological hallmarks are also involved in the generation of tumors. Immunological hallmarks in cancer cells include the ability to induce chronic inflammatory response, evasion of tumor recognition, and ability to induce tolerance (Cavallo et al., 2011). Whether ART may participate in the mechanisms involved in these events has yet to be determined. Overall, the real potential and benefits of the ART drug class remain yet to be uncovered. The imminent possibility of ARTs being included in the arsenal of anti-cancer drugs has opened the door for challenging research in this area, one that seems to fulfill many expectations (Crespo-Ortiz and Wei, 2012).

In conclusion, the inhibition of angiogenesis induced by ART-derived drugs has been shown to be a mechanism of anti-cancer activity *in vitro* and *in vivo*. In particular, cancer angiogenesis plays a key role in the growth, invasion, and metastasis of tumors. ARTs-induced inhibition of angiogenesis could be a promising therapeutic strategy for treatment and prevention of cancer. Other anti-cancer mechanisms induced by ARTs have been recognized recently that have guided various clinical trials in anti-cancer therapy. Since new and alternative angiogenesis mechanisms have been found, further research on the mechanism of efficacy and toxicity could lead us to understand more deeply the possibilities inherent in therapeutic development of ARTs for malaria, cancer, and other indications. The new therapeutic strategies for use of ARTs as anti-angiogenic agents should be considered to avoid problems associated with reproductive toxicity and neurotoxicity. Taken together, ART and its derivatives have been shown to have potent anti-angiogenic and antivasculogenic effects in tumor cells. These observations have many implications in terms of cancer therapy and prevention as well as avoidance of drug toxicity associated with inhibition of angiogenesis.

Acknowledgements

This material has been reviewed by Walter Reed Army Institute of Research. There is no objection to its presentation and/or publication. The opinions or assertions contained herein are the private views of the authors and are not to be construed as official, or as reflecting the views of the Department of the Army or the Department of Defense.

Author details

Qigui Li*, Peter Weina and Mark Hickman

*Address all correspondence to: qigui.li@us.army.mil

Division of Experimental Therapeutics, Walter Reed Army Institute of Research, Silver Spring, USA

References

[1] van Agtmael, MA., Cheng-Qi, S., Qing, JX., Mull, R., van Boxtel, CJ. (1999) Multiple dose pharmacokinetics of artemether in Chinese patients with uncomplicated falciparum malaria. Int J Antimicrob Agents. 12, 151-158.

[2] Alagbala, AA., McRiner, AJ., Borstnik, K., Labonte, T., Chang, W., D'Angelo, JG., Posner, GH., Foster, BA. (2006) Biological mechanisms of action of novel C-10 non-acetal trioxane dimers in prostate cancer cell lines. J Med Chem. 49, 7836-7842.

[3] D'Alessandro, S., Gelati, M., Basilico, N., Parati, EA., Haynes, RK., Taramelli, D. (2007) Differential effects on angiogenesis of two antimalarial compounds, dihydroartemisinin and artemisone: implications for embryotoxicity. Toxicology 241, 66–74.

[4] Alvero, AB., Fu, HH., Holmberg, J., Visintin, I., Mor, L., Marquina, CC., Oidtman, J., Silasi, DA., Mor, G. (2009) Stem-like ovarian cancer cells can serve as tumor vascular progenitors. Stem Cells. 27, 2405–2413.

[5] Andrae, J., Gallini, R., Betsholtz, C. (2008) Role of platelet-derived growth factors in physiology and medicine. Genes Dev. 22, 1276-1312.

[6] Anfosso, L., Efferth, T., Albini, A., Pfeffer, U. (2006) Microarray expression profiles of angiogenesis-related genes predict tumor cell response to artemisinins. Pharmacogenomics J. 6, 269-278.

[7] Ashton, M., Sy, ND., Gordi, T., Hai, TN., Thach, DC., Huong, NV., Johansson, M., Coeng, LD. (1996) Evidence for time-dependence artemisinin kinetics in adults with uncomplicated malaria. Pharm Pharmacol Lett. 6, 127-130.

[8] Ashton, M., Hai, TN., Sy, ND., Huong, DX., Van Huong, N., Nieu, NT., Cong, LD. (1998) Artemisinin pharmacokinetics is time-dependent during repeated oral administration in healthy male adults. Drug Metab Dispos. (1998). 26, 25-27.

[9] Aung, W., Sogawa, C., Furukawa, T., Saga, T. (2011) Anti-cancer effect of dihydroartemisinin (DHA) in a pancreatic tumor model evaluated by conventional methods and optical imaging. Anti-cancer Res. 31, 1549-1558.

[10] Baluk, P., Morikawa, S., Haskell, A., Mancuso, M., McDonald, DM. (2003) Abnormalities of basement membrane on blood vessels and endothelial sprouts in tumors. Am J Pathol. 163, 1801-1815.

[11] Batty, KT., Le, AT., Ilett, KF., Nguyen, PT., Powell, SM., Nguyen, CH., Truong, XM., Vuong, VC., Huynh, VT., Tran, QB., Nguyen, VM., Davis, TM. (1998) A pharmacokinetic and pharmacodynamic study of artesunate for vivax malaria. Am. J. Trop. Med. Hyg. 59, 823-827.

[12] Beekman, AC., Wierenga, PK., Woerdenbag, HJ., van Uden, W., Pras, N., Konings, AW., el-Feraly, FS., Galal, AM., Wikstrom, HV. (1998) Artemisinin-derived sesquiter-

pene lactones as potential antitumour compounds: cytotoxic action against bone marrow and tumor cells. Planta Med. 64, 615–619.

[13] Berger, TG., Dieckmann, D., Efferth, T., Schultz, ES., Funk, JO., Baur, A., Schuler, G. (2005) Artesunate in the treatment of metastatic uveal melanoma--first experiences. Oncol. Rep. 14, 1599-1603.

[14] Bergers, G., Hanahan, D. (2008) Modes of resistance to anti-angiogenic therapy. Nat Rev 8, 592–603.

[15] Bhat, TA., Singh, RP. (2008) Tumor angiogenesis--a potential target in cancer chemoprevention. Food Chem Toxicol. 46, 1334-1345.

[16] Biselli-Chicote, PM., Oliveira, AR., Pavarino, EC., Goloni-Bertollo, EM. (2012) VEGF gene alternative splicing: pro- and anti-angiogenic isoforms in cancer. J Cancer Res Clin Oncol. 138, 363-370.

[17] Bosman, A., Mendis, KN. (2007) A major transition in malaria treatment: The adoption and deployment of artemisinin-based combination therapies. Am J Trop Med Hyg. 77(Suppl. 6), 193-197.

[18] Buommino, E., Baroni, A., Canozo, N., Petrazzuolo, M., Nicoletti, R., Vozza, A., Tufano, MA. (2009) Artemisinin reduces human melanoma cell migration by down-regulating alpha V beta 3 integrin and reducing metalloproteinase 2 production. Invest, New Drugs. 27, 412-418.

[19] Bussolati, B., Bruno, S., Grange, C., Ferrando, U., Camussi, G. (2008) Identification of a tumor-initiating stem cell population in human renal carcinomas. FASEB J. 22, 3696–3705.

[20] Bussolati, B., Grange, C., Sapino, A., Camussi, G. (2009) Endothelial cell differentiation of human breast tumor stem/progenitor cells. J. Cell. Mol. Med. 13, 309–319.

[21] Bussolati, B., Grange, C., Camussi, G. (2011) Tumor exploits alternative strategies to achieve vascularization. FASEB J. 25, 2874-2882.

[22] Butler, AR., Gilbert, BC., Hulme, P., Irvine, LR., Renton, L., Whitwood, AC. (1998) EPR evidence for the involvement of free radicals in the iron-catalysed decomposition of qinghaosu (artemisinin) and some derivatives; antimalarial action of some polycyclic endoperoxides. Free Radical Res. 28, 471-476.

[23] Cao, Y., Liu, Q. (2007) Therapeutic targets of multiple angiogenic factors for the treatment of cancer and metastasis. Adv Cancer Res. 97, 203-224.

[24] Cao, Y., Cao, R., Hedlund, EM. (2008) R Regulation of tumor angiogenesis and metastasis by FGF and PDGF signaling pathways. J Mol Med (Berl). 86, 785-789.

[25] Cao, Y. (2009) Tumor angiogenesis and molecular targets for therapy. Front Biosci 14, 3962-3973.

[26] Cao, Y., Zhong, W., Sun, Y. (2009) Improvement of anti-angiogenic cancer therapy by understanding the mechanisms of angiogenic factor interplay and drug resistance. Semin Cancer Biol 19, 338-343.

[27] Cao, Y. (2010) Off-tumor target--beneficial site for anti-angiogenic cancer therapy? Nat Rev Clin Oncol. 7, 604-608.

[28] Cao, Y., Arbiser, J., D'Amato, RJ., D'Amore, PA., Ingber, DE., Kerbel, R., Klagsbrun, M., Lim, S., Moses, MA., Zetter, B., Dvorak, H., Langer, R. (2011) Forty-year journey of angiogenesis translational research. Sci Transl Med. 3, 114rv3.

[29] Cao, Y. (2011) Anti-angiogenic cancer therapy: why do mouse and human patients respond in a different way to the same drug? Int J Dev Biol. 55, 557-562.

[30] Carmeliet, P., Jain, RK. (2011) Principles and mechanisms of vessel normalization for cancer and other angiogenic diseases. Nat Rev Drug Discov. 10, 417-427.

[31] Cavallo, F., De Giovanni, C., Nanni, P., Forni, G., Lollini, PL. (2011) the immune hallmarks of cancer. Cancer Immunol Immunother. 60, 319-326.

[32] Chen, G., Wei, DP., Jia, LJ., Tang, B., Shu, L., Zhang, K., Xu, Y., Gao, J., Huang, XF., Jiang, WH., Hu, QG., Huang, Y., Wu, Q., Sun, ZH., Zhang, JF., Hua, ZC. (2009) Oral delivery of tumor-targeting Salmonella exhibits promising therapeutic efficacy and low toxicity. Cancer Sci 100, 2437–2443.

[33] Chen, HH., Zhou, HJ., Fang, X. (2003) Inhibition of human cancer cell line growth and human umbilical vein endothelial cell angiogenesis by artemisinin derivatives in vitro. Pharmacol. Res. 48, 231–236.

[34] Chen, HH., Zhou, HJ., Wang, WQ., Wu, GD. (2004a) Antimalarial dihydroartemisinin also inhibits angiogenesis. Cancer Chemother. Pharmacol. 53, 423-432.

[35] Chen, HH., Zhou, HJ., Wu, GD., Lou, XE. (2004b) Inhibitory effects of artesunate on angiogenesis and on expressions of vascular endothelial growth factor and VEGF receptor KDR/flk-1. Pharmacology 71, 1–9.

[36] Chen, HH., Zhou HJ. (2004c) Inhibitory effects of artesunate on angiogenesis. Yao Xue Xue Bao. 39, 29-33.

[37] Chen, HX., Cleck, JN. (2009a) Adverse effects of anti-cancer agents that target the VEGF pathway. Nat Rev Clin Oncol 6, 465-477.

[38] Chen, H., Sun, B., Pan, S., Jiang, H., Sun, X. (2009b) Dihydroartemisinin inhibits growth of pancreatic cancer cells In vitro and In vivo. Anti-Cancer Drugs, 20, 131–140.

[39] Chen, T., Li, M., Zhang, R., Wang, H. (2009c) Dihydroartemisinin induces apoptosis and sensitizes human ovarian cancer cells to carboplatin therapy. J Cell Mol Med. 13, 1358-1370.

[40] Chen, CN., Chang, CC., Su, TE., Hsu, WM., Jeng, YM., Ho, MC., Hsieh, FJ., Lee, PH., Kuo, ML., Lee, H., Chang, KJ. (2009d) Identification of calreticulin as a prognosis

marker and angiogenic regulator in human gastric cancer. Ann Surg Oncol. 16, 524–533.

[41] Chen, H., Shi, L., Yang, X., Li, S., Guo, X., Pan, L. (2010a) Artesunate inhibiting angiogenesis induced by human myeloma RPMI8226 cells. Int J Hematol. 92, 587-597.

[42] Chen, H., Sun, B., Wang, S., Pan, S., Gao, Y., Bai, X., Xue, D. (2010b) Growth inhibitory effects of dihydroartemisinin on pancreatic cancer cells: involvement of cell cycle arrest and inactivation of nuclear factor-kappaB. J Cancer Res Clin Oncol. 136, 897-903.

[43] Classen, W., Altmann, B., Gretener, P., Souppart, C., Skelton-Stroud, P., Krinke, G. (1999) Differental effects of orally versus parenterally administered qinghaosu derivatives artemether in dogs. Exp Toxicol Pathol. 51, 507-516.

[44] Creek, DJ., Charman, WN., Chiu, FC., Prankerd, RJ., Dong, Y., Vennerstrom, JL., Charman, SA. (2008) Relationship between antimalarial activity and heme alkylation for spiro- and dispiro-1,2,4-trioxolane antimalarials. Antimicrob Agents Chemother. 52, 1291-1296.

[45] Crespo-Ortiz, MP., Wei, MQ. (2012) Antitumor activity of artemisinin and its derivatives: from a well-known antimalarial agent to a potential anti-cancer drug. J Biomed Biotechnol. 2012:247597

[46] Culotta, E., Koshland, DE Jr. (1994) DNA repair works it works its way to the top. Science. 266, 1926-1929.

[47] Daniele, G., Corral, J., Molife, LR., de Bono, JS. (2012) FGF receptor inhibitors: role in cancer therapy. Curr Oncol Rep. 14, 111-119.

[48] Davis, TM., Phuong, HL., Ilett, KF., Hung, NC., Batty, KT., Phuong, VD., Powell, SM., Thien, HV., Binh, TQ. (2001) Pharmacokinetics and pharmacodynamics of intravenous artesunate in severe falciparum malaria. Antimicrob. Agents Chemother. 45, 181-186.

[49] Dell'Eva, R., Pfeffer, U., Vené, R., Anfosso, L., Forlani, A., Albini, A., Efferth, T. (2004) Inhibition of angiogenesis in vivo and growth of Kaposi's sarcoma xenograft tumors by the anti-malarial artesunate. Biochem. Pharmacol. 68, 2359–2366.

[50] Döme, B., Hendrix, M.J., Paku, S., Tóvári, J., Tímár, J. (2007) Alternative vascularization mechanisms in cancer: Pathology and therapeutic implications. Am. J. Pathol. 170, 1-15.

[51] Du, JH., Zhang, HD., Ma, ZJ., Ji, KM. (2010) Artesunate induces oncosis-like cell death In vitro and has antitumor activity against pancreatic cancer xenografts In vivo. Cancer Chemotherapy and Pharma. 65, 895–902.

[52] Dufraine, J., Funahashi, Y., Kitajewski, J. (2008) Notch signaling regulates tumor angiogenesis by diverse mechanisms. Oncogene. 27, 5132-5137.

[53] Eckstein-Ludwig, U., Webb, RJ., van Goethem, ID., East, JM., Lee, AG., Kimura, M., O'Neill, PM., Bray, PG., Ward, SA., Krishna, S. (2003) Artemisinins target the SERCA of Plasmodium falciparum. Nature, 424, 957-961.

[54] Eder, JP., Vande Woude, GF., Boerner, SA., LoRusso, PM. (2009) Novel therapeutic inhibitors of the c-Met signaling pathway in cancer. Clin Cancer Res. 15, 2207–2214.

[55] Efferth, T., Ruecker, G., Falkenberg, M., Manns, D., Olbrich, A., Fabry, U., Osieka, R. (1996) Detection of apoptosis in KG-1a leukemic cells treated with investigational drugs. Arzneimittelforschung. 46, 196–200.

[56] Efferth, T., Dunstan, H., Sauerbrey, A., Miyachi, H., Chitambar, CR. (2001) The anti–malarial artesunate is also active against cancer. Int. J. Oncol. 18, 767–773.

[57] Efferth, T., Davey, M., Olbrich, A., Rücker, G., Gebhart, E., Davey, R. (2002) Activity of drugs from traditional Chinese medicine toward sensitive and MDR1- or MRP1-overexpressing multidrug-resistant human CCRF-CEM leukemia cells. Blood Cells Mol. Dis., 28, 160-168.

[58] Efferth, T., Sauerbrey, A., Olbrich, A., Gebhart, E., Rauch, P., Weber, HO., Hengstler, JG., Halatsch, ME., Volm, M., Tew, KD., Ross, DD., Funk, JO. (2003) Molecular modes of action of artesunate in tumor cell lines. Mol Pharmacol. 64, 382-394.

[59] Efferth, T., Ramirez, T., Gebhart, E., Halatsch, ME. (2004a) Combination treatment of glioblastoma multiforme cell lines with the anti-malarial artesunate and the epidermal growth factor receptor tyrosine kinase inhibitor OSI-774. Biochem. Pharmacol., 67, 1689-1700.

[60] Efferth, T., Benakis, A., Romero, M.R., Tomicic, M., Rauh, R., Steinbach, D., Häfer, R., Stamminger, T., Oesch, F., Kaina, B., Marschall, M. (2004b) Enhancement of cytotoxicity of artemisinins toward cancer cells by ferrous iron. Free Radic. Biol. Med. 37, 998-1009.

[61] Efferth T. (2005) Mechanistic perspectives for 1,2,4-trioxanes in anti-cancer therapy. Drug Resist Updat. 8, 85-97.

[62] Efferth T. (2006) Molecular pharmacology and pharmacogenomics of artemisinin and its derivatives in cancer cells. Curr Drug Targets. 7, 407-421.

[63] Efferth T. (2007) Willmar Schwabe Award 2006: antiplasmodial and antitumor activity of artemisinin--from bench to bedside. Planta Med. 73, 299-309.

[64] Efferth, T., Giaisi, M., Merling, A., Krammer, P.H., Li-Weber, M. (2007) Artesunate induces ROS-mediated apoptosis in doxorubicin-resistant T leukemia cells. PLoS One. 2, e693.

[65] Efferth, T., Kaina, B. (2010) Toxicity of the antimalarial artemisinin and its derivatives. Crit Rev Toxicol. 40, 405-421

[66] Ellis, LM., Hicklin, DJ. (2008) VEGF-targeted therapy: mechanisms of anti-tumour activity. Nat Rev. 8, 579–591.

[67] Escudier, B., Eisen, T., Stadler, WM., Szczylik, C., Oudard, S., Siebels, M., Negrier, S., Chevreau, C., Solska, E., Desai, AA., Rolland, F., Demkow, T., Hutson, TE., Gore, M., Freeman, S., Schwartz, B., Shan, M., Simantov, R., Bukowski, RM. TARGET Study Group. (2007) Sorafenib in advanced clear-cell renal-cell carcinoma. N Engl J Med. 356, 125-134.

[68] Feng, FS., Guantai, EM., Nell, MJ., van Rensburg, CE., Hoppe, H., Chibale, K. (2000) Antiplasmodial and antitumor activity of dDHA analogs derived via the aza-Michael addition reaction. Bioorganic and Medicinal Chemistry Letters, 21, 2882–2886.

[69] Ferrara, N., Gerber, HP., LeCouter, J. (2003) The biology of VEGF and its receptors. Nat Med. 9, 669-676.

[70] Ferrara, N. (2009) Vascular endothelial growth factor. Arterioscler Thromb Vasc Biol 29, 789–791.

[71] Ferrara, N. (2010) Pathways mediating VEGF-independent tumor angiogenesis. Cytokine Growth Factor Rev. 21, 21-26.

[72] Firestone, GL., Sundar, SN. (2009) Anti-cancer activities of artemisinin and its bioactive derivatives. Expert Rev Mol Med. 30, 11:e32.

[73] Galal, AM., Gul, W., Slade, D., Ross, SA., Feng, S., Hollingshead, MG,, Alley, MC., Kaur, G., ElSohly, MA. (2009) Synthesis and evaluation of dihydroartemisinin and dihydroartemisitene acetal dimers showing anti-cancer and antiprotozoal activity. Bioorg Med Chem. 17, 741-751.

[74] Galustian, C., Dalgleish, A. (2009) Lenalidomide: a novel anti-cancer drug with multiple modalities. Expert Opin. Pharmacother. 10, 125-133.

[75] Garcia, A., Kandel, JJ. (2012) Notch: a key regulator of tumor angiogenesis and metastasis. Histol Histopathol. 27, 151-156.

[76] Gardlik, R., Celec, P., Bernadic, M. (2011a) Targeting angiogenesis for cancer (gene) therapy. Bratisl Lek Listy. 112, 428-434.

[77] Gardlik, R., Behuliak, M., Palffy, R., Celec, P., Li, CJ. (2011b) Gene therapy for cancer: bacteria-mediated anti-angiogenesis therapy. Gene Ther. 18, 425-431.

[78] Gatter, KC., Brown, G., Trowbridge, IS., Woolston, RE., Mason, DY. (1983) Transferrin receptors in human tissues: their distribution and possible clinical relevance J. Clin. Pathol., 36, 539-545.

[79] Geyer, HJ., Scheuntert, I., Rapp, K., Kettrup, A., Korte, F., Greim, H., Rozman, K. (1990) Correlation between acute toxicity of 2,3,7,8-tetrachlorodibenzo-p-dioxin (TCDD) and total body fat content in mammals. Toxicology 65, 97-107.

[80] Gordon, MS., Mendelson, DS., Kato, G. (2010) Tumor angiogenesis and novel antiangiogenic strategies. Int J Cancer. 126, 1777-1787.

[81] Gravett, AM., Liu, WM., Krishna, S., Chan, WC., Haynes, RK., Wilson, NL., Dalgleish, AG. (2011) In vitro study of the anti-cancer effects of artemisone alone or in com-

bination with other chemotherapeutic agents. Cancer Chemother Pharmacol. 67, 569-577.

[82] Hait, NC., Allegood, J., Maceyka, M., Strub, GM., Harikumar, KB., Singh, SK., Luo, C., Marmorstein, R., Kordula, T., Milstien, S., Spiegel, S. (2009) Regulation of histone acetylation in the nucleus by sphingosine-1-phosphate. Science 325, 1254–1257.

[83] El Hallani, S., Boisselier, B., Peglion, F., Rousseau, A., Colin, C., Idbaih, A., Marie, Y., Mokhtari, K., Thomas, JL., Eichmann, A., Delattre, JY., Maniotis, AJ., Sanson, M. (2010) A new alternative mechanism in glioblastoma vascularization: tubular vasculogenic mimicry. Brain 133, 973–982.

[84] Handrick, R., Ontikatze, T., Bauer, KD., Freier, F., Rubel, A., Durig, J., Belka, C., Jendrossek, V. (2010) Dihydroartemisinin induces apoptosis by a Bak-dependent intrinsic pathway. Mol Cancer Ther. 9, 2497-2510.

[85] He, Q., Shi, J., Shen, XL., An, J., Sun, H., Wang, L., Hu, YJ., Sun, Q., Fu, LC., Sheikh, MS., Huang, Y. (2010) Dihydroartemisinin upregulates death receptor 5 expression and cooperates with TRAIL to induce apoptosis in human prostate cancer cells. Cancer Biol Ther. 9, 819-824.

[86] He, Y., Fan, J., Lin, H., Yang, X., Ye, Y., Liang, L., Zhan, Z., Dong, X., Sun, L., Xu, H. (2011) The anti-malaria agent artesunate inhibits expression of vascular endothelial growth factor and hypoxia-inducible factor-1α in human rheumatoid arthritis fibroblast-like synoviocyte. Rheumatol. Int. 31, 53-60.

[87] Hou, J., Wang, D., Zhang, R., Wang, H. (2008) Experimental therapy of hepatoma with artemisinin and Its derivatives: In vitro and In vivo activity, chemosensitization, and mechanisms of action. Clinical Cancer Research, 14, 5519–5530.

[88] Hsu, E. (2006) The history of qinghao in the Chinese materia medica. Trans. R. Soc. Trop. Med. Hyg. 100, 505-508.

[89] Huan-Huan, C., Li-Li, Y., Shang-Bin, L. (2004) Artesunate reduces chicken chorioallantoic membrane neovascularisation and exhibits anti-angiogenic and apoptotic activity on human microvascular dermal endothelial cell. Cancer Lett. 211, 163–173.

[90] Huang, XJ., Li, CT., Zhang, WP., Lu, YB., Fang, SH., Wei, EQ. (2008) Dihydroartemisinin potentiates the cytotoxic effect of temozolomide in rat C6 glioma cells. Pharmacology. 82, 1-9.

[91] Hurwitz, H., Fehrenbacher, L., Novotny, W., Cartwright, T., Hainsworth, J., Heim, W., Berlin, J., Baron, A., Griffing, S., Holmgren, E., Ferrara, N., Fyfe, G., Rogers, B., Ross, R., Kabbinavar, F. (2004) Bevacizumab plus irinotecan, fluorouracil, and leucovorin for metastatic colorectal cancer. N Engl J Med. 350, 2335-2342.

[92] Hwang, YP., Yun, HJ., Kim, HG., Han, EH., Lee, GW., Jeong, HG. (2010) Suppression of PMA-induced tumor cell invasion by dihydroartemisinin via inhibition of PKCalpha/Raf/MAPKs and NF-kappaB/AP-1-dependent mechanisms. Biochem Pharmacol. 79, 1714-1726.

[93] Ichihara, E., Kiura, K., Tanimoto, M. (2011) Targeting angiogenesis in cancer therapy. Acta Med Okayama. 65, 353-362.

[94] Jefford, CW. (2007) New developments in synthetic peroxidic drugs as artemisinin mimics," Drug Discovery Today, 12, 487–495.

[95] Jeong, SJ., Itokawa, T., Shibuya, M., Kuwano, M., Ono, M., Higuchi, R., Miyamoto, T. (2002) Costunolide, a sesquiterpene lactone from Saussurea lappa, inhibits the VEGFR KDR/Flk-1 signaling pathway. Cancer Lett. 187, 129-133.

[96] Ji, Y., Zhang, YC., Pei, LB., Shi, LL., Yan, JL., Ma, XH. (2011) Anti-tumor effects of dihydroartemisinin on human osteosarcoma," Molecular and Cellular Biochemistry, 351, 99–108.

[97] Jiao, J., Ge, CM., Meng, QH., Cao, JP., Tong, J., Fan, SJ (2007) Dihydroartemisinin is an inhibitor of ovarian cancer cell growth," Acta Pharmacologica Sinica, 28, 1045–1056.

[98] Jorgensen, RJ. (1980) Dictyocaulus viviparous: Migration in agar of larvae subjected to a variety of physicochemical exposure. Exp. Parasit. 49, 106-115.

[99] Jung, M., Lee, S., Ham, J., Lee, K., Kim, H., Kim, SK. (2003) Antitumor activity of novel deoxoartemisinin monomers, dimers, and trimer. J Med Chem. 46, 987-994.

[100] Khanh, NX., de Vries, PJ., Ha, LD., van Boxtel, CJ., Koopmans, R., Kager, PA. (1999) Declining concentrations of dihydroartemisinin in plasma during 5-day oral treatment with artesunate for falciparum malaria. Antimicrob Agents Chemother. 43, 690-692.

[101] Kim, SH., Kim, HJ., Kim, TS. (2003) Differential involvement of protein kinase C in human promyelocytic leukemia cell differentiation enhanced by artemisinin. Eur. J. Pharmacol. 482, 67–76.

[102] Kim, SJ., Kim, MS., Lee, JW., Lee, CH., Yoo, H., Shin, SH., Park, MJ., Lee, SH. (2006) Dihydroartemisinin enhances radiosensitivity of human glioma cells in vitro. J Cancer Res Clin Oncol. 132, 129-135.

[103] Kim, YC., Lee, MK., Sung, SH., Kim, SH. (2007) Sesquiterpenes from Ulmus davidiana var. japonica with the inhibitory effects on lipopolysaccharide-induced nitric oxide production. Fitoterapia. 78, 196-199.

[104] Kimbrough, RD. (1990) How toxic is 2,3,7,8-tetrachlorodibenzodioxin to humans? J. Toxicol. Environ. Health. 30, 261-271.

[105] Korc, M., Friesel, RE. (2009) The role of fibroblast growth factors in tumor growth. Curr Cancer Drug Targets. 9, 639-651.

[106] Krishna, S., Uhlemann, AC., Haynes, RK. (2004) Artemisinins: mechanisms of action and potential for resistance. Drug Resist Updat. 7, 233-244.

[107] Krishna, S., Bustamante, L., Haynes, RK., Staines, HM. (2008) Artemisinins: their growing importance in medicine. Trends Pharmacol Sci. 29, 520-527.

[108] Lai, H., Singh, NP. (1995) Selective cancer cell cytotoxicity from exposure to dihydroartemisinin and holotransferrin. Cancer Lett. 91, 41-46.

[109] Lai, H., Sasaki, T., Singh, NP., Messay, A. (2005) Effects of artemisinin-tagged holotransferrin on cancer cells. Life Sci., 76, 1267-1279.

[110] Lai, H., Nakase, I., Lacoste, E., Singh, NP., Sasaki, T. (2009) Artemisinin-transferrin conjugate retards growth of breast tumors in the rat. Anti-cancer Res. 29, 3807-3810.

[111] Lee, CH., Hong, H., Shin, J., Jung, M., Shin, I., Yoon, J., Lee, W. (2000) NMR studies on novel antitumor drug candidates, deoxoartemisinin and carboxypropyldeoxoartemisinin. Biochem Biophys Res Commun. 274, 359-369.

[112] Lee, J., Zhou, HJ., Wu, XH. (2006) Dihydroartemisinin downregulates vascular endothelial growth factor expression and induces apoptosis in chronic myeloid leukemia K562 cells. Cancer Chemother. Pharmacol. 57, 213-220.

[113] Li, JL., Harris, AL. (2009) Crosstalk of VEGF and notch pathways in tumor angiogenesis: therapeutic implications. Front Biosci. 14, 3094–3110.

[114] Li, PC., Lam, E., Roos, WP., Zdzienicka, MZ., Kaina, B., Efferth, T. (2008) Artesunate derived from traditional Chinese medicine induces DNA damage and repair. Cancer Research. 68, 4347-4351.

[115] Li, Q., Peggins, JO., Fleckenstein, LL., Masonic, K., Heiffer, MH., Brewer, TG. (1998) The pharmacokinetics and bioavailability of dihydroartemisinin, arteether, artemether, artesunic acid and artelinic acid in rats. J Pharm Pharmacol. 50, 173-182.

[116] Li, QG., Mog, SR., Si, YZ., Kyle, DE., Gettayacamin, M., Milhous, WK. (2002) Neurotoxicity and efficacy of arteether related to its exposure times and exposure levels in rodents. Am. J. Trop. Med. Hyg. 66, 516-525.

[117] Li, Q., Milhous, WK., Weina, PJ. (2006) Fatal neurotoxicity of the artemisinin derivatives is related to drug pharmacokinetic profiles in animal species. Curr. Topics. Toxicol, 3, 1-16.

[118] Li, Q., Milhous, WK., Weina, PJ. Eds. (2007a) Antimalarial in Malaria Therapy. Nova Science Publishers Inc, New York; 1st edition. pp.1-133.

[119] Li, Q., Si, Y., Smith, KS., Zeng, Q., Weina, PJ. (2008) Embryotoxicity of artesunate in animal species related to drug tissue distribution and toxicokinetic profiles. Birth Defects Res. B Dev. Reprod. Toxicol. 83, 435-445.

[120] Li, Q., Si, YZ., Xie, LH., Zhang, J., Weina, P. (2009) Severe embryolethality of artesunate related to pharmacokinetics following intravenous and intramuscular doses in pregnant rats. Birth Defects Res. B Dev. Reprod. Toxicol. 86, 385–393.

[121] Li, Q., Weina, P. (2010a) Artesunate: the best drug in the treatments of severe and complicated malaria. Pharmaceuticals. 3, 2322-2332.

[122] Li, Q., Weina, P. (2010b) Severe embryotoxicity of artemisinin derivatives in experimental animals, but possibly safe in pregnant women. Molecules. 15, 40-57.

[123] Li Q, Hickman M. (2011) Toxicokinetic and toxicodynamic (TK/TD) evaluation to determine and predict the neurotoxicity of artemisinins. Toxicology. 279, 1-9.

[124] Li, Q., Weina P. (2011) Antimalarial in Drugs: Age of the Artemisinins. Edited by Qigui Li & Peter Weina. Nova Science Publishers Inc, New York; 1st edition (August 2011), 1-645 pages. ISBN-978-1-61761-851-2.

[125] Li, Q, Hickman, M., Weina, P. (2011) Chapter 8: Therapeutic and Toxicological Inhibition of Vasculogenesis and Angiogenesis Mediated by Artesunate, a Compound with both Antimalarial and Anti-cancer Efficacy. Eds. Dan T. Simionescu and Agneta Simionescu. in "Vasculogenesis and Angiogensis" InTech Open Access Publisher, Rijeka. Page 145-184

[126] Li, Y., Shan, F., Wu, JM., Wu, GS., Ding, J., Xiao, D., Yang, WY., Atassi, G., Leonce, S., Caignard, DH., Renard, P. (2001) Novel antitumor artemisinin derivatives targeting G1 phase of the cell cycle. Bioorg. Med. Chem. Lett., 11, 5-8.

[127] Lijuan, W. (2010) Effect of artesunate on human endometrial carcinoma. Journal of-Medical Colleges of PLA, 25, 143–151.

[128] Liu, WM. (2008) Enhancing the cytotoxic activity of novel targeted therapies--is there a role for a combinatorial approach? Curr. Clin. Pharmacol. 3, 108-117

[129] Liu, WM., Gravett, AM., Dalgleish, AG. (2011) The antimalarial agent artesunate possesses anti-cancer properties that can be enhanced by combination strategies. Int. J. Cancer. 128, 1471-1480.

[130] Lobov, IB., Renard, RA., Papadopoulos, N., Gale, NW., Thurston, G., Yancopoulos, GD., Wiegand, SJ. (2007) Delta-like ligand 4 (Dll4) is induced by VEGF as a negative regulator of angiogenic sprouting. Proc Natl Acad Sci U S A. 104, 3219-3224.

[131] Longo, M., Zanoncelli, S., Torre, PD., Riflettuto, M., Cocco, F., Pesenti, M., Giusti, A., Colombo, P., Brughera, M., Mazué, G., Navaratman, V., Gomes, M., Olliaro, P. (2006a) In vivo and in vitro investigations of the effects of the antimalarial drug dihydroartemisinin (DHA) on rat embryos. Reprod. Toxicol. 22, 797-810.

[132] Longo, M., Zanoncelli, S., Manera, D., Brughera, M., Colombo, P., Lansen, J., Mazué, G., Gomes, M., Taylor, WR., Olliaro, P. (2006b) Effects of the antimalarial drug dihydroartemisinin (DHA) on rat embryos in vitro. Reprod. Toxicol. 21, 83-93.

[133] Longo, M., Zanoncelli, S., Torre PD., Rosa, F., Giusti, A., Colombo, P., Brughera, M., Mazué, G., Olliaro, P. (2008) Investigations of the effects of the antimalarial drug dihydroartemisinin (DHA) using the Frog Embryo Teratogenesis Assay-Xenopus (FETAX). Reprod. Toxicol. 25, 433-441.

[134] Lu, JJ., Meng, LH., Cai, YJ., Chen, Q., Tong, LJ., Lin, LP., Ding, J. (2008) Dihydroartemisinin induces apoptosis in HL-60 leukemia cells dependent of iron and p38 mitogen-activated protein kinase activation but independent of reactive oxygen species. Cancer Biol Ther. 7, 1017-1023.

[135] Lu, JJ., Meng, LH., hankavaram, UT., Zhu, CH., Tong, LJ., Chen, G., Lin, LP., Weinstein, JN., Ding, J. (2010) Dihydroartemisinin accelerates c-MYC oncoprotein degradation and induces apoptosis in c-MYC-overexpressing tumor cells. Biochem Pharmacol. 80, 22-30.

[136] Lu, JJ., Chen, SM., Zhang, XW., Ding, J., Meng, LH. (2011) The anti-cancer activity of dihydroartemisinin is associated with induction of iron-dependent endoplasmic reticulum stress in colorectal carcinoma HCT116 cells. Invest New Drugs. 29, 1276-1283.

[137] Lu, YY., Chen, TS., Qu, JL., Pan, WL., Sun, L., Wei, XB. (2009) Dihydroartemisinin (DHA) induces caspase-3-dependent apoptosis in human lung adenocarcinoma ASTC-a-1 cells," Journal of Biomedical Science, 16, 16.

[138] Makrilia, N., Lappa, T., Xyla, V., Nikolaidis, I., Syrigos, K. (2009) The role of angiogenesis in solid tumours: an overview. Eur J Intern Med. 20, 663-671.

[139] McDonald 3rd., ER., El-Deiry, WS. (2000) Cell cycle control as a basis for cancer drug development (Review)," International Journal of Oncology, 16, 871–886.

[140] Mercer, AE., Copple, IM., Maggs, JL., O'Neill, PM., Park, BK. (2011) The role of heme and the mitochondrion in the chemical and molecular mechanisms of mammalian cell death induced by the artemisinin antimalarials. J Biol Chem. 286, 987-996.

[141] Molinari, AJ., Pozzi, EC., Monti, Hughes. A., Heber, EM., Garabalino, MA., Thorp, SI., Miller, M., Itoiz, ME., Aromando, RF., Nigg, DW., Trivillin, VA., Schwint, AE. (2012) Tumor blood vessel "normalization" improves the therapeutic efficacy of boron neutron capture therapy (BNCT) in experimental oral cancer. Radiat Res. 177, 59-68.

[142] Moore, JC., Lai, H., Li, JR., Ren, RL., McDougall, JA., Singh, NP., Chou, CK. (1995) Oral administration of dihydroartemisinin and ferrous sulfate retarded implanted fibrosarcoma growth in the rat. Cancer Lett., 98, 83-87.

[143] Morrissey, C., Gallis, B., Solazzi, JW., Kim, BJ., Gulati, R., Vakar-Lopez, F., Goodlett, DR., Vessella, RL., Sasaki, T. (2010) Effect of artemisinin derivatives on apoptosis and cell cycle in prostate cancer cells. Anti-cancer Drugs. 21, 423-432.

[144] Motzer, RJ., Michaelson, MD., Redman, BG., Hudes, GR., Wilding, G., Figlin, RA., Ginsberg, MS., Kim, ST., Baum, CM., DePrimo, SE., Li, JZ., Bello, CL., Theuer, CP., George, DJ., Rini, BI. (2006) Activity of SU11248, a multitargeted inhibitor of vascular endothelial growth factor receptor and platelet-derived growth factor receptor, in patients with metastatic renal cell carcinoma. J Clin Oncol 24, 16-24.

[145] Motzer, RJ., Hutson, TE., Tomczak, P., Michaelson, MD., Bukowski, RM., Rixe, O., Oudard, S., Negrier, S., Szczylik, C., Kim, ST., Chen, I., Bycott, PW., Baum, CM., Figlin, RA. (2007) Sunitinib versus interferon alfa in metastatic renal-cell carcinoma. N Engl J Med. 356, 115–124.

[146] Munaut, C., Colige, AC., Lambert, CA. (2010) Alternative splicing: a promising target for pharmaceutical inhibition of pathological angiogenesis? Curr Pharm Des. 16, 3864-3876

[147] Muramatsu, M., Yamamoto, S., Osawa, T., Shibuya, M. (2010) Vascular endothelial growth factor receptor-1 signaling promotes mobilization of macrophage lineage cells from bone marrow and stimulates solid tumor growth. Cancer Res. 70, 8211-8221.

[148] Navaratnam, V., Mansor, SM., Sit, NW., Grace, J., Li, QG., Olliaro, P. (2000) Pharmacokinetics of artemisinin-type compounds. Clin. Pharmacokinet. 39, 255-270.

[149] Nissen, LJ., Cao, R., Hedlund, EM., Wang, Z., Zhao, X., Wetterskog, D., Funa, K., Bråkenhielm, E., Cao, Y. (2007) Angiogenic factors FGF2 and PDGF-BB synergistically promote murine tumor neovascularization and metastasis. J Clin Invest. 117, 2766-2777.

[150] Nosten, F., vanVugt, M., Price, RN., Luxemburger, C., Thway, KL., Brockman, A., McGready, R., ter Kuile, F., Looareesuwan, S., White, NJ. (2000) Effects of artesunate-mefloquine combination on incidence of Plasmodium falciparum malaria and mefloquine resistance in western Thailand: A prospective study. Lancet. 356, 297-302.

[151] Oh, S., Jeong, IH., Ahn, CM., Shin, WS., Lee, S. (2004) Synthesis and anti-angiogenic activity of thioacetal artemisinin derivatives. Bioorg. Med. Chem. 12, 3783–3790.

[152] Ohgami, Y., Elstad, CA., Chung, E., Shirachi, DY., Quock, RM., Lai, HC. (2010) Effect of hyperbaric oxygen on the anti-cancer effect of artemisinin on molt-4 human leukemia cells. Anti-cancer Res. 30, 4467-4470.

[153] Olsson, AK., Dimberg, A., Kreuger, J., Claesson-Welsh, L. (2006) VEGF receptor signalling - in control of vascular function. Nat Rev Mol Cell Biol. 7, 359-371.

[154] O'Neill, PM., Posner, GH. (2004) A medicinal chemistry perspective on artemisinin and related endoperoxides. J. Med. Chem., 47, 2945-2964.

[155] Oon, CE., Harris, AL. (2011) New pathways and mechanisms regulating and responding to Delta-like ligand 4-Notch signalling in tumour angiogenesis. Biochem Soc Trans. 39, 1612-1618.

[156] Opsenica, D., Pocsfalvi, G., Juranic, Z., Tinant, B., Declercq, JP., Kyle, DE., Milhous, WK., Solaja, BA. (2000) Cholic acid derivatives as 1,2,4,5-tetraoxane carriers: structure and antimalarial and antiproliferative activity. J Med Chem. 43, 3274-3282.

[157] O'Reilly, MS., Holmgren, L., Shing, Y., Chen, C., Rosenthal, RA., Cao, Y., Moses, M., Lane, WS., Sage, EH., Folkman, J. (1994) Angiostatin: a circulating endothelial cell in-

hibitor that suppresses angiogenesis and tumor growth. Cold Spring Harb Symp Quant Biol. 59, 471-482.

[158] Park, BK., O'Neill, PN., Maggs, JL., Pirmohamed, M. (1998) Safety assessment of peroxide antimalarials: Clinical and chemical perspectives. Br J Clin Pharmacol. 46, 521-529.

[159] Parapini, S., Basilico, N., Mondani, M., Olliaro, P., Taramelli, D., Monti, D. (2004) Evidence that haem iron in the malaria parasite is not needed for the antimalarial effects of artemisinin. FEBS Lett., 575, 91-94.

[160] Pardali, E., ten Dijke, P. (2009) Transforming growth factor-beta signaling and tumor angiogenesis. Front Biosci. 14, 4848-4861.

[161] Payne, AG. (2003) Exploiting intracellular iron and iron-rich compounds to effect tumor cell lysis Med. Hypotheses, 61, 206-209.

[162] Pezzolo, A., Parodi, F., Marimpietri, D., Raffaghello, L., Cocco, C., Pistorio, A., Mosconi, M., Gambini, C., Cilli, M., Deaglio, S., Malavasi, F., and Pistoia, V. (2011) Oct-4+/Tenascin C+ neuroblastoma cells serve as progenitors of tumor-derived endothelial cells. Cell Res. 21, 1470-1486.

[163] Price, RN. (2000) Artemisinin drugs: Novel antimalarial agents. Expert Opin. Investig. Drugs. 9, 1815-1827.

[164] Radloff, PD., Philipps, J., Nkeyi, M., Sturchler, D., Mittelholzer, ML., Kremsner, PG. (1996) Arteflene compared with mefloquine for treating Plasmodium falciparum malaria in children. Am J Trop Med Hyg. 55, 259-262.

[165] Ramirez, AP., Thomas, AM., Woerpel, KA. (2009) Preparation of bicyclic 1,2,4-trioxanes from γ,δ-unsaturated ketones. Organic Letters, 11, 507–510.

[166] Rangan, U., Hedli, C., Gallo, M., Lioy, P., Snyder, R. (1997) Exposure and risk assessment with respect to contaminated soil: Significance of biomarkers and bioavailability. Int. J. Toxicol. 16, 419-432.

[167] Rasheed, SA., Efferth, T., Asangani, IA., Allgayer, H. (2010) First evidence that the antimalarial drug artesunate inhibits invasion and in vivo metastasis in lung cancer by targeting essential extracellular proteases. Int J Cancer. 127, 1475-1485.

[168] Ribatti, D. (2008) The discovery of the placental growth factor and its role in angiogenesis: a Historical review. Angiogenesis. 11, 215–221.

[169] Ribatti, D. (2011) Vascular normalization: a real benefit? Cancer Chemother Pharmacol. 68, 275-278.

[170] Ridgway, J., Zhang, G., Wu, Y., Stawicki, S., Liang, WC., Chanthery, Y., Kowalski, J., Watts, RJ., Callahan, C., Kasman I., Singh, M., Chien, M., Tan, C., Hongo, JA., de Sauvage, F., Plowman, G., Yan, M. (2006) Inhibition of Dll4 signalling inhibits tumour growth by deregulating angiogenesis. Nature. 444, 1083-1087.

[171] Rivard, A., Fabre, JE., Silver, M., Chen, D., Murohara, T., Kearney, M., Magner, M., Asahara, T., Isner, JM. (1999) Age-dependent impairment of angiogenesis. Circulation. 99, 111-120.

[172] Roll Back Malaria. (2008) The RBM partnership's global response; a programmatic strategy 2004–2008. Available at: http://rbm.who.int/partnership/board/meetings/docs/strategy_rev.pdf (accessed December 2010).

[173] Rolny, C., Mazzone, M., Tugues, S., Laoui, D., Johansson, I., Coulon, C., Squadrito, ML., Segura, I., Li, X., Knevels, E., Costa, S., Vinckier, S., Dresselaer, T., Åkerud, P., De Mol, M., Salomäki, H., Phillipson, M., Wyns, S., Larsson, E., Buysschaert, I., Botling, J., Himmelreich, U., Van Ginderachter, JA., De Palma, M., Dewerchin, M., Claesson-Welsh, L., Carmeliet, P. (2011) HRG inhibits tumor growth and metastasis by inducing macrophage polarization and vessel normalization through downregulation of PlGF. Cancer Cell. 19, 31-44.

[174] Rozman, KK. (1998) Quantitative definition of toxicity: a mathematical description of life and death with dose and time as variables. Med. Hypotheses. 51, 175-178.

[175] Rozman, KK., Doull, J. (2000) Dose and time as variable of toxicity. Toxicology. 144, 169-178.

[176] Sadava, D., Phillips, T., Lin, C., Kane, SE. (2002) Transferrin overcomes drug resistance to artemisinin in human small-cell lung carcinoma cells. Cancer Lett. 179, 151-156.

[177] Scehnet, JS., Jiang, W., Kumar, SR., Krasnoperov, V., Trindade, A., Benedito, R., Djokovic, D., Borges, C., Ley, EJ., Duarte, A., Gill, PS. (2007) Inhibition of Dll4-mediated signaling induces proliferation of immature vessels and results in poor tissue perfusion. Blood. 109, 4753-4760.

[178] Schmidt, T., Carmeliet, P. (2011) Angiogenesis: a target in solid tumors, also in leukemia? Hematology Am Soc Hematol Educ Program. 2011, 1-8.

[179] Schmuck, G., Klaus, AM., Krötlinger, F., Langewische, FW. (2009) Developmental and reproductive toxicity studies on artemisone. Birth Defects Res. B Dev. Reprod Toxicol. 86, 131-143.

[180] Semenov, A., Olson, JE., Rosenthal, PJ. (1998) Antimalarial synergy of cysteine and aspartic protease inhibitors Antimicrob. Agents Chemother., 42, 2554-2558.

[181] Sertel, S., Eichhorn, T., Sieber, S., Sauer, A., Weiss, J., Plinkert, PK., Efferth, T. (2010) Factors determining sensitivity or resistance of tumor cell lines towards artesunate. Chem Biol Interact. 185, 42-52.

[182] Shenai, BR., Sijwali, PS., Singh, A., Rosenthal, PJ. (2000) Characterization of native and recombinant falcipain-2, a principal trophozoite cysteine protease and essential hemoglobinase of Plasmodium falciparum J. Biol. Chem., 275, 29000-29010.

[183] Shirakawa, K., Takara, K., Tanigawara, Y., Aoyama, N., Kasuga, M., Komada, F., Sakaeda, T., Okumura, K. (1999) Interaction of docetaxel ("Taxotere") with human P-glycoprotein. Jpn. J. Cancer Res., 90, 1380-1386.

[184] Shterman, N., Kupfer, B., Moroz, C. (1991) Comparison of transferrin receptors, iron content and isoferritin profile in normal and malignant human breast cell lines. Pathobiology, 59, 19-25.

[185] Sieber, S., Gdynia, G., Roth, W., Bonavida, B., Efferth, T. (2009) Combination treatment of malignant B cells using the anti-CD20 antibody rituximab and the anti-malarial artesunate. Int. J. Oncol. 35, 149-158.

[186] Singh, H., Milner, CS. (2009) Aguilar Hernandez MM, Patel N, Brindle NP. Vascular endothelial growth factor activates the Tie family of receptor tyrosine kinases. Cell Signal. 21, 1346-1350.

[187] Singh, NP., Lai, H. (2001) Selective toxicity of dihydroartemisinin and holotransferrin toward human breast cancer cells. Life Sci., 70, 49-56.

[188] Singh, NP., Lai, HC. (2004) Artemisinin induces apoptosis in human cancer cells. Anti-cancer Res., 24, 2277-2280.

[189] Singh, NP., Lai, HC. (2005) Synergistic cytotoxicity of artemisinin and sodium butyrate on human cancer cells. Anti-cancer Res. 25, 4325-4331.

[190] Singh, NP., Panwar, VK. (2006) Case report of a pituitary macroadenoma treated with artemether. Integr. Cancer Ther. 5, 391-394.

[191] Singh, NP., Verma, KB. (2002) Case report of a laryngeal squamous cell carcinoma treated with artesunate. Arch Oncol. 10, 279-280.

[192] Soomro, S., Langenberg, T., Mahringer, A., Konkimalla, VB., Horwedel, C., Holenya, P., Brand, A., Cetin, C., Fricker, G., Dewerchin, M., Carmeliet, P., Conway, EM., Jansen, H., Efferth, T. (2011) Design of novel artemisinin-like derivatives with cytotoxic and anti-angiogenic properties. J Cell Mol Med. 15, 1122-1135.

[193] Stockwin, LH., Han, B., Yu, SX., Hollingshead, MG., ElSohly, MA., Gul, W., Slade, D., Galal, AM., Newton, DL., Bumke, MA. (2009) Artemisinin dimer anti-cancer activity correlates with heme-catalyzed reactive oxygen species generation and endoplasmic reticulum stress induction. Int J Cancer. 125, 1266-1275.

[194] Sutherland, R., Delia, D., Schneider, C., Newman, R., Kemshead, J., Greaves, M. (1981) Proc. Natl. Acad. Sci. U.S.A., 78, 4515-4519.

[195] Tan, W., Lu, J., Huang, M., Li, Y., Chen, M., Wu, G., Gong, J., Zhong, Z., Xu, Z., Dang, Y., Guo, J., Chen, X., Wang, Y. (2011) Anti-cancer natural products isolated from chinese medicinal herbs. Chin Med. 6, 27.

[196] Tang, HS., Feng, YJ., Yao, LQ. (2009) Angiogenesis, vasculogenesis, and vasculogenic mimicry in ovarian cancer.

[197] Int J Gynecol Cancer. 19, 605-610.

[198] Taylor, DK., Avery, TD., Greatrex BW., Tiekink, ER., Macreadie, IG., Macreadie, PI., Humphries, AD., Kalkanidis, M., Fox, EN., Klonis, N., Tilley, L. (2004) Novel endoperoxide antimalarials: synthesis, heme binding, and antimalarial activity," Journal of Medicinal Chemistry, 47, 1833–1839.

[199] Teicher, BA., Fricker, SP. (2010) CXCL12 (SDF-1)/CXCR4 pathway in cancer. Clin Cancer Res. 16, 2927–2931.

[200] Teicher, BA. (2011) Anti-angiogenic agents and targets: A perspective. Biochem Pharmacol. 81, 6-12.

[201] Thomas, M., Augustin, HG. (2009) The role of the Angiopoietins in vascular morphogenesis. Angiogenesis. 12, 125-137.

[202] Thurston, G. (2002) Complementary actions of VEGF and angiopoietin-1 on blood vessel growth and leakage. J Anat. 200, 575-580.

[203] Tischer, E., Mitchell, R., Hartman, T., Silva, M., Gospodarowicz, D., Fiddes, JC., Abraham, JA. (1991) The human gene for vascular endothelial growth factor. Multiple protein forms are encoded through alternative exon splicing. J Biol Chem. 266, 11947-11954.

[204] Turner, N., Grose, R. (2010) Fibroblast growth factor signalling: from development to cancer. Nat Rev Cancer. 10, 116-129.

[205] Van de Veire, S., Stalmans, I., Heindryckx, F., Oura, H., Tijeras-Raballand, A., Schmidt T. (2010) Further pharmacological and genetic evidence for the efficacy of PlGF inhibition in cancer and eye disease. Cell, 141, 178–190.

[206] Vogelstein, B., Kinzler, KW. (2004) Cancer genes and the pathways they control. Nature Medicine. 10, 789–799.

[207] Wang, J., Guo, Y., Zhang, BC., Chen, ZT., Gao, JF. (2007) Induction of apoptosis and inhibition of cell migration and tube-like formation by dihydroartemisinin in murine lymphatic endothelial cells. Pharmacology. 80, 207-218.

[208] Wang, J., Zhang, B., Guo, Y., Li, G., Xie, Q., Zhu, B., Gao, J., Chen, Z. (2008) Artemisinin inhibits tumor lymphangiogenesis by suppression of vascular endothelial growth factor C. Pharmacology. 82, 148-155.

[209] Wang, Q., Wu, LM., Zhao, Y., Zhang, XL., Wang, NP. (2002) The anti-cancer effect of artesunate and its mechanism. Yao Xue Xue Bao, 37, 477-478.

[210] Wang, R., Chadalavada, K., Wilshire, J., Kowalik, U., Hovinga, K. E., Geber, A., Fligelman, B., Leversha, M., Brennan, C., Tabar, V. (2010) Glioblastoma stem-like cells give rise to tumor endothelium. Nature. 468, 829–833

[211] Wang, SJ., Gao, Y., Chen H. (2010) Dihydroartemisinin inactivatesNF-κB and potentiates the anti-tumor effect of gemcitabine on pancreatic cancer both In vitro and In vivo. Cancer Letters, 293, 99–108.

[212] Wang, SJ., Sun, B., Cheng, ZX., Zhou, HX., Gao, Y., Kong, R., Chen, H., Jiang, HC., Pan, SH., Xue, DB., Bai, XW. (2011) Dihydroartemisinin inhibits angiogenesis in pancreatic cancer by targeting the NF-κB pathway. Cancer Chemother Pharmacol. 68, 1421-1430.

[213] Wang, TY. (1989) Follow-up observation on the therapeutic effects and remote reactions of artemisinin (Qinghaosu) and artemether in treating malaria in pregnant woman. J. Tradit. Chin. Med. 9, 28-30.

[214] Wartenberg, M., Wolf, S., Budde, P., Grünheck, F., Acker, H., Hescheler, J., Wartenberg, G., Sauer, H. (2003) The antimalaria agent artemisinin exerts anti-angiogenic effects in mouse embryonic stem cell-derived embryoid bodies. Lab Invest. 83, 1647-1655.

[215] White, CL. (2002) Cancer Smart Bomb, Part I and II: An idea from ancient Chinese medicine. 2002, http://www.mwt.net/~drbrewer/canart1.htm

[216] White, NJ., Olliaro, P. (1998) Artemisinin and derivatives in the treatment of uncomplicated malaria. Med. Trop. (Mars.). 58 (Suppl. 3), 54-56.

[217] White, NJ. (1999a) Antimalarial drug resistance and combination chemotherapy. Philos. Trans. R. Soc. Lond. B. Biol. Sci. 354, 739-749.

[218] White, NJ. (1999b) Delaying antimalarial drug resistance with combination chemotherapy. Parassitologia. 41, 301-308.

[219] White, NJ. (2004) Antimalarial drug resistance. J Clin Invest. 113, 1084-1092.

[220] White, TE., Bushdid, PB., Ritter, S., Laffan, SB., Clark, RL. (2006) Artesunate-induced depletion of embryonic erythroblasts precedes embryolethality and teratogenicity in vivo. Birth Defects Res. B Dev. Reprod. Toxicol. 77, 413-429.

[221] WHO. (2006a) Guidelines for the treatment of malaria. Geneva, Switzerland: World Health Organization, November 8, 2006. http://www.who.int/malaria/publications/atoz/9789241547925/en/ (accessed December 2010).

[222] WHO. (2006b) Assessment of the safety of artemisinin compounds in pregnancy. Geneva: The Special Pro-gramme for Research and Training Diseases (TDR) and The Global Malaria Programme of the World Health Organization; 2006. http://malaria.who.int/docs/mip/artemisinin_compounds_pregnan-cy.pdf.

[223] WHO. (2007) WHO informal consultation with manufacturers of artemisinin based pharmaceutical products in use for the treatment of malaria. August 24, 2007. 20 Avenue Appia. World Health Organization, Geneva, Switzerland.at: http://www.who.int/malaria/publications/atoz/manufacturers_artemisinin_products/en/ . (accessed December 2010).

[224] WHO (2010). Guidelines for the treatment of malaria. 2nd Ed. Geneva, World Health Organization 2011

[225] Willoughby, JA., Sundar, SN., Cheung, M., Tin, AS., Modiano, J., Firestone, GL. (2009) Artemisinin blocks prostate cancer growth and cell cycle progression by disrupting Sp1 interactions with the cyclin-dependent kinase-4 (CDK4) promoter and inhibiting CDK4 gene expression," Journal of Biological Chemistry, 284, 2203–2213.

[226] Woerdenbag, HJ., Moskal, TA., Pras N. (1993) Cytotoxicity of artemisinin-related endoperoxides to Ehrlich ascites tumor cells. Journal of Natural Products, 56, 849–856.

[227] Wu, JM., Shan, F., Wu, GS., Li, Y., Ding, J., Xiao, D., Han, JX., Atassi, G., Leonce, S., Caignard, DH., Renard, P. (2001) Synthesis and cytotoxicity of artemisinin derivatives containing cyanoarylmethyl group. Eur J Med Chem. 36, 469-479.

[228] Wu, XH., Zhou, HJ., Lee, J. (2006) Dihydroartemisinin inhibits angiogenesis induced by multiple myeloma RPMI8226 cells under hypoxic conditions via downregulation of vascular endothelial growth factor expression and suppression of vascular endothelial growth factor secretion. Anti-cancer Drugs. 17, 839-848.

[229] Wu, ZP., Gao, CW., Wu, YG., Zhu, QS., Yan, Chen., Xin, Liu., Chuen, Liu. (2009) Inhibitive effect of artemether on tumor growth and angiogenesis in the rat C6 orthotopic brain gliomas model. Integr Cancer Ther. 8, 88-92.

[230] Xiao, SH., Keiser, J., Chollet, J., Utzinger, J., Dong, Y., Endriss, Y., Vennerstrom, JL., Tanner, M. (2007) In vitro and in vivo activities of synthetic trioxolanes against major human schistosome species. Antimicrob Agents Chemother. 51, 1440-1445.

[231] Xue, Y., Religa, P., Cao, R., Hansen, AJ., Lucchini, F., Jones, B., Wu, Y., Zhu, Z., Pytowski, B., Liang, Y., Zhong, W., Vezzoni, P., Rozell, B., Cao, Y. (2008) Anti-VEGF agents confer survival advantages to tumor-bearing mice by improving cancer-associated systemic syndrome. Proc Natl Acad Sci U S A. 105, 18513-18518.

[232] Yang, XP., Pei, ZH., Ren, J. (2009) Making up or breaking up: the tortuous role of platelet-derived growth factor in vascular ageing. Clin Exp Pharmacol Physiol. 36, 739-747.

[233] Yamachika, E., Habte, T., Oda, D. (2004) Artemisinin: an alternative treatment for oral squamous cell carcinoma. Anti-cancer Res. 24, 2153-2160.

[234] Yao, L., Xie, H., Jin, Q.-Y., Hu, W.-L., Chen, L.-J. (2008) Analyzing anti-cancer action mechanisms of dihydroartemisinin using gene chip," China Journal of Chinese Materia Medica, 33, 1583–1586.

[235] Yao, XH., Ping, YF., Bian, XW. (2011) Contribution of cancer stem cells to tumor vasculogenic mimicry. Protein Cell. 2, 266–272.

[236] Youns, M., Efferth, T., Reichling, J., Fellenberg, K., Bauer, A., Hoheisel, JD. (2009) Gene expression profiling identifies novel key players involved in the cytotoxic effect of Artesunate on pancreatic cancer cells," Biochemical Pharmacology, 78, 273–283.

[237] Zhang, ZY., Yu, SQ., Miao, LY., Huang, XY., Zhang, XP., Zhu, YP., Xia, XH., Li, DQ. (2008)Artesunate combined with vinorelbine plus cisplatin in treatment of advanced non-small cell lung cancer: a randomized controlled trial. Zhong Xi Yi Jie He Xue Bao. 6, 134-138.

[238] Zhang, F., Tang, Z., Hou, X., Lennartsson, J., Li, Y., Koch, AW. (2009) VEGF-B is dispensable for blood vessel growth but critical for their survival, and VEGF-B targeting inhibits pathological angiogenesis. Proc Natl Acad Sci USA 106, 6152–6157.

[239] Zhang, S., Chen, H., Gerhard, GS. (2010) Heme synthesis increases artemisinin-induced radical formation and cytotoxicity that can be suppressed by superoxide scavengers. Chem Biol Interact. 186, 30-35.

[240] Zhou, HJ., Wang, WQ. G., Wu, D., Lee, J., Li, A. (2007) Artesunate inhibits angiogenesis and downregulates vascular endothelial growth factor expression in chronic myeloid leukemia K562 cells," Vascular Pharmacology, 47, 131–138.

[241] Zhou, HJ., JZhang, JL., Li, A., Wang, AZ., Lou, XE. (2010) Dihydroartemisinin improves the efficiency of chemotherapeutics in lung carcinomas In vivo and inhibits murine Lewis lung carcinoma cell line growth In vitro," Cancer Chemotherapy and Pharmacology, 66, 21–29.

Chapter 8

3-D Microvascular Tissue Constructs for Exploring Concurrent Temporal and Spatial Regulation of Postnatal Neovasculogenesis

Mani T. Valarmathi, Stefanie V. Biechler and John W. Fuseler

Additional information is available at the end of the chapter

http://dx.doi.org/10.5772/53118

1. Introduction

Development of postnatal new blood vessels occurs essentially by two temporally distinct but interrelated processes, vasculogenesis and angiogenesis. Vasculogenesis is the process of blood vessel formation occurring by a de novo production of endothelial cells in an embryo (primitive vascular network) or a formerly avascular area when endothelial precursor cells (angioblasts, hemangioblasts or stem cells) migrate and differentiate in response to local cues (such as growth factors and extracellular matrix) to form new intact blood vessels (Risau and Flamme, 1995). Angiogenesis refers principally to the sprouting of new blood vessels from the differentiated endothelium of pre-existing vessels. These vascular trees or plexuses are then pruned, remodeled and extended through angiogenesis to become larger caliber vessels (Carmeliet, 2000). In addition, there exists yet another unique mechanism of neovascularization, the postnatal vasculogenesis, where new blood vessels are formed by the process of fusion and differentiation of endothelial progenitors of bone marrow origin (Valarmathi et al., 2009). This indicates a potential role for bone marrow-derived progenitor cells in postnatal neovasculogenesis and/or neoangiogenesis. This implies that additional mechanisms besides angiogenesis can occur in the adult, and has opened up the possibility to investigate the embryonic origin and development of these putative progenitor cells.

The adult bone marrow contains two subsets of multipotential stem cells, hematopoietic stem cells (HSCs) and bone marrow stromal cells or mesenchymal stem cells (BMSCs/MSCs). BMSCs are a readily available heterogeneous population of cells that can be directed to differentiate into multiple mesenchymal and non-mesenchymal cells either in vitro or in

INTECH
open science | open minds

© 2013 The Author(s). Licensee InTech. This chapter is distributed under the terms of the Creative Commons Attribution License http://creativecommons.org/licenses/by/3.0), which permits unrestricted use, distribution, and reproduction in any medium, provided the original work is properly cited.

vivo (Wakitani et al., 1995; Pittenger et al., 1999; Makino et al., 1999; Fukuda et al., 2001; Bianco et al., 2001; Valarmathi et al., 2009; 2010). Most noticeably, BMSCs have been induced to undergo maturation and differentiation towards vascular endothelial and smooth muscle cell lineages. Previous reports indicate that BMSCs and bone marrow-derived multipotent adult progenitor cells (MAPCs) can be differentiated into endothelial-like cells in vitro and contribute to neoangiogenesis in vivo (Oswald et al., 2004; Reyes et al., 2002; Al-Khaldi et al., 2003). Additionally, it has been shown that BMSCs can augment collateral remodeling and perfusion in ischemic models through paracrine mechanisms rather than by cellular incorporation upon local delivery (Kinnaird et al., 2004). Therefore, the identification of bone-marrow-derived (hematopoietic and non-hematopoietic stem cells) and non-bone-marrow-derived (tissue-resident stem/progenitor cells – adipose, neural, heart, skeletal muscle; peripheral and cord blood-derived stem cells) endothelial progenitors cells (EPCs) has led to the realization of potential postnatal vasculogenesis (Urbich and Dimmeler, 2004).

A variety of cellular types can be mobilized from the bone marrow reservoir and can home to sites of neovascularization, where they enhance the angiogenic process (Bertolini et al., 2006). While the concept that vascular progenitors are delivered and recruited was initially conceived and based on the circulating endothelial stem/progenitors (EPCs) paradigm, currently, it has become obvious that other classes of vasculogenic cells can also be derived from the in situ de novo differentiation of precursor cells. Among these, a population of Tie2 expressing mesenchymal precursor cells was recently identified, which are capable of in vitro expansion and of generating Tie2 negative but α-SMA positive cells when re-introduced into the tumors (De Palma et al., 2005). On the one hand, the mechanism by which these cells (EPCs) are recruited from the bone marrow to sites of new blood vessel formation remains an area of active study, but on the other hand, the mechanisms of by which EPCs egress from the bone marrow and subsequent recruitment to sites of neovascularization/neoangiogenesis warrants further investigation.

Even though there exists ample evidence for the existence of EPCs, proof of a functional requirement for EPCs mobilization and vascular recruitment in human cancer necessitates further experimentation. In addition, to address the temporal as well as spatial contribution of not only these EPCs but also other marrow-derived stem/progenitors to a specific tumor environment require the generation of novel tumor model systems. And these model systems can be utilized to evaluate the subtle contribution of marrow-derived stem/progenitors during the early phases of the neo-angiogenic switch besides oncogenic transformation.

For the above mentioned reasons, embryonic, fetal and postnatal stem cells as well as various types of progenitor cells, can be a potential cellular source for vascular tissue engineering (Levenberg, 2005). However, the source for the early-stage developmental cells is restricted. The utility of embryonic stem cells (ESCs) and induced pluripotent stem cells (iPSCs) in facilitating vascularized tissue/organ regeneration is still in its incipient stages. A number of issues, including a propensity for some implanted ESCs/iPSCs to form benign teratomas and/or malignant teratocarcinomas in the regenerating tissue/organ, remain to be addressed. In contrast to both ESCs/iPSCs, it has been well established that the adult stem cell, BMSCs exhibit multilineage differentiation potential in a well-controlled, predictable fashion. Moreover, unlike ESCs derivation, obtaining autologous or allogeneic BMSCs is feasible and can potentially be exploited to develop tissue-engineered blood vessel constructs for therapeutic purposes. Similarly, when compared to bone marrow-derived BMSCs, repeated isolation and rapid expansion of sufficient yield of autologous and/or allogeneic non-bone-marrow-derived resident stem cells/progenitors, especially from vital organs for routine therapeutic purposes are highly constrained. On the contrary, to a certain extent, autologous and/or allogeneic bone marrow-derived BMSCs are amenable for repeated isolation and reasonable in vitro expansion from the patients. In addition, the significant advantage of using these BMSCs is their low immunogenicity. And these autologous or allogeneic BMSCs have been reported to be immunomodulatory and immunotolerogenic both in vitro as well as in vivo. (Aggarwal and Pittenger, 2005). Taken together, these data strongly indicate that BMSCs can represent the potential cell of choice for adult autologous and/or allogeneic stem cell based vascularized tissue regeneration.

Extracellular molecules initiate biological signals and play a critical role in the control of cellular proliferation, differentiation, and morphogenesis. Many parameters, such as the presence and amount of soluble factors such as hormones, growth factors, and cytokines or the insoluble factors such as the physical configuration of the matrix which mediates the cell-cell interactions and cell-matrix interactions, exert a strong influence on the success of angiogenic processes in vitro and presumably in vivo (Even-Ram and Yamada, 2005; Carlson, 2007). The likelihood and ultimate success of in vitro cellular differentiation depends on how closer the cell-matrix interactions and relationships' mimic to those found during normal development or regeneration. In vascular tissue engineering, the application of these principles in vivo will be important to ensure that the matrix/scaffold to be implanted can support endothelial cell proliferation and migration resulting in endothelial tube formation (Ingber and Folkman, 1989). The vital issue for realistic clinical application is whether these scaffolds with preformed network of endothelial capillaries/microvessels can survive implantation into tissue defects and subsequently be able to anastomose to the host vasculature.

We therefore hypothesized that under appropriate in vitro physicochemical microenvironmental cues (combination of growth factors and extra cellular matrix, ECM) multipotent adult BMSCs could be differentiated into vascular endothelial and smooth muscle cell lineages. To test this hypothesis, we characterized the intrinsic vasculogenic differentiation potential of adult BMSCs when seeded onto a three-dimensional (3-D) tubular scaffold engineered from aligned type I collagen strands and cultured in both vasculogenic and non-vasculogenic growth media. In these culture conditions, BMSCs differentiated and matured into both endothelial and smooth muscle/pericyte cell lineages and showed microvascular morphogenesis. We also explored the potential of the 3-D model system to undergo postnatal de novo vasculogenesis.

2. Experimental approach

The differentiation of rat BMSCs was carried out on a 3-D tubular scaffold made up of aligned type I collagen-gel fibers. Rat BMSCs were isolated from the tibial and femoral bone marrow of adult rats. The BMSCs isolated from the bone marrow were expanded, maintained and passaged to make sure that the attached marrow stromal cells were devoid of any non-adhering populations of cells. Phenotypic characterization of the BMSCs for cell surface markers was performed by confocal microscopy (qualitative evaluation) and single-color flow cytometry (quantitative analysis). This adherent population of cells was further purified and enriched by indirect magnetic cell sorting. The cells were subjected to CD90 positive selection. The resultant enriched $CD90^{+}/CD34^{-}/CD45^{-}$ fractions were expanded by subculturing and subjected to flow cytometric analysis to validate the proper phenotype. This population of purified BMSCs was used in all experiments. For vasculogenic differentiation of BMSCs, the expanded and purified population of $CD90^{+}$ BMSCs were seeded into the collagen-gel tubular scaffold and cultured either in vasculogenic or non-vasculogenic culture medium for 28 days. At regular intervals of 7, 14, 21 and 28 days the tube cultures were assayed by RT-qPCR, immunofluorescence, ultrastructural and biochemical analyses for various endothelial and smooth muscle differentiation markers as shown in table 1, 2 and 3. The time points at which these analyses were carried out cover the optimal range of both vasculogenesis and angiogenic processes seen in vivo and/or in vitro and mimic the progression of microvascular development.

3. Research methods

3.1. Fabrication of tubular scaffold

The 3-D collagen type I tube served as a scaffold on which rat BMSCs differentiation cultures were carried out (Figure 1). The details of the production and properties of the collagen tubular scaffolds have previously been described (Yost et al., 2004). Briefly, a 25 mg/ml solution of bovine collagen type I was extruded with a device that contained two counter-rotating cones. The liquid collagen was fed between the two cones and forced through a circular annulus in the presence of an NH_3-air (50-50 vol/vol) chamber. This process results in a hollow cylindrical tube of aligned collagen fibrils with an inner central lumen. The dimensions of tubes produced for this set of experiments had a length of 30 mm with a luminal diameter of 4 mm and an external diameter of 5 mm, leaving a wall thickness of 0.5 mm. The collagen tubes had a defined fiber angle of 18° relative to the central axis of the tube and had pores ranging from 1 to 10 μm. The rationale for the particular orientation of collagen fibers was based on our previous work on cardiovascular tissue engineering (Yost et al., 2004). When proepicardial organ (PE) cells were seeded onto this scaffold, they underwent maturation and differentiation and produced elongated vessel-like structures reminiscent of in vivo-like phenotype (Valarmathi et al., 2008). The tubes were sterilized using gamma radiation 1200 Gy followed by Stratalinker UV crosslinker 1800 (Stratagene) and then placed in Mosconas's solution (in mM: 136.8 NaCl, 28.6 KCl, 11.9 $NaHCO_3$, 9.4 glucose, 0.08 NaH_2PO_4, pH 7.4) (Sigma-Aldrich) containing 1 μl/ml gentamicin (Sigma-Aldrich) and incubated in 5% CO_2 at 37°C until cellular seeding (Valarmathi et al., 2010).

http://dx.doi.org/10.5772/53118

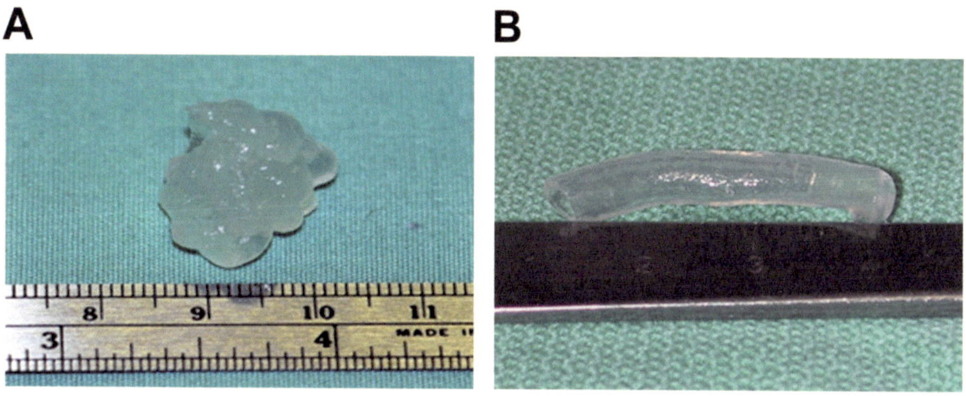

Figure 1. Fabrication of 3-D collagen gel based tubular scaffolds engineered from aligned type I collagen fibers. Type I collagen was extracted from bovine calf hides (A). Bovine collagen type I was extruded with a device that contained two counter-rotating cones to generate the 3-D collagen gel tubular scaffolds. The dimensions of tubes produced for this set of experiments had a length of 30 mm with a luminal diameter of 4 mm and an external diameter of 5 mm, leaving a wall thickness of 0.5 mm. The collagen tubes had a defined fiber angle of 18° relative to the central axis of the tube and had pores ranging from 1 to 10 μm (B). (A and B, courtesy of M.J. Yost)

3.2. BMSCs isolation, expansion and maintenance

The initial step is to isolate the mononuclear cells from the bone marrow by aspiration and centrifugation followed by plating and isolation of the cells based on differential adherence capacity to tissue culture dishes (passage 0 cells). Rat BMSCs were isolated from the bone marrow of adult 300g Sprague Dawley®™ SD®™ rats (Harlan Sprague Dawley, Inc.). Briefly, after deep anesthesia, the femoral and tibial bones were removed aseptically and cleaned extensively to remove associated soft connective tissues. The marrow cavities of these bones were flushed with Dulbecco's Modified Eagle Medium (DMEM; Invitrogen) and combined. The isolated marrow plugs were triturated, and passed through needles of decreasing gauge (from 18 gauge to 22 gauge) to break up clumps and cellular aggregates. The resulting single-cell suspensions were centrifuged at 200g for 5 minutes. Nucleated cells were counted using a Neubauer chamber. Cells were plated at a density of 5×10^6 – 2×10^7 cells per T75 cm^2 flasks in basal media composed of DMEM supplemented with 10% fetal bovine serum (FBS, lot-selected; Hyclone), gentamicin (50 μg/ml) and amphotericin B (250 ng/ml) and incubated in a humidified atmosphere of 5% CO_2 at 37°C for 7 days. The medium was replaced, and changed three times per week until the cultures become ~70% confluent (between 12 and 14 days). Cells were trypsinized using 0.05% trypsin-0.1% EDTA and re-plated at a density of 1×10^6 cells per T75 cm^2 flasks. After three passages, attached marrow stromal cells were devoid of any non-adhering population of cells. These passaged BMSCs were cryopreserved and stored in liquid nitrogen until further use (Valarmathi et al., 2011).

3.3. Immunophenotyping of BMSCs by flow cytometry and confocal microscopy

BMSCs are a heterogeneous population of cells with varying degrees of cell shapes and sizes (Anokhina et al., 2007). Stringent characterization of BMSCs used in experimental procedures is required for various cell surface markers; this is to ensure that the employed population of cells contains solely stem/progenitor cells. This will obviate the possible contamination of marrow-derived endothelial cells and macrophages that are part of the adherent population of cultured cells. Therefore, characterization of BMSCs included qualitative evaluation for various cell surface markers and was performed on cells grown in the Lab-tek™ chamber slide system™ (Nunc) using a Zeiss LSM 510 Meta confocal scanning laser microscope (Carl Zeiss, Inc.), and quantitative analysis of the same set of markers was performed by single-color flow cytometry using a Coulter® EPICS® XL™ Flow Cytometer (Beckman Coulter, Inc.) as previously described (Valarmathi et al., 2009).

Criteria to Identify BMSCs/MSCs			
1.	Adherence to plastic in standard culture conditions		
2.	Phenotype	Positive (≥95%+)	Negative (≤2%+)
		CD73	CD11b or CD14
		CD90	CD34
		CD105	CD45
			CD79α or CD19
			HLA-DR
3.	In vitro differentiation: Osteoblasts, Chondroblasts and Adipocytes. (Demonstrated by staining of in vitro cell culture)		
International Society for Cellular Therapy (ISCT): Mesenchymal and Tissue Stem Cell Committee			

Table 1. Criteria to identify BMSCs/MSCs (Dominici et al., 2006)

Immunophenotyping of passage 3 undifferentiated BMSCs for various cell surface markers by flow cytometry revealed that the fluorescent intensity and distribution of the cells stained for CD11b, CD31, CD34, CD44, CD45 and CD106 were not significantly different from the intensity and distribution of cells stained with isotype controls (Figure 2 A-E, H). In addition, these cells were negative for the rat endothelial cell surface marker OX43 (Figure 2, I), an antigen expressed on all vascular endothelial cells of rat, indicating that these cultures were devoid of any possible hematopoietic stem and/or progenitor cells as well as differentiated bone-marrow-derived endothelial cells. In contrast, BMSCs exhibited high expression of CD73 and CD90 surface antigens (Figure 2, F-G), which is consistent with their undifferentiated state. Furthermore, flow cytometric analysis of the same passage 3 BMSCs for various other vascular endothelial cell surface antigens and smooth muscle cell intracellular antigens revealed that these cells were negative for Flt1, Flk1 and VE-cadherin (Figure 2, J-L) and, were predominantly positive for calponin (Figure 2, M). The expression profiles of these surface molecules were consistent with previous reports and the minimal criteria for defining multipotent mesenchymal stromal cells, enunciated by the international society for cellular therapy (ISCT) position statement (Valarmathi et al., 2009; Reyes et al., 2002; Dominici et al., 2006).

Phenotypic characterization using the same set of markers on passage 3 BMSCs by confocal microscopy also revealed that the cells were negative for CD11b, CD31, CD34, CD44, CD45 and OX43 (Figure 3, A-J, O-P), and strongly positive for CD73 and CD90 (Figure 3, K-N). The permeabilized cells when stained for Vcam1 (CD106), Flt1 (Vegfr1), Flk1 (Vegfr2) and VE-cadherin (Figure 4, A-H) revealed faintly detectable cytoplasmic and/or nuclear signal of these endothelial antigens. While these cells showed abundant cytoplasmic expression of smooth muscle antigen, calponin (Figure 4, I-J). Phenotypic characterization and evaluation of these markers on clonally expanded BMSCs showed similar expression patterns consistent with their parent culture.

Primary Antibodies	**Dilutions**	**Source**	**Cell Target**
BMSCs characterization markers			
CD11b	1:50	BD Pharmingen	Leukocytes
CD31	1:10	Abcam	Endothelial
CD44	1:10	Gene Tex, Inc	Leukocytes
CD45	1:50	BD Pharmingen	Hematopoietic
CD73	1:50	BD Pharmingen	BMSCs
CD90	1:50	BD Pharmingen	BMSCs
CD106	1:50	BD Pharmingen	Endothelial
OX43	1:10	Gene Tex, Inc	Endothelial
Endothelial cell differentiation markers			
CD34	1:100	Santa Cruz Biotechnology	Endothelial
Flt-1	1:100	Santa Cruz Biotechnology	Endothelial
Flk-1	1:100	Santa Cruz Biotechnology	Endothelial
VE- cadherin	1:100	Santa Cruz Biotechnology	Endothelial
Pecam1	1:100	Santa Cruz Biotechnology	Endothelial
Vwf	1:100	Santa Cruz Biotechnology	Endothelial
Tomato lectin	1:50	Vector Laboratories	Endothelial
Fibronectin	1:200	Abcam	Endothelial
Smooth muscle cell differentiation markers			
α-SMA	1:100	Sigma-Aldrich	Smooth Muscle
Calponin	1:5000	Sigma-Aldrich	Smooth Muscle

Table 2. Primary antibodies used in this study (Valarmathi et al., 2009).

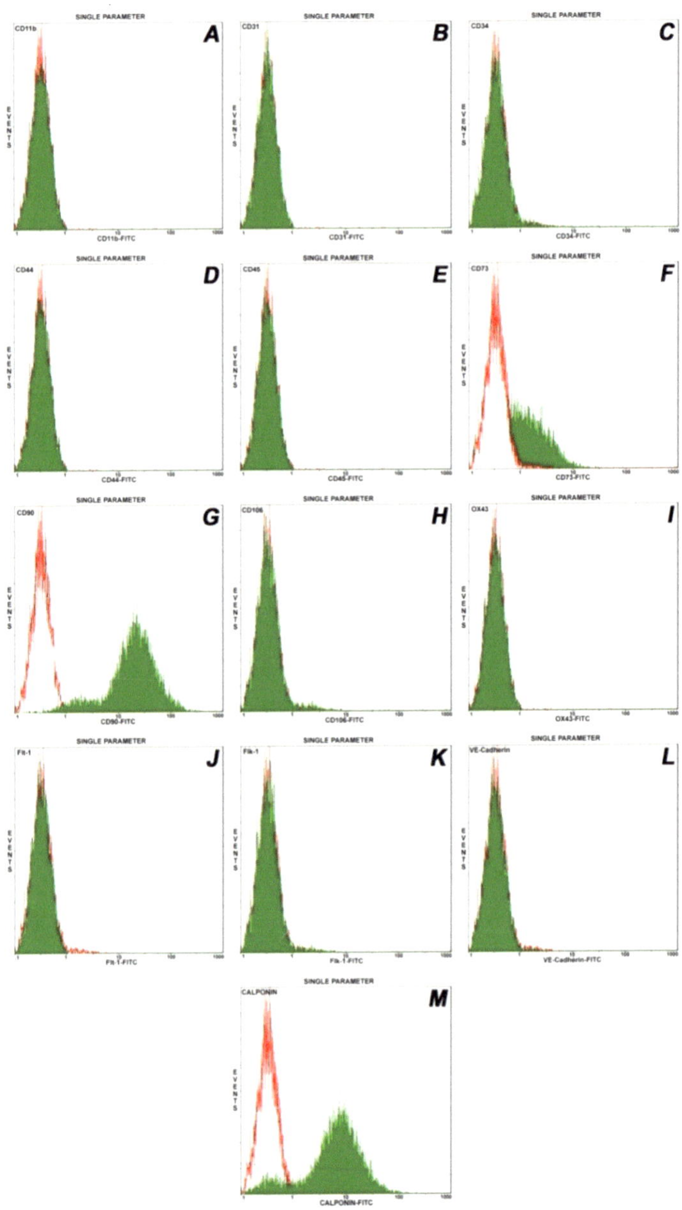

Figure 2. Immunophenotyping of passage 3 undifferentiated rat BMSCs by flow cytometry. Single parameter histograms showing the relative fluorescence intensity of staining (abscissa) and the number of cells analyzed, events (ordinate). Isotype controls were included in each experiment to identify the level of background fluorescence. The intensity and distribution of cells stained for hematopoietic and endothelial markers; CD11b, CD31, CD34, CD44, CD45, CD106, OX43, Flt-1, Flk-1 and VE-cadherin (green, shaded peaks) were not significantly different from those of isotype control (red, open peaks) (Panels A-E, H-L). The fluorescent intensity was greater (shifted to right) when BMSCs were stained with CD73, CD90 and calponin (green) compared to isotype control (red) (Panels F, G, M). The predominant population of BMSCs uniformly expressed CD90 surface molecule, consistent with their undifferentiated state. Adapted from Valarmathi et al., 2009.

http://dx.doi.org/10.5772/53118

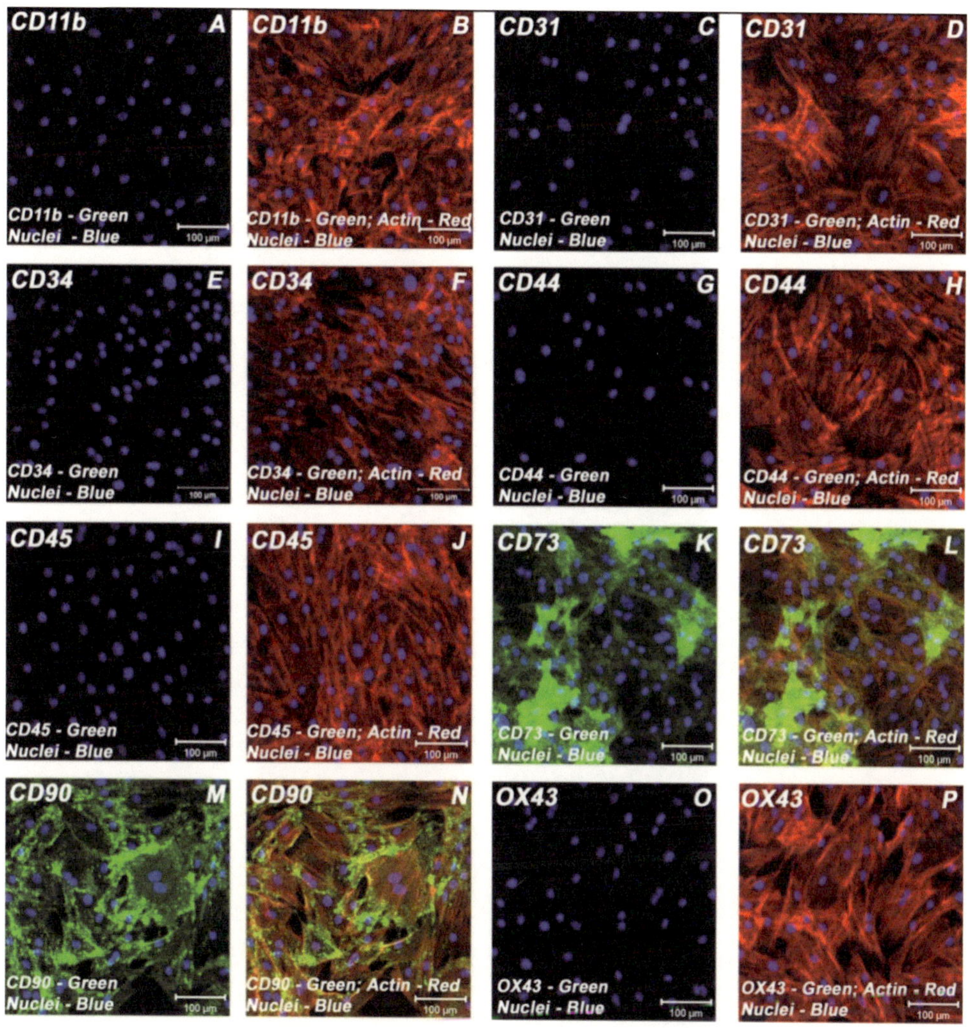

Figure 3. Immunophenotyping of passage 3 undifferentiated rat BMSCs by confocal microscopy. Phenotypic characterization and evaluation revealed that the permeabilized cells were negative for CD11b, CD31, CD34, CD44, CD45 and OX43 (Figure 3, A-J, O-P), indicating that these cultures were devoid of any potential hematopoietic and/or endothelial cells of bone marrow origin. However, the cells consistently expressed both CD73 and CD90 (Figure3, K-N) surface antigens, a property of mesenchymal/stromal stem cells. Isotype controls were included in each experiment to identify the level of background staining. Cells were also stained for nuclei (blue, DAPI) and fibrillar actin (red, rhodamine phalloidin). Merged images (B, D, F, H, J-N, P). (A-P, scale bar 100 µm). Adapted from Valarmathi et al., 2009.

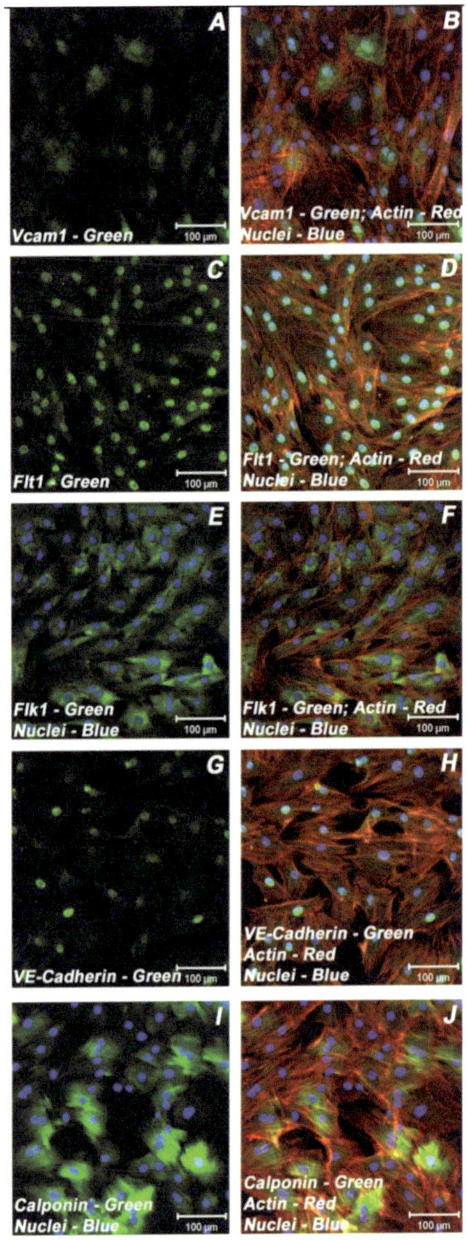

Figure 4. Confocal microscopic analysis of various vascular related antigens on passage 3 undifferentiated rat BMSCs. Evaluation of the permeabilized cells for Vcam1 (CD106), Flt1 (Vegfr1), Flk1 (Vegfr2) and VE-cadherin revealed faintly detectable cytoplasmic and/or nuclear signals of these endothelial antigens (Figure 4, A-H). Whereas, these cells showed abundant cytoplasmic expression of smooth muscle antigen, calponin (Figure 4, I-J). Suggesting that BMSCs constitutively express very low-levels of endothelial associated antigens as well as very high-levels of smooth muscle specific antigens. Isotype and/or negative controls were included in each experiment to identify the level of background staining. Cells were also stained for nuclei (blue, DAPI) and fibrillar actin (red, rhodamine phalloidin). Merged images (B, D-F, H-J). (A-J, scale bar 100 µm). Adapted from Valarmathi et al., 2009.

http://dx.doi.org/10.5772/53118

3.4. Purification and enrichment of $CD90^+$ BMSCs by Magnetic-Activated Cell Sorting (MACS)

Purification and enrichment of input BMSCs (such as CD45-, CD34-, CD105) are mandatory either using MACS (magnetic activated cell sorter) or FACS (fluorescent activated cell sorter). Since the unpurified fraction may contain sizable number of contaminating adherent macrophages and bone marrow-derived endothelial progenitors and differentiated endothelial cells. The adherent populations of BMSCs were further purified by indirect magnetic cell labeling method using an autoMACS™ Pro Separator (Miltenyi Biotech). The cells were subjected to CD90 positive selection by incubating the cells with FITC- labeled anti-CD90 antibodies (BD Pharmingen), followed by incubation with anti-FITC magnetic microbeads (Miltenyi Biotech), and passed through the magnetic columns as per the manufacturer's instructions. The resultant enriched $CD90^+/CD34^-/CD45^-$ fractions were expanded by subcultivation and subjected to flow cytometric analysis as described previously (Valarmathi et al., 2010).

3.5. BMSCs vasculogenic differentiation

For vasculogenic differentiation of BMSCs, the purified population of $CD90^+$ BMSCs were seeded into the collagen-gel tubes at a density of 0.5×10^6 cells/30 mm tube lengths and cultured either in mesenchymal stem cell growth medium supplemented with 10% FBS, penicillin and streptomycin (Poietics® MSCGM™ BulletKit®; Lonza Ltd.) or microvascular endothelial cell growth medium (Clonetics® EGM®-MV Bullet Kit®; Lonza Ltd.) supplemented with 5% FBS, bovine brain extract, human epidermal growth factor (hEGF), hydrocortisone, amphotericin B and gentamicin for 28 days. These BMSCs seeded tubes were cultured either in vasculogenic or non-vasculogenic medium for the defined time periods of 7, 14, 21 and 28 days. In addition, BMSCs were seeded in 65-mm Petri dishes at a density of 3×10^3 cells/cm^2 and cultured in non-vasculogenic (MSCGM) or vasculogenic (EGMMV) media for 7, 14, 21 and 28 days.

4. BMSCs based postnatal de novo vasculogenesis and in situ vascular regeneration

The 3-D collagen-gel tubular scaffold has previously been used to create models of vascularized bone development (Valarmathi et al., 2008a; 2008b). Here we report the utility of a 3-D tubular construct for its ability to support the vasculogenic differentiation of BMSCs culminating into microvascular structures, which are similar to those structures resulting from postnatal de novo vasculogenesis and angiogenesis (Valarmathi et al., 2008a; 2008b).

In the developing vertebrate embryo, the initial event of blood vessel formation is the differentiation of vascular endothelial cells, which subsequently cover the entire interior surface of all blood vessels. Angioblasts are a subpopulation of primitive mesodermal cells that are committed to differentiate into endothelial cells and later on form the primitive vascular labyrinth (Risau and Flamme, 2000). In addition, endothelial cells can also arise from hemangioblasts, a common precursor for both hematopoietic and endothelial cells (His et al., 1900).

In adults, endothelial precursor cells have been identified in bone marrow, peripheral blood and blood vessels (Prater et al., 2007). Two subsets of multipotential stem cells, HSCs and BMSCs/MSCs are resident in the postnatal bone marrow. Of these cells, BMSCs can be differentiated into osteoblasts, chondrocytes, adipocytes, smooth muscle cells and hematopoietic supportive stroma either in vitro or in vivo (Bianco et al., 2001). Previous studies have provided substantial evidence that bone-marrow-derived stem and/or progenitor cells can be differentiated into either endothelial or smooth muscle cells in vitro and in pathological situations are capable of contributing to neoangiogenesis in vivo by cellular integration (Carmeliet and Luttun, 2001).

Although there are a plethora of studies focused on developing viable scaffolds for osteogenic, chondrogenic, adipogenic and musculogenic differentiation of BMSCs (Lanza et al., 2000), the optimal scaffolds that are capable of inducing and supporting the growth and differentiation of BMSCs into vascular cell lineages are yet to be identified and characterized. Despite the much known vasculogenic potential and transgermal plasticity of BMSCs; none of these studies explicitly demonstrated the postnatal de novo vasculogenic potential of BMSCs in vitro (Reyes et al., 2002; Oswald et al., 2004; Brey et al., 2005).

When compared to 2-D planar cultures, the potential 3-D models of vasculogenesis allow us to understand the role of specific factors under more physiological and spatial conditions with respect to dimensionality, architecture and cell polarity. Nevertheless, the molecular composition and the natural complexity and diversity of in vivo extra cellular matrix (ECM) organization cannot be easily mimicked or reproduced in vitro (Vailhe et al., 2001). In addition, even though quite a few in vitro 3-D models of vasculogenesis based on fibrin and collagen gels are in vogue (Folkman and Haudenschild, 1980); none have explored the behavior of BMSCs and their intrinsic vasculogenic differentiation potential on a topographically structured 3-D tubular scaffold made of uniformly aligned type I collagen fibers.

Previous studies demonstrated that the formation of endothelial tubes in vitro was largely influenced by the nature of the substrate (Kleinman et al., 1982). The formation of endothelium lined tubular structures was enhanced when the substrate was rich in laminin (Madri et al., 1988), whereas a matrix rich in type I collagen would not promote rapid tubulogenesis (Montesano et al., 1983; Ingber and Folkman, 1989). Similarly, Ingber and Folkman (1989) documented that under a given cocktail of growth factors, the local physical nature of the interaction between endothelial cells and the underlying matrix/substrate ultimately determined the tubular morphogenesis. Substrates containing abundant fibronectin promoted adhesion, spreading and growth of endothelial cells. In contrast, less adhesive substrate or matrix materials that were arranged three-dimensionally permitted the endothelial cells to retract and form tubes (Ingber and Folkman, 1989).

In general, successful in vitro differentiation of cells depends on cell-cell as well as cell-matrix interactions. Therefore, we hypothesized that under appropriate in vitro local environmental cues (combination of growth factors and ECM) multipotent postnatal BMSCs could be induced to undergo microvascular development. Hence, we developed a 3-D culture system in which a pure population of CD90+ rat BMSCs was seeded and cultured on a highly aligned, porous, biocompatible collagen-fiber tubular scaffold for differentiation purposes. Here, we utilized two types of growth media for vasculogenic differentiation purpose, MSCGM (non-vasculogenic) as control and EGMMV (vasculogenic) preferentially for microvascular differentiation. Both of these culture media consistently promoted the vasculogenic differentiation of BMSCs and also supported the formation of endothelium lined vessel-like structures within the constructs.

A number of early and late stage markers associated with rodent vascular development in vivo were used in this study to characterize the rat BMSCs derived microvascular structures at mRNA and protein levels, which included: CD31/Pecam1, Flt1 (Vegfr1), Flk1 (Vegfr2/Kdr), VE-cadherin (CD144), CD34, Tie1, Tek (Tie2), and Von Willibrand factor (Vwf). Platelet/endothelial cell adhesion molecule, also known as CD31, is a transmembrane protein expressed abundantly early in vascular development that may mediate leukocyte adhesion and migration, angiogenesis, and thrombosis (Albelda et al., 1991). The other early stage differentiation markers Flk1 and Flt1 that are receptors for the vascular endothelial cell growth factor-A (Vegf) essentially play a vital role in embryonic vascular and hematopoietic development (Shalaby et al., 1997). Similarly, VE-cadherin, a member of the cadherin family of adhesion receptors, is a specific and constitutive marker of endothelial cell plays an important role in early vascular assembly. Vascular markers that are expressed at a later stage include CD34 and Tie-2 (Bautch et al., 2000). CD34 is a transmembrane surface glycoprotein that is expressed in endothelial cells and hematopoietic stem cells. Tie1 and Tek are receptor kinases on endothelial cells that are essential for vascular development and remodeling in the embryo and may also mediate maintenance and repair of the adult vascular system. In late phases of vasculogenesis, the mature endothelial cells will synthesize and secrete Vwf homolog, a plasma protein that mediates platelet adhesion to damaged blood vessels and stabilizes blood coagulation factor VIII.

Genes	Forward primer	Reverse primer	Product length (bp)	Annealing temperature (°C)	GenBank accession No
Pecam1	5'–CGAAATCTAGGCCTCAGCAC–3'	5'–CTTTTTGTCCACGGTCACCT–3'	227	56	NM_03159.1
Kdr	5'–TAGCGGGATGAAATCTTTGG–3'	5'–TTGGTGAGGATGACCGTGTA–3'	207	56	NM_013062.1
Tie1	5'–AAGGTCACACACACGGTGAA–3'	5'–TGGTGGCTGTACATTTTGGA–3'	174	56	XM_233462.4
Tek	5'–CCGTGCTGCTGAACAACTTA–3'	5'–AATAGCCGTCCACGATTGTC–3'	201	56	NM_001105737.1
Vwf	5'–GCTCCAGCAAGTTGAAGACC–3'	5'–GCAAGTCACTGTGTGGCACT–3'	163	56	XM_342759.3
Gapdh	5'–TTCAATGGCACAGTCAAGGC–3'	5'–TCACCCCATTTGATGTTAGCG–3'	101	56	XR_007416.1

Table 3. RT-qPCR primer sequences used in this study (Valarmathi et al., 2009; Rozen and Skaletsky, 2000).

In any type of in vitro cellular differentiation, the cytodifferentiated cells need to be critically evaluated for their maturation and differentiation at transcriptional, translational and functional levels. Therefore, to study the expression pattern of key vasculogenic gene transcripts in the 3-D tube constructs; we examined the time-dependent expression pattern of Pecam1, Kdr, Tie1, Tek and Vwf at mRNA level in the tube constructs by real-time PCR (Figure 5 A-D).

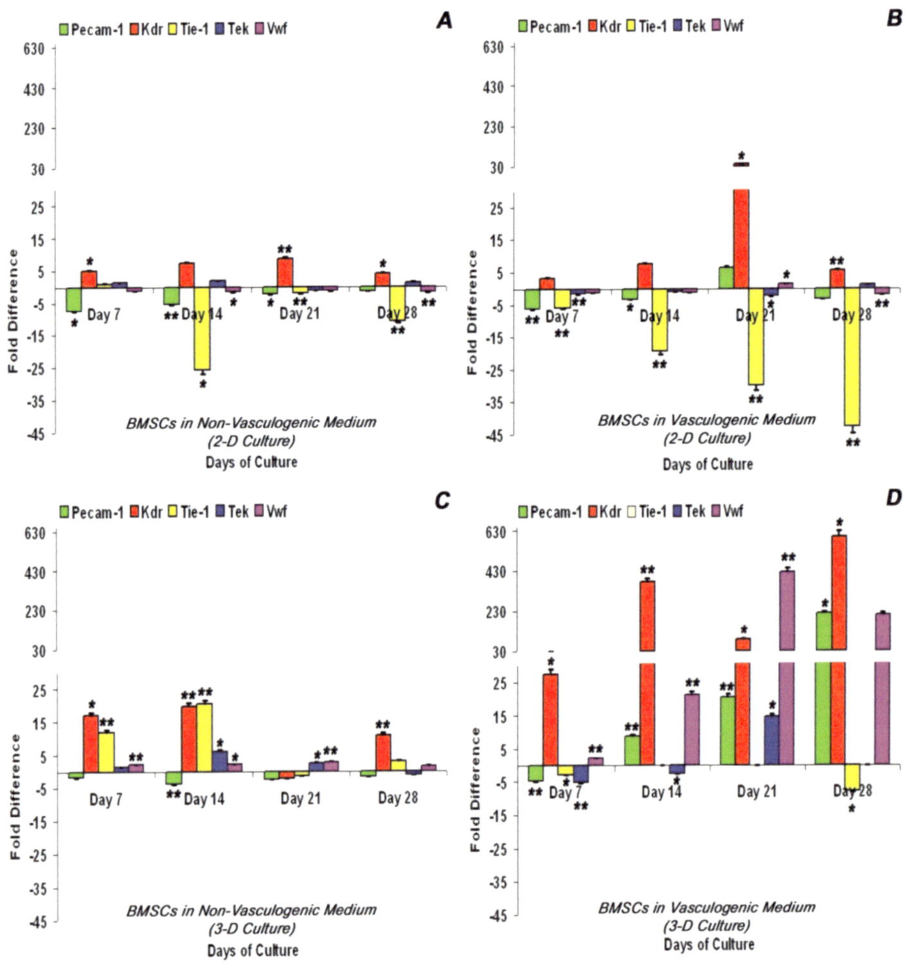

Figure 5. Real-time reverse transcriptase quantitative polymerase chain reaction (RT-qPCR) analysis of various key vasculogenic markers, platelet/endothelial cell adhesion molecule 1 (Pecam1), kinase insert domain protein receptor (Kdr/Flk1/Vegfr-2), tyrosine kinase with immunoglobulin-like and EGF-like domains 1 (Tie1), endothelial-specific receptor tyrosine kinase (Tek/Tie2) and Von Willebrand factor homology (Vwf) as a function of time (abscissa). BMSCs cultured in Petri dishes (2-D culture) in mesenchymal stem cell growth medium (A) and, in microvascular growth medium (B). BMSCs cultured in collagen-gel tubular scaffolds (3-D culture) in mesenchymal stem cell growth medium (C) and, in microvascular growth medium (D). The calibrator control included passage 4 BMSCs day 0 sample and; the target gene expression was normalized by a non-regulated reference gene expression, Gapdh. The expression ratio (ordinate) was calculated using the REST-XL version 2 software (Pfaffl 2001; Pfaffl et al., 2002). The values are means ± standard errors for three cultures (n=3), *p<0.005; **P<0.001. Adapted from Valarmathi et al., 2009.

Constitutive expressions of these markers were detected at low to very low levels in undifferentiated BMSCs. RT-qPCR results showed that differentiation of BMSCs under vasculogenic culture conditions for 28 days resulted in increased expression of transcripts coding for various endothelial cell associated proteins such as Pecam1, Kdr, Tek and Vwf. The peak expression of Vwf, the endothelial specific protein occurred around day 21 (over 400 fold) indicating that the differentiating cells acquired a distinctive phenotype and biosynthetic activity of differentiated and matured endothelial cells. The upregulation of Tek during this period may represent the continual development and remodeling of the developing microvessels. Whereas differentiation of BMSCs under non-vasculogenic conditions for 14 days showed signs of early and rapid induction of transcripts coding for both early and late stage endothelial cell markers such as Kdr, Tie1, Tek and Vwf. The peak expression of Vwf occurred during day 14 (over 20 fold).

As revealed by immunostaining for various vasculogenic markers, day 21 vasculogenic and non-vasculogenic tube cultures showed that BMSCs were able to adhere, proliferate, migrate and, undergo complete maturation and differentiation into microvascular structures (Figure 6 A-C). BMSCs derived microvessel formation is a combination of de novo vasculogenesis i.e., in situ endothelial cell differentiation and endothelium-lined tube formation, and angiogenesis, endothelial sprouting from existing endothelial tubes. In addition, these microvessels are stabilized by association with BMSC-derived smooth muscle cells and/or pericytes.

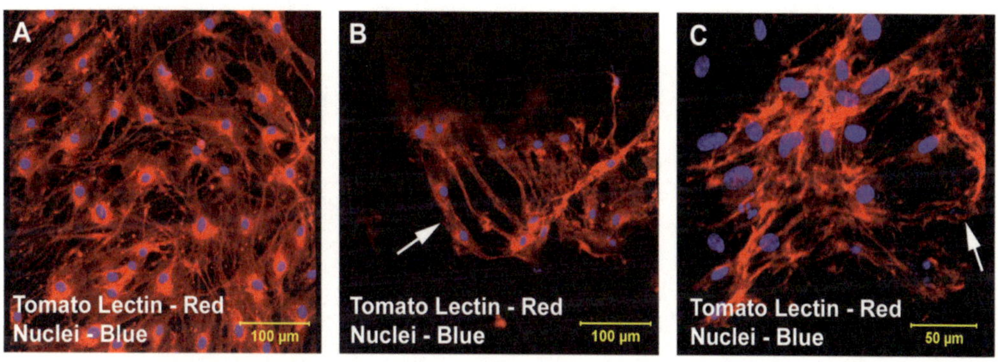

Figure 6. Localization of BMSCs derived endothelial cells by Texas Red labeled Lycopersicon Esculentum lectin/Tomato Lectin (LEL/TL) staining. BMSCs cultured in collagen-gel tubular scaffolds in both vasculogenic and non-vasculogenic culture conditions were incubated with tomato lectin (1:50 in 10 mM N-2-hydroxyethylpiperazine-N'-2-ethanesulfonic acid, pH 7.5; 0.15 M NaCl), and was used to identify endothelial cells. Confocal laser scanning microscopic analysis of sections of day 14 tubular scaffolds in these media conditions demonstrated the typical cobblestone appearance of differentiating endothelial cells (A), fusion and self-assembly (B), and evolving primitive capillary plexus with attempted lumen formation (B-C, white arrows). Cells were also stained for nuclei (blue, DAPI). Image (A) shows a projection representing 19 sections collected at 5.05 µm intervals (90.90 µm). Image (B) shows a projection representing 13 sections collected at 4.05 µm intervals (48.60 µm). Image (C) shows a projection representing 15 sections collected at 6 µm intervals (84.00 µm). Merged images (A-C). (A-B, scale bar 100 µm; C, scale bar 50 µm).

To validate the findings of mRNA expression pattern of important vasculogenic markers in these tube cultures and to determine whether these messages were in fact translated into proteins, immunostaining of the BMSC tube culture was carried out (Figure 7 A-L; Figure 8 A-L).

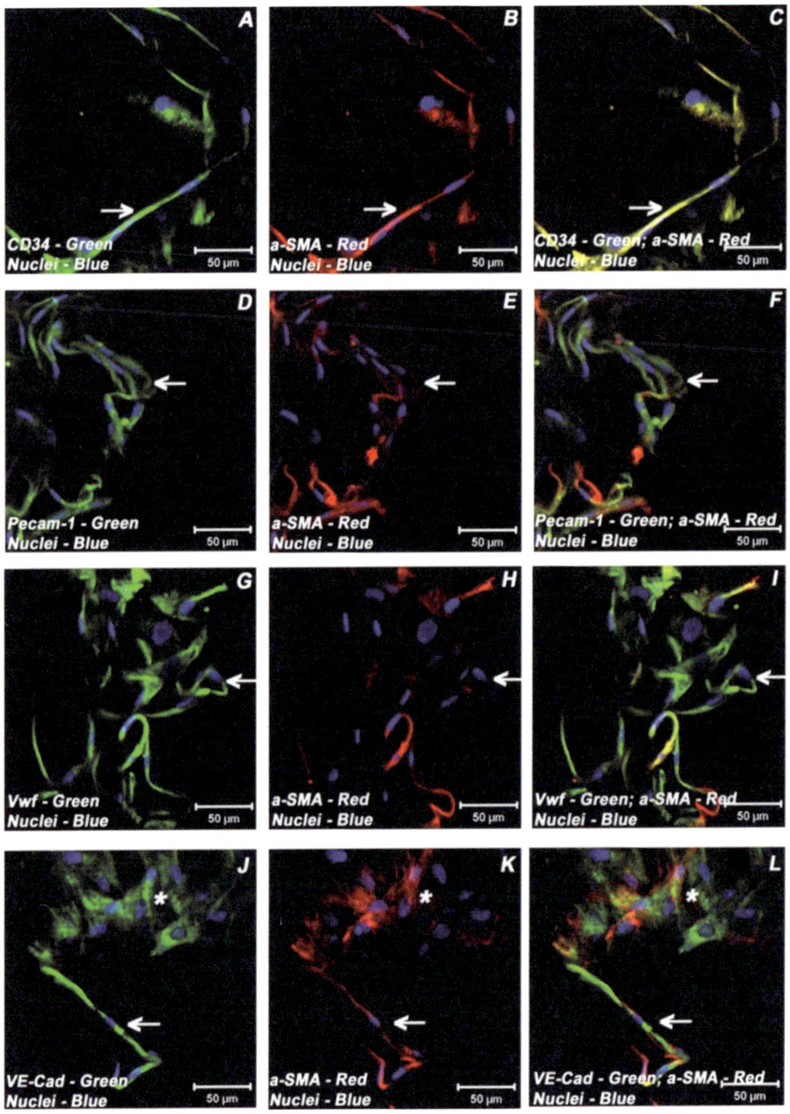

Figure 7. Expression pattern of various vasculogenic markers in tubular scaffold by confocal microscopy. Localization of key endothelial and smooth muscle cell phenotypic markers of day 21 non-vasculogenic tube cultures demonstrated the expression of CD34 (A-C), Pecam1 (D-F), Vwf (G-I), VE-cadherin (J-L) and α-SMA (B-C, E-F, H-I, K-L). Dual immunostainings of non-vasculogenic tube cultures (mesenchymal stem cell growth media, MSCGM) revealed areas of elongated and flattened cells composed of varying degrees of mature endothelial and smooth muscle cells (A-L). These cells were organized into a loose delicate network of nascent capillary-like structures composed of mature endothelial and smooth muscle cells and showed evidence of central lumen formation (white arrows, D-I). In addition, tube-like structures were emanating from the mixed population of vasculogenic cells represented by their distinct morphology and phenotypic expression (white arrows, A-C; white arrows, J-L). Cells were also stained for nuclei (blue, DAPI). Images (A-C) show a projection representing 15 sections collected at 5.05 µm intervals (70.70 µm). Images (D-F) show a projection representing 19 sections collected at 5.05 µm intervals (90.90 µm). Images (J-L) show a projection representing 19 sections collected at 4.04 µm intervals (72.90 µm). Merged images (A-L). (A-L, scale bar 50 µm). Adapted from Valarmathi et al., 2009.

http://dx.doi.org/10.5772/53118

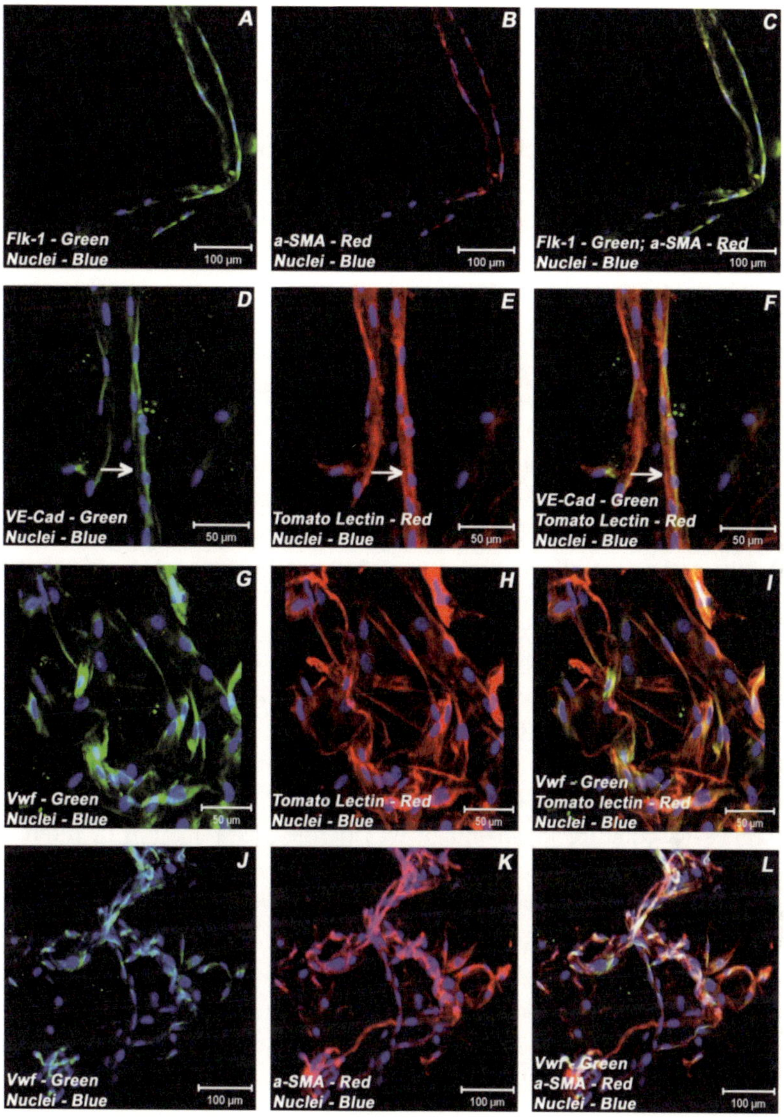

Figure 8. Expression pattern of various vasculogenic markers in tubular scaffold by confocal microscopy. Localization of key endothelial and smooth muscle cell phenotypic markers of day 21 vasculogenic tube cultures demonstrated the expression of Flk1 (A, C), VE-cadherin (D, F), Vwf (G, I; J, L), tomato lectin (E-F; H-I) and α-SMA (B-C, K-L). Dual immunostainings of vasculogenic tube cultures (microvascular endothelial growth medium, EGMMV) revealed areas of elongated cells composed of both mature endothelial and smooth muscle cells (A-L). These cells formed developing microvessl-like structures (A-F, J-L). The linear nascent capillary-like structures showed a translucent central lumen (white arrows, D-F). In addition, the cells were organized into a loose network of vascular cells and were in a ribbon-like configuration (G-I). These aligned vascular cells transformed into thin tube-like structures reminiscent of in vivo microvessel morphogenesis (J-L). Cells were also stained for nuclei (blue, DAPI). Images (D-F) show a projection representing 13 sections collected at 3.05 μm intervals (36.60 μm). Images (G-I) show a projection representing 18 sections collected at 7.05 μm intervals (119.8 μm). Images (J-L) show a projection representing 27 sections collected at 6.05 μm intervals (157.3 μm). Merged images (A-L). (A-C, J-L scale bar 100 μm; D-F, G-I scale bar 50 μm). Adapted from Valarmathi et al., 2009.

It is well known that endothelial cells share a large majority of their characteristic antigenic markers with other types of hematopoietic and mesenchymal cells (Bertolini et al., 2006). Therefore, antigens such as CD31, CD34, CD144 (VE-cadherin), CD146, Vwf or CD105 are not only expressed by endothelial cells but also expressed by hematopoietic cells (specifically HSCs), platelets and certain subpopulations of fibroblasts. Hence to identify the differentiated and matured endothelial cells in the tubular scaffold a battery of various early and late stage vasculogenic markers such as Pecam1, CD34, Flt1, Flk1, VE-cadherin, fibronectin and Vwf were employed. In addition, tomato lectin, another marker specific for rat vascular endothelial cells, was found closely associated with Flk1 and Vwf staining. These endothelial associated markers localized to endothelial cell clusters and capillary-like structures that were present throughout the tubular construct. This suggests that BMSC-derived endothelial cells assembled into endothelium-lined tube-like structures and initiated the process of vasculogenesis, consistent with our previous report (Figure 9 A-H) (Valarmathi et al., 2008a). In addition, the BMSC-derived cells and the microvessel-like structures expressed the smooth muscle antigens, α-SMA and calponin. These α-SMA positive cells were recruited in juxtaposition to the tandemly arranged endothelial cells and, were attached and wrapped around in such a way that is reminiscent of in vivo microvessel morphogenesis.

In order to quantitate the degree of vasculogenesis, image morphometric analyses were used to determine the capillary density, vessel breadth and length (integrated morphometry subroutine of MetaMorph 6.1). In brief, confocal scanning laser microscopic color images were converted to 8-bit monochrome images for both image and fractal analysis (Fuseler et al., 2007; Fernandez et al., 2001; Grizzi et al., 2005; Valarmathi et al., 2012). The fluorescence vasculature in an image was defined as a Region of Interest (ROI) by being thresholded using the "set threshold" subroutine of MetaMorph Image analysis software (v.6.1). The morphological descriptors of fiber breadth were a representative measure of blood vessel diameter. Fiber length was measured using the integrated morphometry algorithm of MetaMorph. Using this technique we were able to reconfirm what our confocal images demonstrated. In microvascular media, the BMSC-derived microvessels were longer (63%) and broader (37%) when compared with microvessels generated in basal media (Figure 10).

Similarly, it is critically important to characterize the ultrastructural morphology of any stem cells that are directed to differentiate into vascular lineage cells. Scanning electron microscopic (SEM) analysis of the tubular constructs depicted the pattern of microvessel morphogenesis and maturity. These formed nascent capillary-like structures and elongated tube-like structures revealed patent lumen-like structures, elucidating the vessel-maturation (Figure 11). Besides, transmission electron microscopic (TEM) analysis (Hanaichi et al., 1986) revealed elongated capillary-like structures lined by differentiating endothelial cells (Figure 12A). These cells showed electron dense bodies as well as numerous small pinocytotic vesicles adjacent to the endothelial cell membranes as well as in their cytoplasm (Figure 12B, small black arrows). In addition these cells exhibited variously sized cell-cell junctions, which have the appearance of typical in vivo endothelial tight junctions (Figure 12C-F).

http://dx.doi.org/10.5772/53118

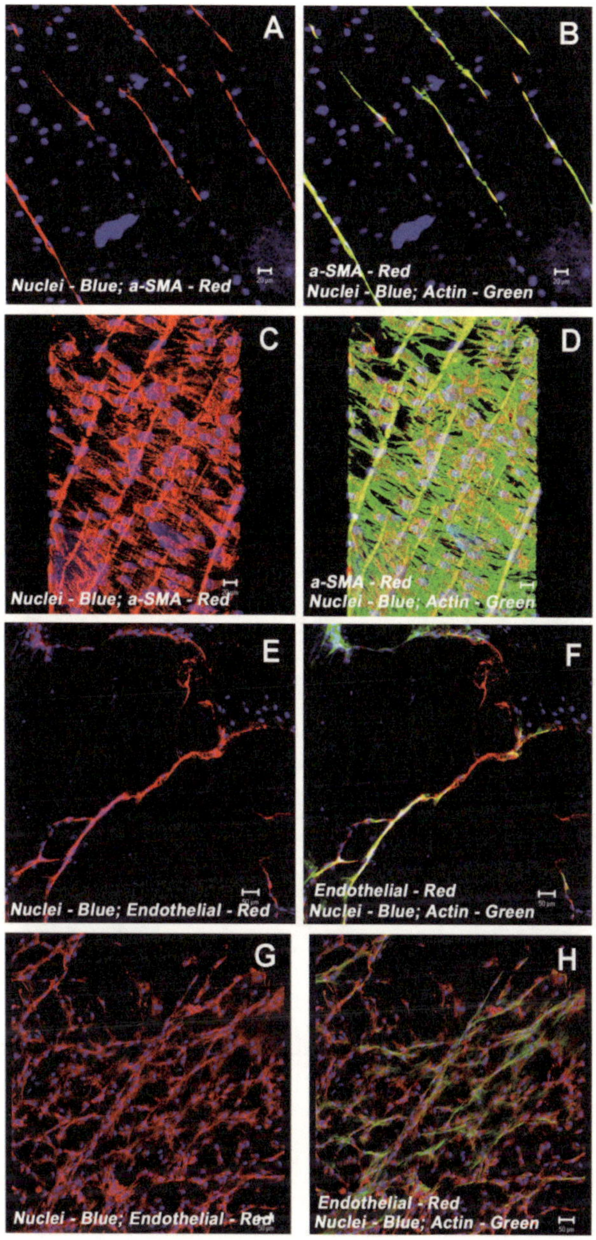

Figure 9. Expression pattern of vasculogenic markers α-SMA and tomato lectin (TL). Localization of BMSC-derived vascular progenitor cells on the collagen tube scaffold by confocal microscopy is seen in panels A, C, E, and G. The merged images showing the actin cytoskeleton are shown in panels B, D,F, and H. Sections of a day 9 osteogenic tube culture demonstrated nascent capillary-like structures positive for α-SMA (red, A). These elongated cord-like structures showed strong colocalization of α-SMA and actin (merged, B). In the tubes nuclei appeared aligned (blue, DAPI). In adjacent fields, abundant sheets of parallel oriented α-SMA positive cells were abutting the nascent vessel-like structures (red, C). The merged image (D) shows actin and α-SMA in vessel-like structures that appear to be in different planes with almost a perpendicular alignment with the underlying α-SMA positive cells (D). Similar sections of osteo-

genic cultured tubes illustrate the sprouting and branching tubular structures positive for the rat endothelial marker tomato lectin (red, E-H). A plexus of arborizing endothelial cells was observed. These plexuses contained capillary-like vessels lined with endothelial cells (red, G). Similarly in the merged panel, the apparent multilayered nature of the vessels was observed. However in these fields, the plexuses of endothelial cells were not in a perpendicular arrangement but rather in a web-like orientation (merged, H). Figures C and D were projections representing 19 sections collected at 2 μm intervals. Figures G and H were projections representing 32 sections collected at 9 μm intervals. Merged images (A-H) (A-D, Scale bar 20 μm; E-H, Scale bar 50 μm). Adapted from Valarmathi et al., 2008a.

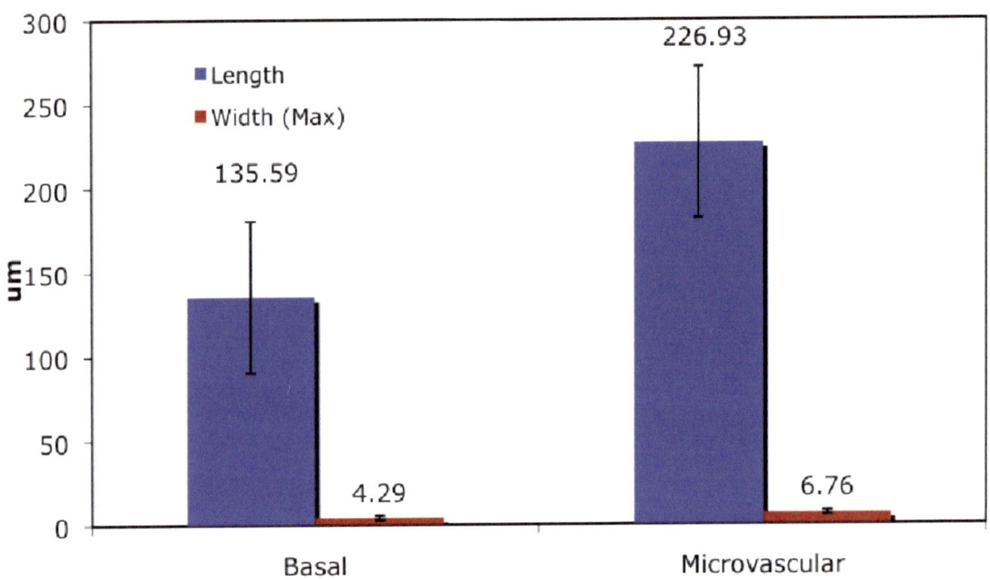

Figure 10. Morphometric analysis of microvessel-like structures generated in the walls of collagen-gel tubular constructs in different culture media, viz., basal or microvascular medium.

http://dx.doi.org/10.5772/53118

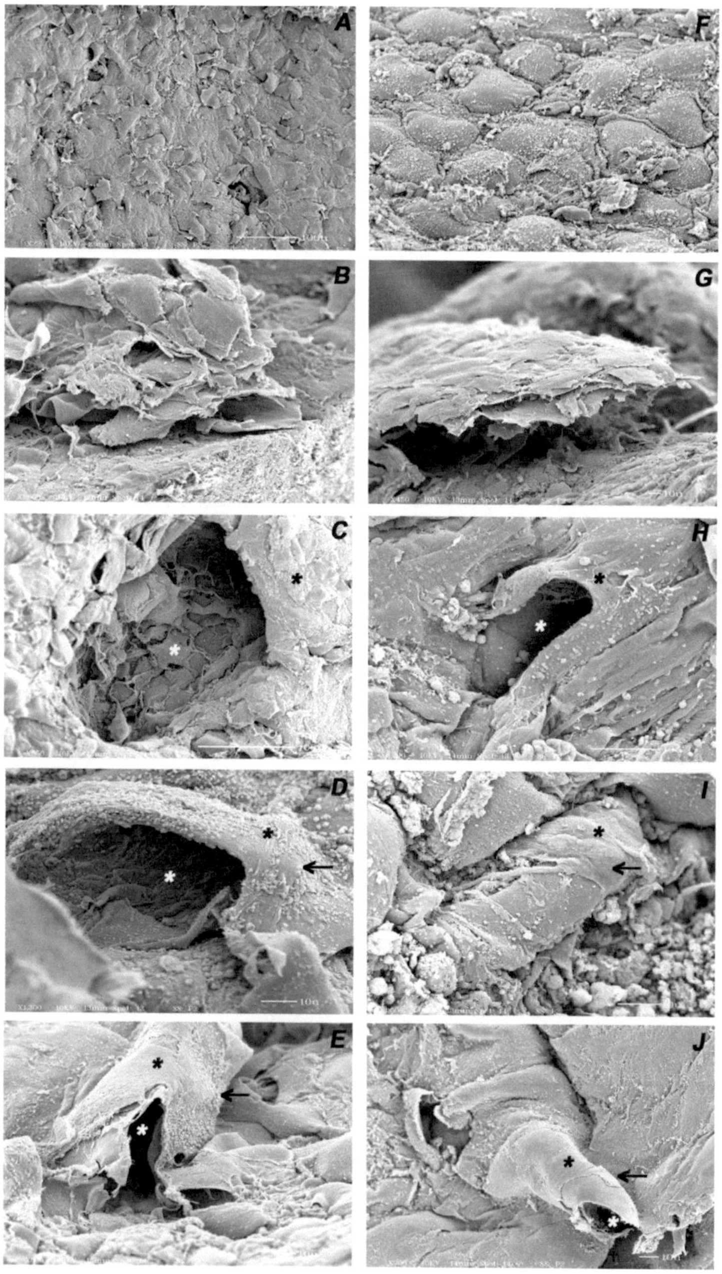

Figure 11. Scanning electron microscopic (SEM) analysis of tubular constructs. SEM analysis of day 28 tubular constructs under both vasculogenic and non-vasculogenic culture conditions showed the typical cobblestone appearance of differentiated endothelial cells (A, F), stratification and networking (B, G), and the presence of smooth-walled tube-like structures with its attached smooth muscle cells and/or pericytes (black arrows, D, E, I, J). Multiple smooth muscle-like cells were wrapping around these tube-like structures (black asterisks, Figure C-E, H-J). These cylindrical structures revealed the presence of evolving patent lumens (white asterisks, C-E, H, J). Some of these luminal surfaces showed the regular cobblestone arrangement of endothelial cells (white asterisks, C, D). Adapted from Valarmathi et al., 2009.

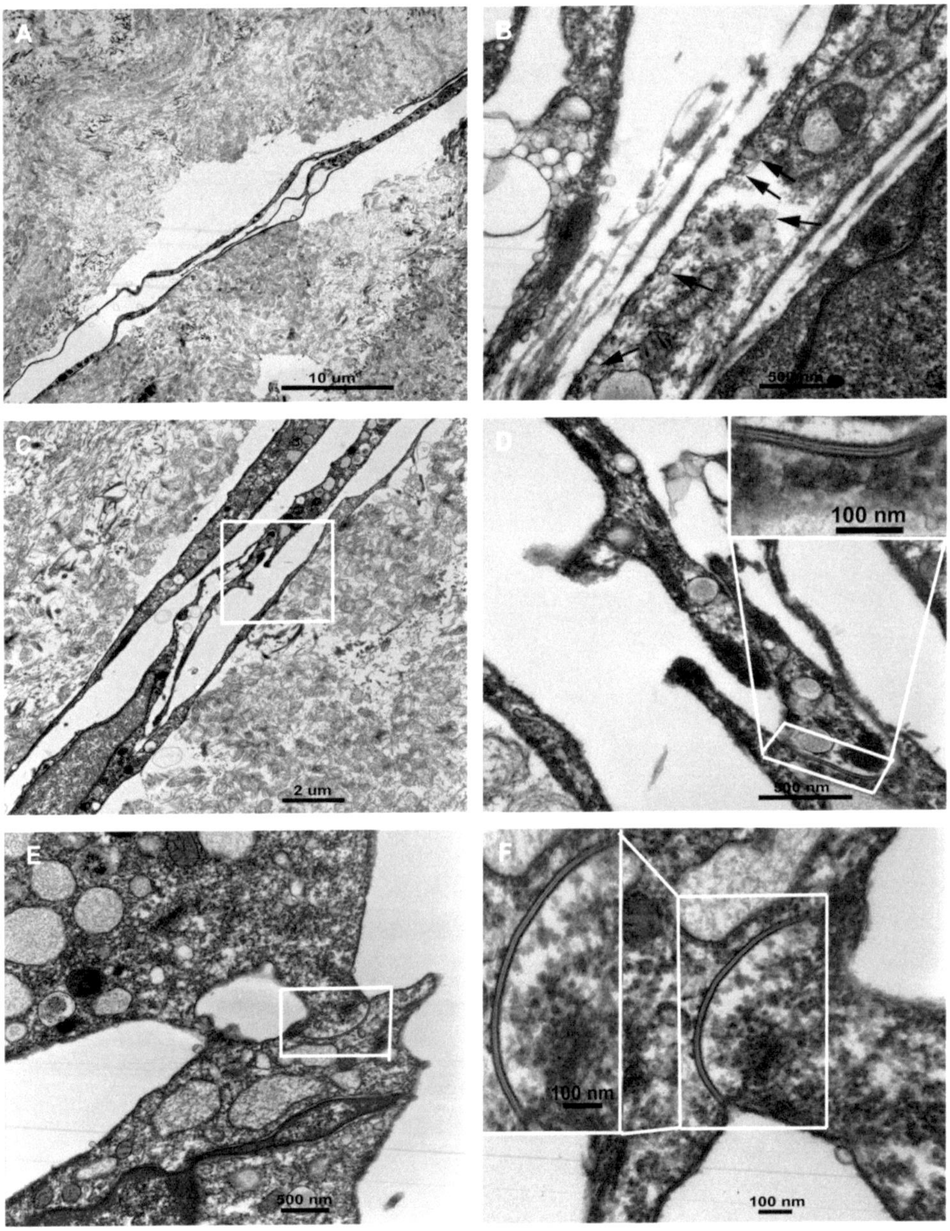

Figure 12. Transmission electron microscopic (TEM) analysis of tubular constructs. TEM analysis of day 28 tubular constructs under both vasculogenic and non-vasculogenic culture conditions showed a vessel-like structure containing many small dense bodies within endothelial cells on either side of the lumen (A). Note the most obvious feature of endothelial cells, the concentration of small vesicles (pinocytotic vesicles) adjacent to the endothelial cell membranes (B, black arrows). The interdigitating endothelial cells showing junctional regions (C, E, inserts, lower magnification). The typical adherent junction could be visualized between two overlapping endothelial cell processes (D, F, inserts, higher magnification).

Furthermore, the ability to identify endothelial cells based on their increased metabolism of Ac-LDL was examined using Ac-LDL tagged with the fluorescent probe (Dil-Ac-LDL) (Voyta et al., 1984). BMSC-derived endothelial cells and the nascent capillary-like structures were brilliantly fluorescent whereas the fluorescent intensity of smooth muscle cells/pericytes was barely detectable as reported previously (Valarmathi et al., 2009). This suggests that the formed endothelial cells were not only fully differentiated but also functionally competent and matured (Figure 13A-J).

This behavior of BMSCs and their exhibition of vasculogenic differentiation potential can be attributed to the nature of microenvironmental factors in this culture conditions. The preconditioned factors in the growth microenvironment rendered by the aligned type I collagen fibers of the tubular scaffold and the soluble differentiating factors provided by the vasculogenic and non-vasculogenic media may be behind the BMSC fate determination. Further work is ongoing to determine whether our prevascularised tubular scaffolds can survive implantation into a tissue defect and is able to anastomose promptly with vascular sprouts emanating from the host. Finally, our morphological, molecular, immunological and biochemical data reveal the intrinsic vasculogenic differentiation potential of BMSCs under appropriate 3-D environmental conditions.

Previously, it has been shown that mature vascular endothelium can give rise to smooth muscle cell (SMC) via endothelial-mesenchymal transdifferentiation, coexpressing both endothelial and SMC-specific phenotypic markers (Frid et al., 2002). Recently, it has been show that Flk1-expressing blast cells derived from embryonic stem cells can act as precursors that can differentiate into both endothelial and mural cell populations of the vasculature (Yamashita et al., 2000). In this study, clonal analyses revealed the bi-lineage potential of BMSCs, suggesting that both endothelial and smooth muscle/pericytes could be derived from single colonies. However, in general, BMSC-derived colonies are clonal or nearly clonal. The colonies of BMSCs resultant from a number of cells may represent co-existence of several subclones, each capable of differentiating into specific lineages. Hence, single cell-derived colonies that are stably transfected with lineage specific markers are needed to gain more meaningful insights and address the origin of both lineages.

Our results indicate that the 3-D tubular scaffold with its unique characteristics provides a favorable microenvironment that permits the development of in situ microvascular structures. Moreover, this is the first ever documentation that explicitly demonstrates that adult BMSCs under appropriate in vitro environmental cues can be induced to undergo vasculogenic differentiation culminating in microvessel morphogenesis. Our model recapitulates many aspects of in vivo de novo vasculogenesis. Thus, this unique culture system provides an in vitro model to investigate the maturation and differentiation of BMSC-derived vascular endothelial and smooth muscle cells in the context of postnatal vasculogenesis. In addition, it allows us to elucidate various molecular mechanisms underlying the origin of both endothelial and smooth muscle cells and especially to gain a deeper insight and validate the emerging concept of 'one cell and two fates' hypothesis of vascular development (Yamashita et al., 2000).

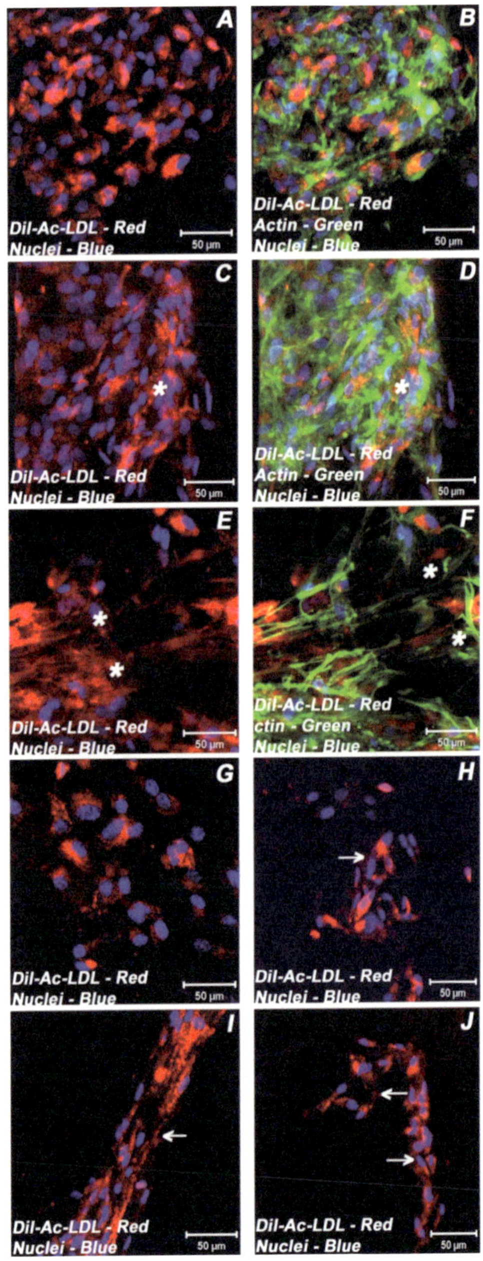

Figure 13. Characterization of BMSC-derived endothelial cells by Dil-Ac-LDL uptake. BMSCs cultured in collagen-gel tubular scaffolds in non-vasculogenic (mesenchymal stem cell growth medium, MSCGM) and vasculogenic (microvascular endothelial cell growth medium, EGMMV) culture conditions were incubated with 10 µg / ml of Dil-Ac-LDL for 4 to 6 hours. Confocal laser scanning microscopic analysis of sections of day 21 tubular scaffolds in MSC growth medium revealed abundant punctate perinuclear bright red fluorescence of the differentiated and matured endothelial cells (A-F). These labeled vascular cells were organized into a discrete cluster (A, B), assembled into tangled capillary-like structures on top of a cluster (white asterisks, C, D) and, transformed into nascent linear and branching capillary-like structures (white asterisks, E, F). Similarly, confocal laser scanning microscopic analysis of sections of day 21 tubular

scaffolds in microvascular endothelial cell growth medium revealed typical abundant punctate perinuclear bright red fluorescence of the differentiated and matured endothelial cells (G-J). These labeled vascular cells were organized into small discrete clusters (G), self-organized into numerous small capillaries with a central lumen (white arrow, H), assembled into solid cord of cells (white arrow, I) and, transformed into tube-like structure with attempted lumen formation (white arrows, J). Cells were also stained for nuclei (blue, DAPI) and fibrillar actin (green, Alexa® 488 phalloidin). Images (A-B) show a projection representing 13 sections collected at 3.05 μm intervals (36.60 μm). Images (C-D) show a projection representing 20 sections collected at 4.05 μm intervals (76.95 μm). Images (E-F) show a projection representing 4 sections collected at 2.05 μm intervals (6.15 μm). Image (H) shows a projection representing 20 sections collected at 5 μm intervals (95.00 μm). Image (I) shows a projection representing 13 sections collected at 4 μm intervals (48.00 μm). Image (J) shows a projection representing 22 sections collected at 5 μm intervals (105.00 μm). Merged images (A-J). (A-J, scale bar 50 μm). Adapted from Valarmathi et al., 2009.

5. Conclusions

Here we report a unique 3-D culture system that recapitulates many aspects of postnatal de novo vasculogenesis and angiogenesis. This is the first comprehensive report that evidently demonstrates that BMSCs under appropriate in vitro environmental conditions can be induced to undergo vasculogenic differentiation culminating in microvessels. Since BMSCs differentiated into both endothelial and smooth muscle cell lineages, this in vitro model system provides a tool for investigating the cellular and molecular origin of both vascular endothelial cells and smooth muscle cells. In addition, this system can potentially be harnessed to develop in vitro engineering of microvascular trees, especially using autologous bone-marrow-derived BMSCs for therapeutic purposes in regenerative medicine.

Acknowledgements

"This work was supported by an award from the American Heart Association." – National Scientist Development Grant (11SDG5280022) as well "This material is based upon work supported by the National Science Foundation/EPSCoR under Grant No. (EPS – 0903795)." – The South Carolina Project for Organ Biofabrication, for Valarmathi Thiruvanamalai.

Author details

Mani T. Valarmathi*, Stefanie V. Biechler and John W. Fuseler

*Address all correspondence to: valarmathi.thiruvanamalai@uscmed.sc.edu or valarmathi64@hotmail.com

Laboratory of Stem Cell Biology and Tissue Engineering, Department of Cell Biology and Anatomy, School of Medicine, University of South Carolina, Columbia, South Carolina, USA

References

[1] Aggarwal S and Pittenger MF. Human mesenchymal stem cells modulate allogeneic immune cell responses. Blood 2005;105:1815-1822.

[2] Albelda SM, Muller WA, Buck CA, Newman PJ. Molecular and cellular properties of PECAM-1 (endoCAM/CD31): a novel vascular cell-cell adhesion molecule. J Cell Biol 1991;114:1059-68.

[3] Al-Khaldi A, Eliopoulos N, Martineau D, Lejeune L, Lachapelle K, Galipeau J. Postnatal bone marrow stromal cells elicit a potent VEGF-dependent neoangiogenic response in vivo. Gene Ther 2003;10:621-29.

[4] Anokhina EB, Buravkova LB. Heterogenecity of stromal cell precursers isolated from rat bone marrow. Cell and Tissue Biology 2007;1:1-7. (Original article in Russian - Tsitologiya 2007;49:40-47.)

[5] Bautch VL, Redick SD, Scalaia A, Harmaty M, Carmeliet P, Rapoport R. Characterization of the vasculogenic block in the absence of vascular endothelial growth factor-A. Blood 2000;95:1979-87.

[6] Bertolini F, Shaked Y, Mancuso P, Kerbel RS. The multifaceted circulating endothelial cell in cancer: towards marker and target identification. Nat Rev Cancer 2006;6:835-45.

[7] Bianco P, Riminucci M, Gronthos S, Robey PG. Bone marrow stromal stem cells: nature, biology, and potential applications. Stem Cells 2001;19:180-92.

[8] Brey EM, Uriel S, Greisler HP, Patrick Jr. CW, McIntire LV. Therapeutic neovascularization: contributions from bioengineering. Tissue Eng 2005;11:567-84.

[9] Carlson BM. Tissue engineering and regeneration In: ed. Principles of regenerative biology. Amsterdam: Elsevier, 2007; pp259-278.

[10] Carmeliet P, Jain RK. Angiogenesis in cancer and other diseases. Nature 2000;407:249-257.

[11] Carmeliet P, Luttun A. The emerging role of the bone marrow-derived stem cells in (therapeutic) angiogenesis. Thromb Haemost 2001;86:289-97.

[12] Carmeliet P. Mechanisms of angiogenesis and arteriogenesis. Nat Med 2000;6:389-95.

[13] De Palma M, Venneri MA, Galli R, Sergi SL, Politi LS, Sampaolesi M, et al. Tie2 identifies a hematopoietic lineage of proangiogenic monocytes required for tumor vessel formation and a mesenchymal population of pericytes progenitors. Cancer Cell 2005;8:211-226.

[14] Dominici M, Le Blanc K, Mueller I, Slaper-Cortenback I, Marini F, Krause D, et al. Minimal criteria for defining multipotent mesenchymal stromal cells. The International Society For Cellular Therapy position statement. Cytotherapy 2006;8:315-7.

[15] Even-Ram S, Yamada KM. Cell migration in 3D matrix. Curr Opin Cell Biol 2005;17:524-32.

[16] Fernández E, Jelinek HF. 2001. Use of fractal theory in neuroscience: methods, advantages, and potential problems. Methods. 2001;24:309-21.

[17] Folkman J, Haudenschild C. Angiogenesis in vitro. Nature 1980;288:551-56.

[18] Frid MG, Kale VA, Stenmark KR. Mature vascular endothelium can give rise to smooth muscle cells via endothelial-mesenchymal transdifferentiation: in vitro analysis. Circ Res 2002;90:1189-96.

[19] Fukuda K. Development of regenerative cardiomyocytes from mesenchymal stem cells for cardiovascular tissue engineering. Artif Organs 2001;25:187-193.

[20] Fuseler JW, Millette CF, Davis JM, Carver W. Fractal and image analysis of morphological changes in the actin cytoskeleton of neonatal cardiac fibroblasts in response to mechanical stretch. Microsc Microanal. 2007;3:133-43.

[21] Fuseler JW, Valarmathi MT. Modulation of the migration and differentiation potential of adult bone marrow stromal stem cells by nitric oxide. Biomaterials 2012;33:1032-43.

[22] Grizzi F, Russo C, Colombo P, Franceschini B, Frezza EE, Cobos E, et al. Quantitative evaluation and modeling of two-dimensional neovascular network complexity: the surface fractal dimension. BMC Cancer. 2005;5:14-23.

[23] Hanaichi T, Sato T, Iwamoto T, Malavasi-Yamashiro J, Hoshino M, Mizuno N. A stable lead by modification of Sato's method. J Electron Microsc (Tokyo). 1986;35:304-06.

[24] His W. Lecithoblast und Angioblast der Wirbeltiere. Abhandl Math-Phys Ges Wiss 1900;26:171-328.

[25] Ingber DE, Folkman J. How does extracellular matrix control capillary morphogenesis? Cell 1989;58:803-05.

[26] Ingber DE, Folkman J. Mechanochemical switching between growth and differentiation during fibroblast growth factor-stimulated angiogenesis in vitro: Role of extracellular matrix. J Cell Biol 1989;109:317-30.

[27] Kinnaird T, Stabile E, Burnett MS, Shou M, Lee CW, Barr S, et al. Local delivery of marrow-derived stromal cells augments collateral perfusion through paracrine mechanisms. Circulation 2004;109:1543-49.

[28] Kleinman HK, McGarvey ML, Liotta LA, Robey PG, Tryggvason K, Martin GR. Isolation and characterization of type IV procollagen, laminin, and heparan sulfate proteoglycan from the EHS sarcoma. Biochemistry 1982;21:6188-93.

[29] Lanza RP, Langer R, Vacanti J. Principles of tissue engineering. San Diego, CA: Academic Press; 2000.

[30] Levenberg S. Engineering blood vessels from stem cells: recent advances and applications. Curr Opin Biotechnol 2005;16:516-23.

[31] Madri JA, Pratt BM, Tucker AM. Phenotypic modulation of endothelial cells by transforming growth factor- depends upon the composition and organization of the extracellular matrix. J Cell Biol 1988;106:1375-84.

[32] Makino S, Fukuda K, Miyoshi S, Konishi F, Kodama H, Pan J, et al. Cardiomyocytes can be generated from marrow stromal cells in vitro. J Clin Invest 1999;103:697-705.

[33] Montesano R, Orci L, Vassalli JD. In vitro rapid organization of endothelial cells into capillary-like network is promoted by collagen matrices. J Cell Biol 1983;97:1648-52.

[34] Oswald J, Boxberger S, Jorgensen B, Feldmann S, Ehninger G, Bornhauser M, et al. Mesenchymal stem cells can be differentiated into endothelial cells in vitro. Stem Cells 2004;22:377-84.

[35] Pfaffl MW, Horgan GW, Dempfle L. Relative expression software tool (REST) for group-wise comparison and statistical analysis of relative expression results in real-time PCR. Nucleic Acids Res 2002;30:e36.

[36] Pfaffl MW. A new mathematical model for relative quantification in real-time RT-PCR. Nucleic Acids Res 2001;29:e45.

[37] Pittenger MF, Mackay AM, Beck SC, Jaiswal RK, Douglas R, Mosca JD, et al. Multilineage potential of adult human mesenchymal stem cells. Science 1999;284:143-147.

[38] Prater DN, Case J, Ingram DA, Yoder MC. Working hypothesis to redefine endothelial progenitor cells. Leukemia 2007;21:1141-49.

[39] Reyes M, Dudek A, Jahagirdar B, Koodie L, Marker PH, Verfaillie CM. Origin of endothelial progenitors in human postnatal bone marrow. J Clin Invest 2002;109:337-46.

[40] Risau W, Flamme I. Vasculogenesis. Annu Rev Cell Dev Biol 1995;11:73-91.

[41] Rozen S, Skaletsky HJ. Primer3 on the WWW for general users and for biologist programmers. In: Krawetz S, Misener S (eds) Bioinformatics Methods and Protocols: Methods in Molecular Biology. Humana Press, Totowa, NJ, 2000; pp 365-386.

[42] Shalaby F, Ho J, Stanford WL, Fischer K-D, Schuh AC, Schwartz L, et al. A requirement for Flk-1 in primitive and definitive hematopoiesis and vasculogenesis. Cell 1997;89:981-90.

[43] Urbich C, Dimmeler S. Endothelial progenitor cells functional characterization. Trends Cardiovasc Med 2004;14:318-22.

[44] Vailhe B, Vittet D, Feige JJ. In vitro models of vasculogenesis and angiogenesis. Lab Invest 2001;81:439-52.

[45] Valarmathi MT, Davis JM, Yost MJ, Goodwin RL, Potts JD. A three-dimensional model of vasculogenesis. Biomaterials 2009;30:1098-112.

[46] Valarmathi MT, Fuseler JW, Goodwin RL, Davis JM, Potts JD. The mechanical coupling of adult marrow stromal stem cells during cardiac regeneration assessed in a 2-D co-culture model. Biomaterials 2011;32:2834-50.

[47] Valarmathi MT, Goodwin RL, Fuseler JW, Davis JM, Yost MJ, Potts JD. A 3-D cardiac muscle construct for exploring adult marrow stem cell based myocardial regeneration. Biomaterials 2010;31:3185-200.

[48] Valarmathi MT, Yost MJ, Goodwin RL, Potts JD. A three-dimensional tubular scaffold that modulates the osteogenic and vasculogenic differentiation of rat bone marrow stromal cells. Tissue Eng 2008a;14:491-504.

[49] Valarmathi MT, Yost MJ, Goodwin RL, Potts JD. The influence of proepicardial cells on the osteogenic potential of marrow stromal cells in a three-dimensional tubular scaffold. Biomaterials 2008b;29:2203-16.

[50] Voyta JC, Via DP, Butterfield CE, Zetter BR. Identification and isolation of endothelial cells based on their increased uptake of acetylated-low density lipoprotein. 1984;6:2034-2040.

[51] Wakitani S, Saito T, Caplan AI. Myogenic cells derived from rat bone marrow mesenchymal stem cells exposed to 5-azacytidine. Muscle Nerve 1995;18:1417-26.

[52] Yamashita J, Itoh H, Hirashima M, Ogawa M, Nishikawa S, Yurugi T, et al. Flk1-positive cells derived from embryonic stem cells serve as vascular progenitors. Nature 2000;408:92-96.

[53] Yost MJ, Baicu CF, Stonerock CE, Goodwin RL, Price RL, Davis M, et al. A novel tubular scaffold for cardiovascular tissue engineering. Tissue Eng 2004;10:273-84.